a practical guide to pediatric respiratory diseases

a practical guide to pediatric respiratory diseases

edited by

DANIEL V. SCHIDLOW, M.D.
Formerly, Professor of Pediatrics
Temple University School of Medicine
Chief, Section of Pulmonology
St. Christopher's Hospital for Children

Presently, Professor and Vice Chairman
Department of Pediatrics
The Medical College of Pennsylvania and
Hahnemann University School of Medicine
Senior Vice President of Clinical Affairs
St. Christopher's Hospital for Children
Philadelphia, Pennsylvania

DAVID S. SMITH, M.D.
Professor, Department of Pediatrics
Temple University School of Medicine
Section of General Pediatrics
St. Christopher's Hospital for Children
Philadelphia, Pennsylvania

HANLEY & BELFUS, INC./ Philadelphia
MOSBY/ St. Louis • Baltimore • Boston • Chicago • London
Philadelphia • Sydney • Toronto

Publisher: HANLEY & BELFUS, INC.
210 S. 13th Street
Philadelphia, PA 19107
(215) 546-7293
FAX (215) 790-9330

North American and worldwide sales and distribution:

MOSBY
11830 Westline Industrial Drive
St. Louis, MO 63146

In Canada: Times Mirror Professional Publishing, Ltd.
130 Flaska Drive
Markham, Ontario L6G 1B8
Canada

Library of Congress Cataloging-in-Publication Data

Schidlow, Daniel V.
A practical guide to pediatric respiratory diseases / Daniel V. Schidlow, David S. Smith.
p. cm.
Includes bibliographical references and index.
ISBN 1-56053-009-X
1. Pediatric respiratory diseases. I. Smith, David S. (David Stickney), 1921- . II. Title.
[DNLM: 1. Respiratory Tract Diseases—in infancy & childhood. WS 280 S331p 1994]
RJ431.S34 1994
618.92′2—dc20
DNLM/DLC
for Library of Congress 94-14803
CIP

A Practical Guide to
Pediatric Respiratory Diseases ISBN 1-56053-009-X

Last digit is the print number : 9 8 7 6 5 4 3 2 1

DEDICATION

To our wives, Sally and Eleanor,
with great love.

DVS
DSS

CONTENTS

CONTRIBUTORS

JULIAN L. ALLEN, MD
Associate Professor of Pediatrics, Temple University School of Medicine, Philadelphia; Director, Pulmonary Function Laboratory, St. Christopher's Hospital for Children, Philadelphia, Pennsylvania

GULNAR R. BALSARA, MD
Associate Professor of Pathology, Medical College of Pennsylvania, Philadelphia, Pennsylvania

ROHINTON K. BALSARA, MD, FACS, FACCP
Professor of Surgery and Pediatrics, Temple University School of Medicine, St. Christopher's Hospital for Children, Philadelphia, Pennsylvania

ROBERT K. BUSH, MD
Professor of Medicine, University of Wisconsin Medical School, Madison; Chief of Allergy, William S. Middleton VA Hospital, Madison, Wisconsin

MICHAEL R. BYE, MD
Formerly, Associate Professor of Pediatrics, Albert Einstein College of Medicine, Bronx; presently, Division of Pediatric Pulmonology, Columbia University College of Physicians and Surgeons, New York, New York

CHARLES W. CALLAHAN, DO
Clinical Assistant Professor of Pediatrics, University of Hawaii School of Medicine, Honolulu; Chief, Pediatric Pulmonology and Critical Care, Tripler Army Medical Center, Honolulu, Hawaii

MICHELLE M. CLOUTIER, MD
Professor of Pediatrics, University of Connecticut School of Medicine, Farmington, Connecticut

ADAMADIA DEFOREST, PhD
Asssociate Professor of Pediatrics, Section of Infectious Diseases, Temple University School of Medicine, Philadelphia; Chief of Virology Section, Department of Laboratories, St. Christopher's Hospital for Children, Philadelphia, Pennsylvania

HENRY L. DORKIN, MD
Associate Professor of Pediatrics, Tufts University School of Medicine, Boston; Chief, Pediatric Pulmonology and Allergy Division, New England Medical Center, Boston, Massachusetts

EDWIN C. DOUGLASS, MD
Professor of Pediatrics, Temple University School of Medicine, Philadelphia; Director, Clinical Oncology, St. Christopher's Hospital for Children, Philadelphia, Pennsylvania

ERIC N. FAERBER, MD
Professor of Diagnostic Imaging, Temple University School of Medicine, Philadelphia; Clinical Professor of Diagnostic Imaging, Medical College of Pennsylvania, Philadelphia; and Director of Radiology, St. Christopher's Hospital for Children, Philadelphia, Pennsylvania

JAMES E. GERN, MD
Assistant Professor of Pediatrics, University of Wisconsin Medical School, Madison, Wisconsin

DONALD P. GOLDSMITH, MD
Professor of Pediatrics, Temple University School of Medicine; Philadelphia; Chief, Section of Rheumatology and Allergy, St. Christopher's Hospital for Children, Philadelphia, Pennsylvania

MARK JOFFE, MD
Assistant Professor of Pediatrics, Temple University School of Medicine, Philadelphia; Director of Emergency Medicine, St. Christopher's Hospital for Children, Philadelphia, Pennsylvania

SUSAN M. KOLB, MSN, RN
Pediatric Pulmonary Clinical Nurse Specialist, and Clinical Nurse Coordinator, Home Ventilation Program, St. Christopher's Hospital for Children, Philadelphia, Pennsylvania

JOHN M. LOISELLE, MD
Assistant Professor of Pediatric Emergency Medicine, Medical College of Pennsylvania, Philadelphia; Section of Pediatric Emergency Medicine, St. Christopher's Hospital for Children, Philadelphia, Pennsylvania

SARAH S. LONG, MD
Professor of Pediatrics, Temple University School of Medicine, Philadelphia; Chief, Section of Infectious Diseases, St. Christopher's Hospital for Children, Philadelphia, Pennsylvania

DAVID A. LOWE, MD, FCCM
Associate Professor of Anesthesiology, Temple University School of Medicine, Philadelphia; Director, Department of Anesthesia and Critical Care, St. Christopher's Hospital for Children, Philadelphia, Pennsylvania

JOEL E. MORTENSEN, PhD
Associate Professor of Pediatrics, Section of Infectious Diseases, Temple University School of Medicine, Philadelphia; Chief of Microbiology Section, Department of Laboratories, St. Christopher's Hospital for Children, Philadelphia, Pennsylvania

BRIAN P. O'SULLIVAN, MD
Assistant Professor of Pediatrics, University of Massachusetts Medical School, Worcester, Massachusetts

RAJ PADMAN, MD
Clinical Associate Professor, Jefferson Medical College of Thomas Jefferson University, Philadelphia; Chief, Division of Pulmonology, Associate Director of Intensive Care Unit, and Director, Cystic Fibrosis Program, Alfred I. duPont Institute, Wilmington, Delaware

HOWARD B. PANITCH, MD
Associate Professor of Pediatrics, Temple University School of Medicine, Philadelphia; Staff Physician, Section of Pediatric Pulmonology, and Medical Director, Home Ventilation Program, St. Christopher's Hospital for Children, Philadelphia, Pennsylvania

CAITLIN PAPASTAMELOS, MD
Assistant Professor of Pediatrics, Temple University School of Medicine, Philadelphia; Attending, Section of Pulmonology, St. Christopher's Hospital for Children, Philadelphia, Pennsylvania

RICHARD J. SCARFONE, MD
Assistant Professor of Pediatrics, Temple University School of Medicine, Philadelphia; Section of Pediatric Emergency Medicine, St. Christopher's Hospital for Children, Philadelphia, Pennsylvania

DANIEL V. SCHIDLOW, MD
Professor, Department of Pediatrics, Temple University School of Medicine, Philadelphia; Chief, Section of Pulmonology, St. Christopher's Hospital for Children, Philadelphia, Pennsylvania

DAVID S. SMITH, MD
Professor of Pediatrics, Temple University School of Medicine, Philadelphia; Section of General Pediatrics, St. Christopher's Hospital for Children, Philadelphia, Pennsylvania

DAVID G. TINKELMAN, MD
Clinical Professor of Pediatrics, Medical College of Georgia, Augusta; Medical Director, Atlanta Allergy Clinic, P.A., Atlanta, Georgia

EILEEN E. TYRALA, MD
Professor of Pediatrics, Temple University School of Medicine, Philadelphia; Director of Neonatology, Temple University Hospital; St. Christopher's Hospital for Children, Philadelphia, Pennsylvania

LAURIE VARLOTTA, MD
Assistant Professor of Pediatrics, Temple University School of Medicine, Philadelphia; Director, Apnea Program, Department of Pulmonology, St. Christopher's Hospital for Children, Philadelphia, Pennsylvania

CHARLES VINOCUR, MD
Professor of Surgery, Temple University School of Medicine, Philadelphia; Attending Pediatric Surgeon, St. Christopher's Hospital for Children, Philadelphia, Pennsylvania

JAMES F. WILEY, II, MD, FAAP, ABMT
Assistant Professor of Pediatrics, Temple University School of Medicine, Philadelphia; Associate Director, Section of Emergency Medicine, St. Christopher's Hospital for Children, Philadelphia; Senior Consultant, The Poison Center, Serving the Greater Philadelphia Area, Philadelphia, Pennsylvania

BARBARA J. WOLFSON, MD
Professor of Diagnostic Imaging, Temple University School of Medicine, Philadelphia; Attending Radiologist, St. Christopher's Hospital for Children, Philadelphia, Pennsylvania

COMMENTATORS

The following individuals have supplied commentaries, which may be found at the ends of selected chapters:

CARLTON DAMPIER, MD
GLEN ISAACSON, MD
THOMAS I. KENNEDY, MD
HOWARD B. PANITCH, MD
DANIEL V. SCHIDLOW, MD
DAVID S. SMITH, MD

PREFACE

This book is intended to provide a practical approach to the understanding, diagnosis, and management of common disorders of the respiratory system in infants and children. Uncommon conditions have been omitted or cursorily mentioned. Repetition has not been totally eliminated because we believe that some overlap is necessary and inevitable.

This text is not all-encompassing. For additional information, each chapter contains a list of suggested readings, primarily review articles. Selected chapters are accompanied by a commentary, which may present an alternative view stemming from the writer's experience, complementary information, or simply a thought about the subject.

The founder of our department of pediatrics at St. Christopher's Hospital for Children, Waldo E. Nelson, M.D., continues to demand of us the duty to break the barriers between "town and gown" and to remember that the learning of pediatrics is a commitment shared by all individuals interested in the welfare of children. The fact that the editorship of this book is shared by a subspecialist, who believes that he is a pediatrician in practice first, and a generalist, who has had extensive experience in the practice of general pediatrics, is not the product of serendipity. It is the product of a strong belief that knowledge and experience are there for everyone to share and enjoy, and that we all have much to learn from one another and from our patients.

This book is offered to the community of pediatric caregivers with great humility and with the hope that it will be useful and enjoyable.

Acknowledgements. The editors would like to thank Phyllis Lewis and Kathleen Rellstab for their expert secretarial help, Frances Pinnel, Librarian at St. Christopher's Hospital for Children, for her most valuable help in locating bibliographic sources, and Linda Belfus, our editor, for her support, patience, and good humor.

Daniel V. Schidlow, MD
David S. Smith, MD
Philadelphia, Pennsylvania

1

HISTORY AND PHYSICAL EXAMINATION

Michelle M. Cloutier, M.D.

Despite major advances in medical technology, the history and physical examination remain the mainstay of medical diagnosis. Respiratory disease is the number-one reason for visits to the physician's office, and most respiratory disease in children can be diagnosed by a careful history and physical examination. In many instances, the history and physical examination are the only information available to the physician. With impending health care reform, today's physician needs to refine further his or her skills in history taking and physical diagnosis (Table 1).

HISTORY

Many pulmonary diseases are missed or misdiagnosed. A careful and complete history is always essential to making a diagnosis. This section concentrates on the important aspects of the respiratory history. These are the questions to be asked and answered, because they are crucial to making an accurate diagnosis of respiratory disease and to implementing appropriate therapy. In obtaining a history of respiratory disease, the physician needs to keep the ten following questions in mind:

1. Is the disorder immediately or eventually life-threatening?

Every physician answers this question within the first 5–10 seconds of seeing a patient. Cyanosis, respiratory distress, or severe stridor—regardless of cause—indicates severe difficulty and the need for immediate action. The cyanotic, pale, limp, or apneic child needs basic life support. Other problems, such as progressive weight loss, recurrent fevers, or a progressive pulmonary opacification, imply a serious problem and require careful, immediate investigation.

2. Is the disorder acute, chronic, or recurrent?

The physician must determine whether the condition is acute and self-limited, chronic (i.e., with symptoms occurring daily for more than 4 weeks), or recurrent (i.e., with disease-free intervals). With chronic or recurrent disorders, the parents may not remember each episode clearly, but they usually can recall—in reasonably good detail—the first time the problem arose. The most difficult history for the physician to obtain is the history of recurrent symptoms. An especially common example is the child with recurrent cough. In this instance, the physician may see the child during an acute exacerbation of the cough, which frequently occurs in association with a viral respiratory illness (cold). The physician may not see the child again until a similar episode occurs later, again in association with a cold. Missing from the history is the observaton that the child's cough lasts 3–4 weeks with each viral respiratory illness. Cough associated with a cold lasts 5–7 days; a cough lasting 3–4 weeks is beyond the normal range and should be investigated further.

3. When did the symptoms begin?

Symptoms that are noted shortly after birth, such as noisy breathing, stridor, or wheezing, suggest a congenital abnormality, such as

TABLE 1. Summary of the History and Physical Examination

History
- Chief complaint
  - Is it life-threatening?
  - Is it acute, chronic, or recurrent?
  - Onset and duration
  - Description of symptoms
  - Previous work-up and results
  - Type of therapy
  - Response to therapy
  - Triggers
- Other accompanying symptoms
- Past medical history
  - History of prematurity
  - History of other respiratory disease, chest trauma
  - History of airway manipulation
  - History of airway surgery (tonsils and adenoids, myringotomy tube placement)
- Environmental history
  - Irritant exposure: Cigarette smoke, woodburning stove, fireplace
  - Allergens: Dust, dust mite, dog, cat, bedroom exposure
- Family history
  - History of similar problems
  - History of any respiratory disease (e.g., asthma, allergy, sinusitis, bronchitis, emphysema, tuberculosis)

Physical examination
- Observation
  - Respiratory rate
  - Respiratory rhythm
  - Work of breathing
    - Flaring
    - Retractions
    - Grunting
    - Snoring
    - Head-bobbing
  - Chest wall appearance and size
  - Skin color
  - Abnormalities outside the chest
    - Signs/symptoms of allergy
    - Nasal polyps
    - Cobblestoning of posterior pharynx
    - Digital clubbing
- Palpation
  - Position of the trachea
- Auscultation
  - Stridor
  - Quality of air exchange
  - Segmental auscultation
    - Crackles
    - Wheezes
    - Rhonchi

laryngomalacia or bronchomalacia. Symptoms associated with feeding suggest gastroesophageal reflux or aspiration. Symptoms that begin after a viral illness suggest postviral airway hyperreactivity. Exercise-related symptoms suggest exercise-induced asthma. Seasonal symptoms suggest allergens, and winter symptoms suggest viral-induced disease.

4. What are the symptoms?

Specific pulmonary symptoms should be sought, such as the presence and characteristics of cough, labored or noisy breathing and its interference with activities, and the presence of wheezing, chest pain, sputum production, or foul breath. Many children deny exercise-induced difficulties. Further questioning, however, reveals that the child has no exercise-induced symptoms because the child does no physical activity. The reason for the inactivity is that exercise results in respiratory symptoms.

For infants with stridor, important questions to ask include what happens to the stridor when the child is asleep (variable lesions that respond to pressure changes, such as laryngomalacia, improve or resolve with sleep) and when the child is crying (variable lesions worsen). The quality of the voice and cry is important. Hoarseness or a muffled, soft cry imply laryngeal disease. Cyanosis or episodes of apnea and failure to thrive or difficulty with eating in an infant with stridor require further evaluation of the airway. Snoring, a common symptom in older children, is frequently not significant unless airway obstruction occurs. The physician needs to ask about obstruction in the snoring child. A history of interrupted snoring associated with vigorous chest wall motion in the absence of air flow and followed by self-arousal is diagnostic of obstructive sleep apnea. The most common cause in children of obstructive sleep apnea is enlarged tonsils and adenoids.

5. What factors affect the severity of symptoms?

It is important to identify factors that improve or worsen symptoms. Asthma is suggested when symptoms are exacerbated by changes in weather, viral infections (colds), exercise, laughing or crying, or exposure to allergens and irritants. A cough that disappears when the child is distracted or at night or on the weekends suggests a psychogenic cough. Symptoms of cough or wheeze that occur only with vigorous activity are diagnostic of exercise-induced asthma. Cough that begins on reclining at night is highly suggestive of postnasal drip. Feeding-related symptoms suggest swallowing discoordination or gastroesophageal reflux with aspiration. Hemoptysis is a frightening symptom for both families and physicians. It is important to try to determine where the blood is coming from. In otherwise healthy children, hemoptysis is seen with a retained foreign body. In children with pallor, hemoptysis may be a sign of pulmonary hemosiderosis, and in children with purulent, chronic bronchitis (e.g., cystic fibrosis, bronchiectasis, and ciliary dyskinesia syndromes), hemoptysis is a sign of acute infection with erosion into the bronchial wall.

6. Are other symptoms present?

The physician should ask about the presence of other symptoms, especially symptoms involving the upper respiratory tract. Specific questions include a history of recurrent otitis media, sinusitis, pharyngitis, and fever. Recurrent lower respiratory tract disease associated with otitis media or sinusitis in the presence of fever suggests an immune deficiency, such as immunoglobulin subclass deficiency. A good review of systems is essential. Questions should stress the head, neck, and skin (presence of eczema or rashes). For children with snoring, a change in school performance and a history of daytime somnolence are symptoms of significant obstructive sleep apnea.

7. Are any enviromental factors involved?

The physician should ask where the child spends his or her day and specifically whether a young child attends daycare. The "sudden" onset of chronic or recurrent respiratory symptoms frequently may be attributed to the recent exposure to other children in a daycare setting. A normal, healthy child may have 8–12 viral infections each year. If the child also has asthma, he or she will be ill continuously. A detailed environmental history is essential. Important questions include smoking in the house, the presence of pets, use of a fireplace or wood-burning stove, presence of carpeting or stuffed animals, presence of a damp basement, and the type of heat in the home.

8. Have any tests been performed? What is the child's immunization status?

The physician should determine which tests have been performed, where they were done, and what the results are. Occasionally, parents seek other opinions, and the physician needs to ask specifically about any type of laboratory evaluation. It is important to know whether immunizations are complete. Even when complete, immunization for diseases such as pertussis provides protection for only approximately 85% of children and adults.

9. Have any treatments been given?

There is frequently a discrepancy between what medication is prescribed and what medication is actually given. Specific questions must be asked about what medications were actually given, how much, and for what period of time. It is also important to ask whether a child received any other medications at the same time. A single daily dose of a medication for 1–2 days/week is unlikely to be effective if the medication is normally prescribed 3–4 times/day.

10. Is there a family history of pulmonary disease?

A family history is particularly helpful for certain types of chronic lung disease, especially asthma. A positive family history of asthma, cystic fibrosis, emphysema at an early age, drug abuse, or tuberculosis, to name a few, puts the child at increased risk for pulmonary disease. Here it is important to ask about asthma in all of its different names, including reactive airway disease, bronchial asthma, asthmatic bronchitis, chronic bronchitis (in a nonsmoker), and wheezing episodes as a child. It is also important to ask about allergic disease, such as recurrent sinusitis, seasonal allergies, and hay fever.

PHYSICAL EXAMINATION

The best indicator of pulmonary function in young infants is the respiratory rate. We breathe at a respiratory rate and tidal volume that provide adequate alveolar ventilation and minimize the work of breathing. Work of breathing is the sum of resistance work and compliance of the respiratory system work. Airway resistance and resistance work increase with increasing respiratory frequency (for this reason we change from nose to mouth breathing with exercise), and compliance work (work of lung inflation) decreases with increasing respiratory frequency. In children with certain kinds of disease of the central nervous system (encephalopathy or metabolic acidosis) and no respiratory tract disease, respirations are deep and rapid. In children with decreased compliance (pneumonia, pulmonary edema, interstitial fibrosis) respirations are very rapid and shallow, whereas in children with increased airway resistance (asthma), respirations are relatively slow and deep, thus minimizing the high resistance work.

Respiratory rate, however, is influenced by the status of the child and is more variable when the child is awake. Therefore, the most reliable and reproducible rate is the sleeping respiratory rate. Sleeping respiratory rates are determined by age (Table 2). In obtaining a sleeping respiratory rate, the child must be in a quiet sleep and cannot be disturbed (e.g., a stethoscope cannot be put on the chest or the side rails of the crib lowered). Respiratory rate can be used by the physician in two ways. In the infant with acute respiratory disease, the sleeping respiratory rate can be used to tract the course of the disease. For example, a child with acute bronchiolitis may have a respiratory rate in the 50s or even 60s. As the child improves, the respiratory rate will decrease toward the normal rate for age. For babies in the hospital, the nursing staff can be asked to circle a respiratory rate that is obtained with the child sleeping quietly. There is then no question about the child's status when the respiratory rate was taken. For the infant with chronic lung disease, such as bronchopulmonary dysplasia (BPD), parents can be instructed in how to take a sleeping respiratory rate and can monitor the rate nightly when they check the infant before going to bed. As the BPD improves, the infant's sleeping respiratory rate decreases toward the normal range for age. If the rate increases by more than 4 breaths/minute, the child may be developing a respiratory illness. Families are instructed to increase their observation of the child the following day to look for signs and symptoms of an acute respiratory illness.

TABLE 2. Sleeping Respiratory Rates in Children

Age (years)	Mean ± SEM
0–1	30.4 ± 0.71
1–2	26.5 ± 0.35
2–3	25.0 ± 0.22
4–5	22.3 ± 0.19
6–8	20.6 ± 0.21
9–10	19.0 ± 0.13
11–13	18.9 ± 0.13
14–16	18.1 ± 0.21
17–18	16.3 ± 0.40

Adapted from Ileff A, Lee VA: Child Dev 23:237–245, 1952, with permission.

While giving the history of a young infant or during the physical examination, parents may report and the physician may observe changes in respiratory rhythm. **Apnea**, which is defined as cessation of airflow for longer than 20 seconds, is a significant finding that requires further evaluation. Cessation of airflow for less than 20 seconds also requires evaluation if it is associated with pallor, limpness, or cyanosis. Most infants experience **respiratory pauses**—cessation of airflow for less than 10 seconds. These pauses are normal and in the absence of pallor, limpness, cyanosis, or other symptomatology are no cause for alarm or further investigation.

Parents also may observe and report **periodic breathing**, which is defined as respiratory pauses of 3–5 seconds' duration with 3–5 episodes occurring in clusters separated by no more than 20 seconds. Periodic breathing is especially common in premature infants. A normal infant of 30 weeks' gestation may spend up to 25% of sleep time in periodic breathing. By term the percentage of periodic breathing has decreased to approximately 3–4% and by 3 months of age to less than 1% of sleep time.

Uncommon patterns of breathing include (1) Cheyne-Stokes breathing, which occurs as cycles of increasing and decreasing tidal volumes, separated by apnea, in children with congestive heart failure and increased intracranial pressure, and (2) Biot breathing, which consists of irregular cycles of respiration at variable tidal volumes interrupted by apnea. Biot breathing is an ominous finding in patients with severe brain damage.

Another important abnormality in respiratory pattern is **paradoxical breathing**, in which the rib cage is drawn in during inspiration. Paradoxical breathing occurs when the rib cage loses its stability and becomes distorted by the action of the diaphragm. It is frequently seen in infants who have a highly compliant chest wall and upper airway obstruction, in infants with intercostal muscle paralysis, and in infants and children with impending respiratory failure.

In addition to respiratory rate and rhythm, work of breathing is an extremely useful clue to respiratory pathology. **Flaring of the alae nasi** is a sign of increased airway resistance. The infant prefers nasal breathing (so-called obligate nose breather). With breathing through the nose, 50% of the resistance to airflow occurs in the nose, whereas the other 50% occurs in the large airways. With obstruction in the airways, the infant can decrease total airway resistance by flaring the alae nasi and thus decreasing the resistance in the nose. You can demonstrate this phenomenon for yourself by sniffing and noting how little air is actually moved through the nose. After flaring the alae nasi, however, the physician will observe that the same maneuver results in a marked increase in nasal airflow and a decrease in resistance.

Retractions are signs of increased work of breathing. Normally, tidal-volume breathing generates a negative intrathoracic pressure of 4–5 cm water. Retractions occur when the negative intrathoracic pressure is increased, as in individuals with airway obstruction or poorly compliant lungs. Retractions are especially striking in extrathoracic airway obstruction, in which the large negative intrathoracic pressure that attempts to overcome the obstruction results in collapse of extrathoracic airways. **Intercostal retractions** are a sign of increased lung stiffness or increased work of breathing due to airway obstruction.

Subcostal retractions are always a sign of hyperinflation and a flattened diaphragm due to small airway obstruction. Normally, when the dome-shaped diaphragm contracts and moves into the abdomen, the lower edge of the rib cage, to which the anterior edge of the diaphragm is attached, moves upward and outward. In the presence of hyperinflation, the diaphragm is depressed, and when it contracts and moves further into the abdomen, it pulls the lower edge of the rib cage inward, resulting in subcostal retractions. Clinically, the presence of subcostal retractions means hyperinflation; when retractions are worsening, small airway obstruction is worsening; when retractions are decreasing in severity, the degree of air trapping is lessening.

Grunting, a sign of loss of lung volume, is a form of self-induced positive end-expiratory pressure (PEEP). Pediatricians most often hear grunting in neonates with respiratory distress syndrome. Grunting is also present in infants with pulmonary edema, and in older children is frequently a sign of chest pain and suggests an acute pneumonic process with pleural involvement. By grunting, the infant closes the glottis and applies positive pressure to the airway to increase the resting volume of the lung. Infants with grunting who subsequently require intubation should be given positive airway pressure immediately. It is not uncommon for such children to arrest on intubation, because they become hypoxemic quickly on removal of self-induced PEEP.

Head-bobbing is a sign of dyspnea in an exhausted or sleeping infant. The head bobs forward because of neck flexion from contraction of the sternocleidomastoid muscle with each inspiration. Head-bobbing is best observed when the child rests with the head supported slightly at the occipital area. Head-bobbing in the absence of pulmonary disease is sometimes seen in infants with disorders of the central nervous system, such as cysts involving the third ventricle.

In children suspected of trauma, the **symmetry of chest wall excursion** is important. Trauma to the rib cage may cause fractures and a so-called flail chest that has paradoxical movement. Splinting and decreased movement of the affected side are seen in children with rib fractures and in children with pneumonia with pleural involvement.

The size of the chest wall also should be assessed as part of the respiratory physical examination. Although nomograms for chest dimensions are available, the physician must decide whether the chest size is too small or whether there is an increase in the anteroposterior (AP) diameter of the chest. It may be helpful to remember that up to 6 months of age, the head circumference is larger than the chest circumference. After 6 months of age, chest circumference is larger than head circumference. A small chest also frequently has a characteristic bell shape with a small, narrow apex and flaring at the bases. An increase in the AP diameter of the chest is best observed from the side, with older children in the standing position. A ratio of the AP diameter to the lateral diameter of the chest (throacic index) of greater than 1 is a sign of increased AP diameter.

Skin color should be assessed in all children with lung disease. Examination of the color of the mucous membranes, conjunctivae, soft palate, lips, and tongue is especially useful in separating cyanosis from paleness. Cyanosis is caused by decreased oxygen content of the blood, whereas pallor suggests anemia or chronic illness.

Signs of respiratory disease also can be found outside the chest. Allergic shiners (bluish discoloration of the lower eyelid), a Dennie crease (a bilateral fold of skin just below the lower lid), a transverse nasal crease from an allergic salute, and blue, boggy nasal mucosa are signs of allergy that may play a role in the patient's respiratory disease. Nasal polyps are frequently seen in children with cystic fibrosis and occasionally in children with aspirin-sensitive asthma. Cobblestoning of the posterior pharynx is due to lymphoid hyperplasia secondary to chronic stimulation by postnasal drip. Although digital clubbing may be seen in various diseases, the two most important diseases associated with clubbing are cystic fibrosis and cyanotic congenital heart disease. Digital clubbing also may be seen in other pulmonary diseases, such as pulmonary abscess, empyema, and certain neoplasms, and in nonpulmonary diseases, including subacute bacterial endocarditis, biliary cirrhosis, chronic ulcerative colitis, and regional enteritis.

TABLE 3. Characteristics of Abnormal Breath Sounds

Crackles
Primarily inspiratory
Rhythmic
Repetitive
Not altered by coughing (usually)
Sensitive to postural changes
Wheezes
Primarily expiratory
Musical
Pitch depends on gas velocity
When inspiratory, a sign of a rigid airway
Rhonchi
Inspiratory and expiratory
Nonrepetitive
Nonmusical
Low-pitched

Although palpation is particularly important in examining many organ sytems, it is not particularly useful in examination of the pediatric respiratory system. It is, however, important to palpate the position of the trachea. Tracheal deviation from the midline in children is seen primarily with atelectasis (usually involving a significant portion of one lung) and with pneumothorax. The trachea is displaced toward a lung that is atelectatic, and the displacement is exaggerated during inspiration. In a pneumothorax, the trachea is deviated to the opposite side during exhalation and toward the side of the pneumothorax during inspiration.

Auscultation

Auscultation of the lungs has received much less attention than auscultation of the heart. The considerable uncertainty about the terms used to describe breath sounds has contributed to the mystique of lung auscultation. After fashioning the first stethoscope in 1816, Laennec set out to describe lung sounds. In 1819 he published his famous treatise in which he defined the term "râle" as "all the sounds, besides those of health, which the act of respiration gives rise to. . . ." The major pulmonary disease of Laennec's time was tuberculosis, and what he described are the sounds of pulmonary edema associated with end-stage tuberculosis.

Approximately 2 years later Laennec's work was translated into English, and the term râle was translated as rhonchus. Laennec, according to historians, agreed with the translation; he never used the term râle at bedside because patients understood it to mean the "death rattle" of pulmonary tuberculosis. Ten years later, Laennec's work was again translated into English, and this time the term râle was translated as wheeze. Thus a râle is the same as a wheeze, which is the same as a rhonchus. Is it any wonder that such confusion surrounds lung sounds?

To complicate the issue further, in 1876 Latham characterized breath sounds as dry or wet. His idea was to qualify râles and wheezes according to an acoustic impression—not to imply a physiologic abnormality. Unfortunately, the original intention has been lost with time, and wet sounds have been attributed to fluid in the lungs.

In 1957 Robertson and Coope proposed describing breath sounds as either crackles or wheezes (Table 3). **Crackles** are the sounds produced by the explosive opening of airways in territories of the lungs deflated to residual volume. They are primarily inspiratory, rhythmic and repetitive, usually unaltered by coughing, sensitive to postural changes, and best heard in dependent areas of the lung.

The physiology of crackles is important to an understanding of why they are heard in various diseases. During exhalation, the driving pressure for gas movement out of the lung is the sum of the elastic recoil pressure of the lung and the intrathoracic pressure. As gas moves out of the lung, this pressure force is dissipated. At a certain point inside the chest, the pressure inside the airway is equal to the pressure outside the airway (the equal pressure point). For airways beyond that point, the pressure inside the airway is less than the pressure outside; these airways narrow during exhalation (dynamic compression). In normal individuals, the equal pressure point occurs in airways that contain cartilage and resist deformation. In individuals with airway obstruction of any cause or in individuals with a loss of elastic recoil (emphysema), the pressure head for gas flow out of the lung becomes dissipated in an airway closer to the alveolus. If this airway does not contain cartilage, it will collapse. During the following inspiration, traction on the airways produced by a fall in intrathoracic pressure due to contraction of the diaphragm pulls open the collapsed airways. This opening of the airways during inspiration produces the sound that we call crackles.

Any disease process that increases peripheral airway resistance, obstructs the peripheral airway, or causes a loss of elastic recoil will produce crackles. All of these processes result in premature airway closure. Crackles are most copious in the interstitial fibrosis diseases, in which the fibrosis results in airway narrowing, an increase in peripheral airway resistance, and movement of the equal pressure point toward the alveolus. In congestive heart failure, an increase in the size of the interstitium results in narrowing of the airway lumen, dissipation of the pressure head earlier in exhalation, and, again, movement of the equal pressure point toward the alveolus. In children with cystic fibrosis, the combination of mucus retention, airway inflammation, and bronchospasm produces airway narrowing and premature closure during exhalation. Children with asthma have bronchospasm, airway edema, and increased mucus production, all of which can result in airway obstruction and premature airway closure. The presence of crackles in a child with an acute asthma attack does not mean that the child has pneumonia. Crackles may be heard as part of the acute asthma attack. Children with pneumonia, however, may present with localized crackles, because the infiltrate compromises the caliber of small airways and results in airway closure.

Wheezes are the sounds generated by air passing at high velocity through an airway narrowed to the point of closure. They are heard primarily during exhalation when airways inside the chest normally get smaller. Essential to the production of a wheeze is sufficient airflow through a sufficiently narrowed orifice. If airflow is decreased, as in the child with severe airway obstruction, few wheezes may be appreciated. On the other hand, high flow through a normal orifice also may produce a wheeze, just as water rushing through pipes may produce a sound. Wheezes are musical, and the pitch of the wheeze depends on gas velocity rather than on the size or caliber of the involved airway. An inspiratory wheeze is heard in children with fixed airway obstruction. These rigid airways are not sensitive to pressure changes around them. Inspiratory wheezes are heard most often in children with asthma who have airway edema. Inspiratory wheezes in this setting are best treated with steroids or other antiinflammatory drugs to reduce the airway inflammation.

The third important breath sound is the **rhonchus**, which is generated by turbulent air passing through secretions in large airways. The rhonchus is nonmusical (white noise), tends to be low pitched, is nonrepetitive, and occurs during both inspiration and expiration. Rhonchi are frequently referred to as transmitted upper airway sounds.

At the beginning of every auscultation it is important to assess the quality of air exchange. All of the breath sounds discussed above depend on air movement. It is immaterial whether a child has crackles or wheezes if the child is not moving air. Therefore, every auscultation begins with an assessment of whether the overall air exchange is good, fair, or poor. Numerous conditions affect the quality of air exchange in addition to poor air movement. Any condition that increases the distance between the airway and the stethoscope affects air exchange, including pneumothorax, pleural effusion, and obesity. Of all the conditions routinely seen by the pediatrician, however, asthma with fair-to-poor air exchange is the most common—and frequently unappreciated. Affected children may appear pale and ill, but on auscultation they have few wheezes because of insufficient air movement. Frequently it is only after bronchodilator inhalation, when wheezing begins with improved air movement, that the degree of obstruction is appreciated in retrospect.

Stridor is a breath sound appreciated best by the ear and not by the stethoscope. It is a harsh, grating, whistling sound produced by turbulent air flow through laryngeal or tracheal obstruction. In contrast to intrathoracic airways, extrathoracic airways always decrease in caliber during inspiration and increase in caliber during exhalation. The most common cause of inspiratory stridor in children is laryngomalacia. Increases in respiratory effort or rate, such as with crying or excitement, result in greater dynamic narrowing of the airway and increases in inspiratory stridor. Inspiratory stridor in a child who is growing well and in a setting typical of laryngomalacia, without cyanosis or apnea, requires no further evaluation. In contrast, the presence of biphasic stridor always requires further evaluation. Biphasic stridor may be seen in children with vocal cord paralysis, subglottic stenosis, and subglottic granulomas, to name a few etiologies. In addition, stridor associated with any degree of hoarseness or altered voice quality should be evaluated further because of the presence of laryngeal disease (see chapter 8).

Finally, auscultation should proceed in an orderly fashion. Segmental auscultation is a technique for comparing breath sounds of homologous segments. During the auscultation the stethoscope should be moved from one segment to the homologous segment on the other side. Quality of breath sounds should be equal on both sides in the absence of disease. The only segment of the lung that has no topographic relationship to the chest wall and therefore cannot be auscultated is the hilar segment of the lower lobes. Significant disease in either hilum cannot be appreciated by auscultation. The lateral basal segment of the lower lobe is the only lower segment that can be auscultated anteriorly. This point is particularly important in a child who is lying on his or her back and cannot be moved.

In summary, a careful respiratory history and physical examination can lead the physician to an accurate diagnosis and appropriate therapy.

SUGGESTED READING

1. Forgacs P: Lung Sounds. London, Bailliere Tindall, 1978.
2. Murray JF: The Normal Lung, 2nd ed. Philadelphia, W.B. Saunders, 1986.
3. Pasterkamp H: The history and physical examination. In Chernick V, Kendig EL Jr (eds): Disorders of the Respiratory Tract in Children, 5th ed. Philadelphia, W.B. Saunders, 1990, pp 56–77.
4. Polgar G: Practical pulmonary physiology. Pediatr Clin North Am 20:303–322, 1973.
5. Scarpelli EM, Auld PAM, Goldman HS: Pulmonary Disease of the Fetus, Newborn and Child. Philadelphia, Lea & Febiger, 1978.

2

EPISTAXIS

David S. Smith, M.D.

Most children experience epistaxis at some moment in their lives. **Because the nose is in a vulnerable position, trauma is by far the most common cause of nasal bleeding throughout childhood.** Most often hemorrhage originates from the anterior nasal septum, which is richly endowed with terminal branches from the external and internal carotid arteries (Kiesselbach plexus). Contraction of traumatized vessels is limited by a paucity of elastic submucosa along the cartilaginous septum. **Most nosebleeds are self-limited.** An attempt should be made to identify the source of bleeding, particularly if the problem is recurrent or has resulted in substantial blood loss. **Although the majority of children with epistaxis can be adequately cared for by parents or managed in the physician's office or emergency department, hemorrhage from the posterior nasal cavity or nasopharynx should be managed by an otolaryngologist.**

CAUSES (Table 1)

Without question, crusting and drying of the nasal mucosa during the winter months in an overheated home with low environmental humidity increase the likelihood of bleeding. Most children are experts at picking their noses. The child with allergic rhinitis is equally proficient at forcefully wiping the nose, which not only itches but also is engorged and often secondarily infected. The allergic child, if old enough, spends much time blowing the nose, often in vain, as if attempting to expel the edematous mucosa. This exercise often precipitates nasal bleeding.

Although epistaxis is occasionally observed as a complication of childbirth, it is unusual in the neonate. Trauma inflicted with the intranasal use of cotton applicators is the most frequent cause of blood-tinged mucosa from the nares. **Significant bleeding from the nose in infants mandates a careful search for local as well as systemic causes.** A profuse, purulent, and bloodstained nasal discharge often accompanies congenital syphilis and usually is manifested during the second week of life. Most often other manifestations are present, such as mucocutaneous involvement, adenopathy, and hepatosplenomegaly.

A unilateral bloody and foul nasal discharge should always suggest foreign body. Young infants with group A streptococcal infection often have rhinitis accompanied by a serous nasal discharge, which may be blood-tinged. One often sees an associated excoriation at the external nares with tiny satellite impetiginous lesions in the adjacent area. A low-grade fever is often present. After the age of 1 year and through the third year of life, irritability, anorexia, and cervical adenitis complicate the picture and are far more common than the classic pharyngitis due to group A streptococci in the older child. Excoriation of the nares with a foul serosanguinous, mucopurulent discharge may be seen in nasal diphtheria. Few systemic symptoms may be present because of slow absorption of toxin; a white membrane may be seen on the nasal septum. This form of diphtheria most often occurs in infants; it is extremely rare in the United States.

Minor episodes of bleeding may accompany a number of childhood diseases. **Significant**

TABLE 1. Causes of Epistaxis

Common causes
Trauma
External
Nose-picking
Environmental
Winter months—dry heat
Upper respiratory tract infections
Allergic rhinitis
Group A streptococcal infections (particularly infants)
Uncommon causes
Platelet abnormalities
Salicylates
Thrombocytopenia
von Willebrand disease
Foreign body
Rare causes
Angiofibroma
Osler-Weber-Rendu disease
Congenital syphilis
Nasal diphtheria
Rheumatic fever
Mucormycoses

nasal hemorrhage complicating exanthemata, such as rubeola, should always raise the question of an associated thrombocytopenia or an underlying problem, either local or systemic. One should always ask about the use of salicylates if platelet dysfunction is suspected.

In past years I was impressed by the frequency of spontaneous epistaxis in patients with rheumatic fever, even during convalescence. In retrospect, the universal use of aspirin therapy in this disease may be at least partially responsible for the problem.

Nasal congestion, epistaxis, and facial numbness in children with poorly controlled diabetes, leukemia, or other diseaes affecting the immune system should raise the question of mucormycosis. Demonstration of hyphae by biopsy is superior to culture for diagnosis. Black eschar may be seen on the turbinates or hard palate.

Children with platelet defects have superficial bleeding from skin and mucous membranes. Although not common, von Willebrand disease, usually inherited in autosomal dominant fashion, results from an abnormality in the production of a glycoprotein responsible for adhesion of platelets to subendothelial surfaces. Epistaxis may present early in life. Menorrhagia and easy bruising follow in adolescence. Bleeding time is prolonged secondary to abnormal plasma thromboplastin time and platelet dysfunction. Autoimmune and other thrombocytopenic states are usually associated with other clinical signs of capillary bleeding when epistaxis is a presenting symptom.

Tumors of vascular origin include hemangiomas and angiofibromas. Angiofibromas appear to arise from the sphenoethmoid recess and are composed of masses of large blood vessels deficient in contractile elastic tissue. Symptoms usually appear in adolescence; the majority of patients are male. Nasal obstruction, hyponasality, and epistaxis are common symptoms. Occasionally, anosmia is present. Growth rate varies, but the tumor has a propensity to invade adjacent structures. Surgical removal is usually difficult.

TREATMENT

Bleeding from the anterior nares usually can be controlled by simple compression or pinching the nose, preferably with the child in an upright position and with the head forward. Positioning the head minimizes drainage of blood posteriorly into the airway or esophagus. Parents may be instructed to insert a small amount of cotton into the nasal vestibule while pinching the nostrils for 5–10 minutes. If this therapy fails, the child should be seen by the physician, and the bleeding should be localized by removing any clots. Use of a head mirror has the advantage of freeing both hands. Suction is essential. A cotton pledget soaked with 1:1,000 epinephrine or 0.5% phenylephrine solution with external compression for 5–6 minutes usually controls the bleeding. This may be followed by gently touching the bleeding area with a silver-nitrate–tipped applicator after applying a local anesthetic. If oozing continues, further investigation is recommended, including possible referral to an otolaryngologist. Bleeding from the posterior nares or nasopharynx, as previously stated, is probably best managed by the surgeon.

SUGGESTED READING

1. Culbertson MC Jr: Epistaxis. In Bluestone CD, Stool SE (eds): Pediatric Otolaryngology. Philadelphia, W.B. Saunders, 1983, pp 719–728.
2. Juselius H: Epistaxis: A clinical study of 1734 patients. J Laryngol Otol 88:317, 1974.

3

RHINITIS

David S. Smith, M.D.

COMMON COLDS

Few if any medical problems are associated with as much frustration as the common cold. More than 200 viruses are responsible for upper respiratory tract infection; immunity appears largely type-specific. The major reservoirs for community and household spread are children. Infections peak after school convenes in the fall. Small groups living in relative isolation—as, for example, crews of ships at sea—remain free of infection, despite frequent severe exposures to the elements, until people-to-people contacts are made in port. Day care has become a major contributor to the problem. Virus appears to be spread by droplets and, perhaps more often than suspected, from contaminated hands. Children appear to shed more virus than adults with colds and for longer periods of time. In experiments with young adults, aspirin therapy also has been found to be associated with prolonged shedding of virus compared with controls infected with rhinoviruses. Complications in infants and preschool children are common, particularly in the middle ear. Treatment of the common cold is symptomatic and has little influence on duration of illness.

Prevention and Cause

Folklore about acquisition and treatment of colds continues through generations. Unfortunately, little evidence indicates that the frequency of respiratory tract infections can be reduced in relatively closed populations, such as a day-care center or a classroom, by any intervention, including exclusion. It is also not feasible to isolate children with respiratory tract infections from their peers unless a specific etiology demands separation. Handwashing by the caretaker and frequent cleansing of surfaces and toys may be the best interventions.

Viruses that usually cause the common cold include over 100 antigenic types of rhinovirus, at least four groups of respiratory coronavirus, respiratory syncytial virus, parainfluenza viruses, enteroviruses, and others. Usually, nasal symptoms in children largely subside in approximately 2 weeks. Secondary elevations in temperature, cough, persistent rhinorrhea, and irritability or drowsiness require evaluation by the physician. Sinusitis, otitis media, pneumonia, and other secondary and potentially serious bacterial complications must be excluded.

Treatment

No antiviral drugs presently exist for treating the common cold. **Antibiotics have no place in the management of the uncomplicated illness.** Nasal obstruction is a problem particularly in infants, most of whom are obligate nasal breathers in the first few weeks of life. Sneezing may be the best method of spontaneously clearing nasal mucous. Elevating the head of the crib or even holding an infant in an upright position for a few minutes is helpful. Attention to room temperature is important. Normal ciliary movement of the so-called mucous blanket that lines the airway functions most efficiently around

69–70°F. An overheated, dry bedroom in the winter months does much to inhibit this mechanism. Provision of cool moisture may aid in liquefying secretions; a vaporizer or humidifier should be washed daily to minimize contamination with molds and bacteria.

Normal saline is commonly used intranasally to aid in the mechanical removal of secretions by bulb syringe, but the effect is probably undercut by the crying that accompanies the act. **The topical use of vasoconstrictors should be discouraged.** Most of the drops end up on either the infant's or the parent's shirt. Many bottles that have been hidden in the medicine cabinet are contaminated; rebound regularly follows whatever vasoconstriction is attained. Use of oral, so-called nasal decongestants has not been evaluated fully in small children. Inclusion of antihistamine drugs further complicates management because of the atropine-like drying effect on nasal secretions. Antihistamine-containing mixtures have emerged as an occasional cause of hallucinations in small children. Cough medicines are largely prescribed for patients whose sleep has been interrupted. Parents have been unable to differentiate between the therapeutic effects in their children of cough suppressant and placebo.

Controversy also surrounds the use of large doses of vitamin C in the prevention of colds. **Few scientific data justify the administration of vitamin C to children for this purpose in excess of normal daily requirements.**

ALLERGIC RHINITIS

Seasonal pollenosis, or **hay fever**, affects nearly 1 in 20 to 1 in 10 children in secondary school and appears to increase in frequency with age. The syndrome is relatively uncommon in preschool children, and early onset in this age group seems most often to be related to grass pollen. Much geographic variation exists, from heavy exposure to grass pollen over relatively few weeks in the spring and early summer along the middle Atlantic coast of the United States to relatively light exposure in areas of Florida over much of the calendar year. On the other hand, exposure to tree pollen in the spring is relatively short for a specific species, and the heavy pollen is wind-borne for relatively short distances. Ragweed pollen begins to disseminate into the atmosphere in the middle Atlantic states in mid-August and continues unabated until frost has killed the weed in late fall. The pollen is light and carried by the wind for several miles. Molds, carried at high altitudes, are a year-round problem for sensitized individuals. Exposure is heaviest in damp basements, along creek beds, and in hot and humid climates. Young children with grass pollenosis often have seasonal conjunctivitis for a year or two before the development of nasal symptoms, such as sneezing; itching of nose, ears, and palate; and congestion. Epistaxis is not unusual, particularly since the nose is easily traumatized because of itching.

In children with *perennial allergic rhinitis* symptoms are present year round. Causative antigens are not always easily identified but usually involve dust mites, feathers, danders of household pets, and molds.

Nasal obstruction is bilateral. The mucosa may be somewhat bluish with an edematous boggy appearance, and a transverse nasal crease may result from rubbing in an upward manner. Mouth breathing is common; dark circles under the eyes are usually present, probably as the consequence of venous stasis from obstruction of blood flow through the edematous nasal mucosa. Nasal polyps are somewhat unusual in children with seasonal or perennial allergic rhinitis; their presence is more suggestive of cytsic fibrosis.

Symptoms of **vasomotor rhinitis** simulate perennial allergic rhinitis, although allergic mechanisms cannot be identified. Nasal congestion follows moving from areas of differing temperatures or humidity or from exposure to irritants such as tobacco smoke. **In contrast to the allergic child, children with vasomotor rhinitis do not have eosinophils in nasal secretions and experience minimal itching, sneezing, and rhinorrhea.**

Treatment

Management of seasonal or perennial rhinitis primarily involves minimizing or avoiding exposure to the offending allergens. Obviously, complete avoidance may be impossible, particularly of airborne pollens. Much benefit, however, can be derived from keeping bedroom windows closed during specific seasons, from ensuring that the filter in hot-air heating systems are cleansed or changed frequently, from providing a relatively dust-free environment, and from measures to control mold growth, such as the use of a 1:750 solution of benzalkonium chloride. The elimination of exposure to animal dander is difficult in families who already have house dogs or cats. Control of exposure to tobacco smoke is an even greater problem. On relatively unusual occasions, the elimination of milk or wheat from an infant's diet may relieve nasal obstruction.

Despite the cost, risks, and inconveniences, selected patients with allergic rhinitis and asthma benefit from immunotherapy, particularly those with pollen and mold allergy. The injection or other use of bacterial vaccines, dog or house dander, food extracts, or occupational allergens, in addition to being hazardous, has not been demonstrated to alter the clinical course of allergic rhinitis or asthma. Immunotherapy should always be carried out in the physician's office; children should be observed for at least 30 minutes after injections.

Antihistamine therapy is the cornerstone for managing seasonal hay fever. Children often tolerate such drugs with minimal side effects; sedation is particularly uncommon. Although itching and rhinorrhea may be well controlled, there is often little relief of nasal congestion. One should not get trapped into the chronic use of topical vasoconstrictor nosedrops. Rebound congestion and dependence quickly develop. Cromolyn nasal solution may be helpful in children with seasonal pollenosis as well in children with perennial allergic rhinitis. Therapy should be started before the specific pollen season. The topical use of corticosteroids may be quite helpful in children who do not respond to antihistamine therapy. Beclomethasone or flunisolide is administered in 1–2 inhalations once or twice daily until relief is obtained. Eye symptoms may be treated with 4% cromolyn eyedrops or with topical corticosteroids. Although the topical use of corticosteroids provokes burning and irritation, mucosal atrophy and fungal or candidal overgrowth have not been problems. Secondary persistent purulent rhinitis and/or sinusitis shold be treated with an appropriate antibiotic systemically.

Many other causes for nasal obstruction in children and adolescents may need to be considered, including cocaine abuse or use of reserpine, foreign body, angiofibroma, hypothyroidism, Wegener granulomatosis, and rhinitis medicamentosa.

SUGGESTED READING

1. Meltzer EO, Zeiger RS, Schatz M, et al: Chronic rhinitis in infants and children: Etiologic, diagnostic and therapeutic considerations. Pediatr Clin North Am 30:847, 1983.
2. Simons FE: Allergic rhinitis: Recent advances. Pediatr Clin North Am 35:1053, 1988.

4

SINUSITIS

David S. Smith, M.D.

An understanding of the embryology and development of the sinuses is important to the clinician confronted with possible pathology of these respiratory structures in the infant, small child, and adolescent. The paranasal sinuses are irregular air-filled cavities that develop as outpouchings of the nasal cavity, usually during the second trimester of pregnancy. Growth of the paranasal sinuses influences the size and shape of the face during infancy and childhood. Their somewhat limited function includes the addition of resonance to the voice during adolescence; contributions to warming and humidifying inspired air are probably relatively minor.

According to the generally accepted view, the **ethmoid and maxillary sinuses** are present at birth. Recent data, however, have identified hypoplasia of both in the first 2 months of life in one-third of normal infants examined by computed tomography. Development of the remaining sinuses is staggered throughout the first decade and into adolescence.

The maxillary sinus measures 7–8 mm in diameter in the majority of full-term infants; at maturity it has a capacity of 8–12 ml of air and occupies most of the space inferior to the orbit and superior to the hard palate. Because the maxillary sinus must accommodate two sets of teeth in the developing skull, growth of the maxillary antrum is most rapid after the age of 6 years. The first and second molar teeth and the second bicuspid remain closely approximated to the floor of the sinus. Periapical dental pathology may affect the health of the maxillary sinus. Drainage of the sinus is against gravity and into the middle meatus.

The ethmoid sinus consists of multiple air cells, usually 5–15. Each cell has a separate ostium, with an anterior component draining into the middle meatus and posterior cells draining into the posterior portion of the middle turbinate. Ethmoid cells are present at birth in approximately two-thirds of normal infants. The lateral wall of the ethmoid sinus, which is in close proximity to the orbit, is paper-thin. Infections of the ethmoid cells may lead to retroorbital abscess and cellulitis.

The **frontal sinus** lies above the roof of the orbit and varies greatly in size and shape. Anterior ethmoid cells contribute to the development of the frontal sinus; first radiographic recognition is around 6 or 7 years of age. Rapid development and clinical relevance await the onset of puberty. Patients who experience disease of the ethmoids early in life, such as children with cystic fibrosis, appear in some instances to have underdeveloped frontal sinuses.

The **sphenoid sinus** is the last to develop fully and remains rudimentary until the sixth or seventh year. Growth of the sinus continues for another 7–8 years.

The paranasal sinuses are lined by pseudostratified, ciliated columnar epithelial cells, goblet cells, and submucosal glands that produce a mucous blanket identical to that found throughout the respiratory tract. Abnormal mucus production, dysfunctional motility of the cilia, or obstruction of the ostia may contribute to disease of the sinuses (Table 1). **Sinusitis is a common problem in pediatric practice and complicates 5–10% of upper respiratory tract infections.**

TABLE 1. Predisposing Factors for Development of Sinusitis

Upper respiratory tract infections
Allergic rhinitis
Barotrauma
Nasal polyps
Anatomic variants (e.g., deviated nasal septum)
Tumor (intranasal or intrasinus)
Dental pathology
Cystic fibrosis
Ciliary dyskinesia syndromes
Immunodeficiency
Foreign body

DIAGNOSIS

Sinusitis should be suspected in small children by the presence of mucopurulent rhinorrhea persisting beyond the usual 7–10 days for uncomplicated upper respiratory infections. The breath often has a fetid odor. Low-grade fever and cough are expected. Intermittent painless periorbital edema may be noted. Headache and facial pain are infrequently encountered in preadolescent patients. Percussion over the sinuses or upper dentition is equally nonrewarding in the younger age group. The use of an intranasal vasoconstrictor may help to visualize pus exiting from the middle meatus, although this technique may be difficult in a preschool child. Gagging the patient with a tongue depressor may allow one to observe mucopurulent material appearing from the postnasal space.

Transillumination, if carried out correctly in a darkened room, may be helpful in the adolescent. It is usually of no value in the younger child.

Differences of opinion exist as to the relative merits of plain radiography or a coronal computed tomogram in the diagnosis of acute sinusitis. Varying degrees of mucosal thickening (2–6 mm), frank opacification, or air–fluid levels have been accepted as criteria for diagnosis. Problems in interpretation include the following: (1) mucosal thickening is often caused by an allergic response rather than by infection; (2) opacification may be a developmental variation rather than evidence of fluid collection; and (3) the lack of cooperation in small children may preclude visualization of air–fluid levels. In addition, the frequency of normal radiographs has been high in studies of children with confirmed sinusitis. Some centers recommend forgoing plain radiography in favor of presumptive treatment for children who are suspected clinically of having acute sinusitis. In routine practice, computed tomography (CT) and sinus endoscopy are impractical in children unless complications such as orbital cellulitis or brain abscess are suspected.

MICROBIOLOGY AND TREATMENT OF ACUTE SINUSITIS

The bacteriology of acute sinusitis is virtually identical with organisms recovered from children with acute otitis media. *Streptococcus pneumoniae*, nontypable *Hemophilus influenzae*, and *Moraxella catarrhalis* predominate. Beta-lactamase production presents the same problem as in the treatment of otitis media. Patients with prolonged symptoms or patients who have had surgical intervention generally harbor *Staphylococcus aureus* and various anaerobes, such as *Peptostreptococcus* and *Bacteroides* species. Respiratory viruses such as rhinoviruses, influenza virus, parainfluenza virus, and adenovirus have been reported in approximately 10% of children with acute sinusitis.

Amoxicillin is the drug of choice for effectiveness, cost and safety in the treatment of a condition that is self-limited in most children. Second-line antibiotics are the same as for the treatment of middle-ear disease: amoxicillin-clavulanate, erythromycin-sulfisoxazole, trimethoprim-sulfamethoxazole, cefaclor, and cefuroxime axetil. Therapy should be continued for a minimum of 14 days, although no studies have been carried out to date on the appropriate duration of treatment. Study of the effectiveness of systemic administration of decongestants is also incomplete. Investigation of children with recurrent episodes of sinusitis should include an allergy work-up, a sweat test, measurement of serum immunoglobulin subclasses, and assessment of ciliary function and structure. The use of endoscopic techniques, including surgery, awaits prospective study that compares efficacy and safety with the use of prophylactic antibiotics, antral lavage, and nasal-antral windows. The practicing physician is advised to consult with an experienced otolaryngologist before recommending a surgical approach to children

TABLE 2. Complications of Sinusitis

Cellulitis of the orbit; retroorbital abscess
Osteomyelitis (frontal most common)
Cavernous sinus thrombosis
Meningitis
Epidural abscess (through penetrating veins of posterior table)
Brain abscess (nearly all in frontal lobe)
Mucocele and pyocele

with recurrent or chronic sinusitis. Many children with chronic sinusitis have either allergy or unrecognized immunodeficiency.

Major complications of acute sinusitis (Table 2) include extension of ethmoiditis and maxillary sinusitis into the retroorbital area. Orbital infections are associated with exophthalmos and eventually with impaired extraocular eye movement. In our experience, most children have responded well to antimicrobial therapy without surgical drainage. The majority of centers, however, surgically drain most, if not all, children with acute sinusitis. More aggressive therapy has coincided with the advent of computed tomography.

In recent years multiple theories have linked sinusitis and asthma, but none has withstood scientific scrutiny. At present sinusitis and asthma appear to be concurrent inflammatory disease in two areas of respiratory mucosa—sinus and bronchial tube. Chronic sinus disease does not appear to be a factor in the pathogenesis of asthma, although some authorities may disagree.

SUGGESTED READINGS

1. Glasier C, Mallory G, Steele R: Significance of opacification of the maxillary and ethmoid sinuses in infants. J Pediatr 114:45–50, 1989.
2. Lusk R, Lazar R, Muntz H: The diagnosis and treatment of recurrent and chronic sinusitis in children. Pediatr Clin North Am 36:1411–1421, 1989.
3. Ott N, O'Connell E, Hoffman A, et al: Childhood sinusitis. Mayo Clin Proc 66:1238–1247, 1991.
4. Wald E: Current concepts: Sinusitis in children. N Engl J Med 326:319–323, 1992.

COMMENTARY

by Glen Isaacson, M.D.

Recurrent purulent nasal discharge, which appears to be a problem of increasing prevalence, is highest among children in large day-care settings and their siblings. Recurrent upper respiratory infection and adenoiditis are certainly common causes of this symptom, but many affected children have abnormal sinus radiographs as well. Despite the lack of large-scale studies, many clinicians have approached recurrent sinusitis much as they approach recurrent otitis media. When recurrent sinusitis is established by CT, long-term antibiotic prophylaxis—half a daily dose of amoxicillin or sulfamethoxazole once a day—is often used, generally throughout the winter and early spring. Endoscopic sinus surgery is seldom suggested for this indication.

Sinusitis that persists for several months, despite appropriate antibiotic therapy for acute disease, is considered chronic. The incidence of chronic sinusitis in the general population of children is unknown; studies are confounded by the high prevalence of abnormal sinus radiographs in all children during the winter months. Microbiologic studies of children with chronic sinusitis demonstrate an increased incidence of *Staphylococcus aureus*, gram-negative organisms, and anaerobes compared with studies of acute sinusitis. Treatment with long courses (4–8 weeks) of broad-spectrum antibiotics, often followed with long-term antibiotic prophylaxis, is usually effective in controlling even these refractory cases. When sinusitis fails to clear—and in any case of pansinusitis or sinusitis with polyposis—cystic fibrosis should be suspected and appropriate testing conducted.

The organisms found in the maxillary sinuses of children with acute sinusitis are the same organisms that cause acute otitis media (i.e., *Streptococcus pneumoniae, Moraxella catarrhalis,* and *Hemophilus influenzae*). Choice of antibiotic is logically similar, although good clinical studies are lacking. Amoxicillin remains the drug of choice except in areas with a high prevalence of resistant pathogens. Trimethoprim/sulfamethoxazole is a good alternative drug. For resistant cases, erythromycin-sulfisoxazole, amoxicillin-clavulanate, or second-generation cephalosporin are suggested. A duration of therapy of at least 2 weeks—and longer, if symptoms persits—has been most effective in clinical practice.

Children with inhalant allergy or asthma seem to have a higher incidence of both acute and chronic sinusitis. The pathogens recovered from their sinuses are the same as in unaffected children. Immunosuppressed children and children with AIDS tend to be infected by normal pathogens of sinusitis, but they are also at risk for infection by fungi and other opportunistic agents.

Endoscopic sinus surgery is emerging as a useful modality in the treatment of chronic, symptomatic sinusitis. The technique consists of enlarging the natural openings of the maxillary sinuses and converting the ethmoid sinuses into a common cavity that opens widely into the nose. The surgery is performed through the nose under the guidance of long quartz telescopes. In the hands of experienced pediatric otolaryngologists at children's hospitals, endoscopic sinus surgery appears safe and effective in improving the symptoms of up to three-quarters of children with refractory chronic sinusitis. The long-term effect of this surgery on mid-face and sinus growth is unknown. Severe intracranial and orbital complications have been reported in adults.

5

OTITIS MEDIA

David S. Smith, M.D.

ACUTE OTITIS MEDIA

The highest prevalence of acute otitis media occurs during the first 2 years of life. Most episodes complicate infections of the upper respiratory tract, and up to one-third of infants experience 3 or more bouts of otitis media before the age of 2 years. **Basic to the pathophysiology of acute otitis media is eustachian tube dysfunction, usually due to inflammatory edema and obstruction.** Anatomically, the eustachian tube is horizontal and short in infants and lacks bony development in preschool children; thus it is relatively more compliant. With tubal obstruction and with subsequent absorption of gases from the closed middle ear from development of negative pressure, effusions occur, posing additional problems to the infant and the physician.

Perhaps even more fundamental to the occurrence of otitis media in early life is the susceptibility of the infant to repeated respiratory tract infections. The presence of siblings, attendance in day care, bottle feeding, passive exposure to cigarette smoking, allergic edema, and the presence of nasopharyngeal masses, including adenoidal hypertrophy, may influence the development of otitis media in some children. Anatomic defects, such as those accompanying cleft palate, contribute to malfunction of the eustachian tube. Most common is hypoplasia of the tensor and levator palatini muscles.

Otitis media represents one-fifth of all office and outpatient visits; over two billion dollars are spent annually on physicians' fees and for antibiotics. Middle-ear disease is obviously a major health problem for children. Despite numerous studies and publications, many controversies continue to plague students and practitioners, including choice of antibiotics; duration of therapy; indications for myringotomy, tympanostomy tubes, and adenoidectomy; the role of intranasal and systemic corticosteroid therapy; the role of viruses in pathogenesis; concerns for speech and academic development in the presence of effusions; and the choice and duration of prophylactic antibiotic therapy. Despite the differences of opinion that may confuse the physician, we may have lost sight of the fact that over the past several decades we have been doing something right. A few generations ago chronic otorrhea and mastoiditis were not uncommon; we have forgotten that most children with otitis media recover completely with no therapy.

Acute suppurative otitis media eventually results in a collection of pus in a closed space. An erythematous, bulging, poorly mobile eardrum with indistinct landmarks is usually, but not always, extremely painful. Some infants are amazingly indifferent to the condition. Parents may remember only that the baby was a little fussy a few nights previously when exudate is discovered pulsating through a fresh perforation of an eardrum at a well-baby visit. **High fevers (40°C) are quite unexpected with uncomplicated otitis media; the infant may be bacteremic with such an association.** Infants with otitis media may be more comfortable in an upright position. It is best to leave the ear examination until last, because infants and small children hate to have any body orifice violated, let alone by a stranger. Adequate immobilization is crucial; it is preferable to have one of the parents restrain the infant or small child on the examining table rather than in the lap. The use of positive and negative pressure to the sealed external auditory canal with an insufflation bulb is important to demonstrate mobility of the tympanic membrane and to confirm the presence of effusion. The presence of pus in the external canal nearly always indicates middle-ear disease in a sick infant. **It is important to visualize the site of perforation, which may offer a prognosis for spontaneous healing.**

The most common cause of otitis media is *Streptococcus pneumoniae,* followed by nontypable *Hemophilus influenzae, Moraxella catarrhalis,* and occasionally *Streptococcus pyogenes.* Bacteria may be isolated from middle-ear aspirates in approximately 70% of cases. Recent studies have confirmed the presence of viruses or viral antigens in middle-ear fluid from 8–25% of patients with acute otitis media. Not surprisingly, both bacteria and virus have been recovered from the same specimen. Types of viruses include respiratory syncytial virus, parainfluenza virus, cytomegalovirus, enteroviruses, and adenovirus, among others. At this time it is unknown whether the presence of virus in the middle ear is required to predispose the infant to acute otitis media or whether it affects the outcome. Preliminary data suggest that viral replication in the middle ear may delay clinical response to therapy, although these observations need confirmation. Currently eight antibiotics are licensed for the treatment of acute otitis media (Table 1).

TABLE 1. Antibiotics Licensed for the Treatment of Acute Otitis Media

Beta-lactam
Amoxicillin
Amoxicillin–clavulanate
Cephalosporins
Cefalcor
Cefprozil
Cefixime
Cefuroxime
Sulfonamide combinations
Erythromycin–sulfisoxazole
Trimethoprim–sulfamethoxazole

TABLE 2. Importance of Amoxicillin Resistance in Acute Otitis Media

	% Cases	% Isolates Resistant to Amoxicillin
S. pneumoniae	30–40	0
H. influenzae	10–20	10–30
M. catarrhalis	10–20	20–80
Group A streptococcus	5	0
Sterile	25	—

Older physicians recall that most cases of acute otitis media resolve without specific therapy. Perhaps fewer than one-fourth of children require antibiotic therapy. Predicting outcome, however, is impossible; it is therefore reasonable to treat all children with otitis media. At the present time amoxicillin remains the drug of choice, despite concern over increasing beta-lactamase resistance of nontypable *H. influenzae* and *M. catarrhalis* organisms (Table 2). Until recently penicillin-resistant pneumococci have been considered to be rare in the United States. Continuing surveillance has indicated an increase in penicillin-resistant pneumococci to 13% of isolates from middle-ear fluid at Texas Children's Hospital in Houston. Alternative antibiotic therapy may be indicated in selected areas as patterns of resistance change.

Alternative therapies may increase cost and side effects without necessarily changing outcome. Cephalosporins and amoxicillin–clavulanate cause diarrhea. Cefaclor is associated with a serum sickness reaction in about 5% of recipients. Sulfonamides are occasionally associated with severe hypersensitivity reactions. All therapies should be continued for 10–14 days. The choice of a so-called second-line antibiotic is indicated in children who have had a recent illness treated with an antibiotic or who have developed otitis media while attending day care. The use of nasal decongestants has not been demonstrated to prevent the development of otitis media with onset of the common cold or to influence the frequency or persistence of middle-ear effusions.

OTITIS MEDIA WITH EFFUSION

Children should be reexamined 2 weeks after onset of acute otitis media. Approximately

one-half of patients will demonstrate evidence of middle-ear effusions. Most pediatricians choose not to treat the child unless symptoms, such as otalgia, persist. However, spontaneous resolution of effusion occurs in 90% of children by 12 weeks. Other treatment options—such as topical or systemic decongestants, intranasal or systemic corticosteroids, insufflation of the eustachian tube, or another course of antibiotics—have demonstrated inconsistent efficacy in carefully controlled studies.

Resolution of chronic otitis media with effusion of at least 8 weeks' duration appears to be influenced favorably by administration of an antibiotic, but the relapse rate is high. For children who fail therapy and who experience hearing loss or demonstrate retraction pockets of the tympanic membrane, tympanostomy tubes should be considered after consultation with an otolaryngologist. Substantial controversy continues in regard to the management of such children, including the performance of adenoidectomy in selected patients.

Most physicians agree, however, that antibiotic prophylaxis is effective in prevention of recurrent acute otitis media. Choices include a single dose (20 mg/kg) of amoxicillin at bedtime or a single dose (75 mg/kg) of sulfisoxazole. Prophylaxis should be continued throughout the susceptible season, at least during the school year. Attention should be directed at controlling passive exposure to cigarette smoke; in some circumstances, alternative strategies to day-care attendance should be considered. Polyvalent pneumococcal vaccine may be useful in children older than 2 years, but currently available data do not support its routine use.

SUGGESTED READING

1. Casselbrant M, Kaleida P, Rockette H, et al: Efficacy of antimicrobial prophylaxis and of tympanostomy tube insertion for prevention of recurrent acute otitis media: Results of a randomized clinical trial. Pediatr Infect Dis J 11:278–286, 1992.
2. Chonmaitre T, Owen M, Patel J, et al: Effect of viral respiratory tract infection on outcome of acute otitis media. J Pediatr 120:856–862, 1992.
3. Ford K, Mason E, Kaplan S, et al: Factors associated with middle ear isolates of *Streptococcus pneumoniae* resistant to penicillin in a children's hospital. J Pediatr 119:941–946, 1991.
4. Paradise J, Bluestone C, Rogers K, et al: Efficacy of adenoidectomy for recurrent otitis media in children previously treated with tympanostomy-tube placement. JAMA 263:2066–2073, 1990.
5. Rosenfeld R, Mandel E, Bluestone C: Systemic steroids for otitis media with effusion in children. Arch Otolaryngol Head Neck Surg 117:984–989, 1991.

6

PHARYNGITIS

David S. Smith, M.D.

GROUP A BETA-HEMOLYTIC STREPTOCOCCI

Dramatic declines in the prevalence of rheumatic fever in the United States in the latter half of the twentieth century led to complacency in the differential diagnosis of actue pharyngitis in children. In 1984–1986 major outbreaks of rheumatic fever were reported in a number of areas, including Salt Lake City, Columbus and Akron, Ohio, and Pittsburgh. In contrast to previous experience, up to one-half of the children had no identifiable episode of sore throat or illness preceding onset of rheumatic fever. Furthermore, the majority of patients came from middle-income and often rural families, contradicting the stereotypic view of a disease confined largely to the poor and disadvantaged urban household. Ninety percent of the children developed carditis; Sydenham chorea was observed in nearly one-third of the patients in Utah. **These events, together with the recognition of a severe group A streptococcal infection associated with a toxic shocklike syndrome and scarlet fever toxin A, have reinforced the need for accurate diagnosis and treatment of streptococcal infections.**

Most patients with acute pharyngitis suffer from a viral disease. Except during epidemics, group A beta-hemolytic streptococci account for fewer than 15% of cases. **It is very difficult for experienced clinicians to differentiate streptococcal pharyngitis from a viral-related infection on a clinical basis.** Nevertheless, many clues are helpful, including both positive (Table 1) and negative (Table 2) risk factors.

Streptococcal pharyngitis occurs most frequently in fall, winter, and spring and is nearly always spread by contact with respiratory secretions. Group A streptococci are divided into approximately 80 distinct "M protein" types. The virulence of the streptococcus appears to be conferred by the type and amount of M protein and hyaluronic acid in the capsule. M types 1, 3, and 18 produce large amounts of hyaluronic acid and have been linked to outbreaks of rheumatic fever. **The cross-reactivity of some M proteins with myosin, DNA, and certain alpha-helically coiled proteins in heart tissue supports the likelihood of rheumatogenic strains of group A streptococci.**

Swab specimens from the tonsils and posterior pharynx cultured on sheep-blood agar remain the gold standard for the diagnosis of streptococcal pharyngitis (Table 3). Unfortunately, recovery of group A streptococci does not differentiate the patient from a streptococcal carrier who has pharyngitis from another cause. The degree of positivity is likewise not reliable in distinguishing carriage from infection. For a discussion of rapid antigen detection tests, see chapter 40.

Positivity of throat cultures decreases over time after initial infections. Contagiousness of the infected host is related inversely to duration of carriage. Although the transition from true infection to the carrier stage is incompletely explained by alterations in the production of M proteins, the asymptomatic carrier is at low risk for nonsuppurative complications and is unlikely to spread disease. **Obsession with treating the carrier appears unwarranted**

TABLE 1. Positive Risk Factors for Group A Streptococcal Pharyngitis

Acute onset, fever, nausea, and vomiting
Tender cervical nodes
Beefy red and swollen uvula
Yellow tinge to swab used for culture, often admixed with blood
Excoriated nares with secondary impetiginous lesions
Scarlatiniform rash ("sunburned sandpaper")
Palatal petechiae

except when the epidemiologic setting is unusual. Nearly one-half of patients carry the organism from 1–5 months after infection (Table 4).

Group A streptococci remain uniformly susceptible in vitro to penicillin despite recent reports of an apparent increase in treatment failures. Speculation about cause of the inability of penicillin to eradicate the organism includes beta-lactamase production by pharyngeal flora and tolerance of group A streptococci to penicillin. **Although various antimicrobial agents are effective in attaining bacteriologic cure, penicillin V administered orally for 10 days or benzathine penicillin G given as a single intramuscular injection is the treatment of choice.** Erythromycin is preferred in patients who are allergic to penicillin. Although resistance to erythromycin is a problem in Japan, it remains uncommon in the United States. **Rheumatic fever is a preventable disease, even when penicillin therapy is delayed for as long as 9 days after the onset of illness.**

In contrast to the relatively rapid development of antistreptolysin 0 titers in untreated patients with streptococcal pharyngitis, type-specific antibodies develop relatively slowly and appear to be important in protecting against mucosal invasion but not against colonization. Although the issue is somewhat controversial, delays in initiating therapy for 48 hours in the hope of promoting a better immune response are not recommended (Table 5). There is inadequate documentation to prove that early or delayed therapy for streptococcal pharyngitis has an impact on symptomatic recurrence rates.

TABLE 2. Negative Risk Factors for Group A Streptococcal Pharyngitis

Multiple mucosal surface involvement
Conjunctivitis, diarrhea, cough, rhinitis, hoarseness
Crackles, rhonchi, wheezes
Morbilliform rash
Ulcerative exanthem (e.g., Coxsackie group A, Herpes simplex)
Children under the age of 3 years (usually exhibit cervical adenitis, rhinitis, protracted low-grade fever)

TABLE 3. Indications for Performing Throat Cultures in Pharyngitis

Do not perform in children less than 3 years of age. Group A streptococci are an uncommon cause for pharyngitis; risk for rheumatic fever is extremely low.
Do not perform if negative risk factors are present (see Table 2)
Do perform in siblings of children who have developed rheumatic fever or glomerulonephritis, symptomatic or not.
Do perform in family members when recurrent infections occur.
Do perform in school contacts if outbreak of streptococcal disease, rheumatic fever, or glomerulonephritis is clearly occurring.

DIFFERENTIAL DIAGNOSIS OF PHARYNGITIS

Group C beta-hemolytic streptococci colonize approximately 3% of healthy humans and are recovered from skin and mucosal surfaces such as the nose, throat, vagina, and rectum. On rare occasions, meningitis, endocarditis, subdural empyema, and pericarditis have been reported. Food-borne outbreaks of group C streptococcal pharyngitis have been described. Group C streptococci do not cause false-positive results with rapid antigen detection tests for group A. **Rheumatic fever is not a**

TABLE 4. Posttreatment Throat Cultures

Do not perform unless:
(1) Child is symptomatic, or
(2) Child is at unusually high risk for rheumatic fever

TABLE 5. Advantages of Early Antibiotic Treatment

Limits spread to susceptible children
Patient recovery accelerated
Earlier return to school or day care
Working parents return to jobs sooner

consideration with rare outbreaks of group C pharyngitis.

Arcanobacterium hemolyticum (formerly *Corynebacterium hemolyticum*) has received scant attention as a cause of acute pharyngitis and scarlatiniform rash. Numerous reports in Great Britain and Greece describe throat infection due to this organism in otherwise healthy young adults and children as well as osteomyelitis, pneumonia, endocarditis, and septicemia in immunocompromised hosts. Clinical symptoms and signs closely mimic group A streptococcal infections, including tonsilar exudate and scarlet feverlike rash. Hoarseness, cough, and palatal petechiae have been noted in some patients, along with chills and cervical adenopathy. Relative resistance to penicillin has been demonstrated; erythromycin is the drug of choice.

Infections with *Corynebacterium diphtheriae* are a rarity in the United States, although in 1984 and 1986 outbreaks of disease occurred in Sweden and Denmark, countries with high rates of immunizations. Initially the diphtheric membrane is white and resembles a spider web on the surface of the tonsil. The membrane becomes grayish and extends to the uvula, palate, and posterior pharynx. It becomes thick and tenacious and emits a foul odor that can be detected at a distance. There is surprisingly little surrounding erythema. Laryngeal diphtheria usually results from extension of the membrane from the pharynx and presents a serious threat to the airway. The diagnosis of diphtheria must be made on clinical grounds without delay since early administration of antitoxin is crucial.

Infections of the pharynx with *Neisseria gonorrhoeae*, which are acquired by orogenital contact, result in an asymptomatic state or in pharyngitis resembling that caused by streptococci. Consideration should be given to the disease in homosexual males, teenagers with proved or suspected genital gonorrhea, and sexually abused children. **All pediatric patients with gonorrhea should be tested for syphilis at the outset and 6–8 weeks later.** Children with uncomplicated gonococcal pharyngitis should be treated with a single does of ceftriaxone, 250 mg intramuscularly. **Genital, rectal, and pharyngeal cultures should be obtained before initiating therapy.** Selective media, such as Thayer-Martin, should be inoculated immediately, because *N. gonorrhoeae* are extremely sensitive to drying and changes in temperature.

Chlamydia pneumoniae, formerly known as TWAR, has recently been identified as distinct genetically and antigenically from other *Chlamydia* species. In addition to nonexudative pharyngitis, children frequently demonstrate hoarseness and cough accompanied with fever and rales. Illness is usually of mild-to-moderate severity and may be prolonged. Recurrent infections are common. A specific IgM titer $\geq$ 1:16 or an IgG titer of 1:512 constitutes presumptive evidence of recent infection. Erythromycin is the preferred therapy in children younger than 9 years. Tetracycline is a therapeutic option in the older child or adolescent.

Chlamydia trachomatis has been long recognized as a common cause of conjunctivitis in neonates as well as a common cause of an afebrile pneumonia in infants presenting between 3 and 19 weeks after birth. Fortunately, it is a poor colonizer of the oropharynx with low recovery rates in homosexual males, women known to have had orogenital contact with men with *Chlamydia trachomatis* urethritis, and sexually active college students, whether symptomatic or not. Testing for this organism is not indicated in teenagers with pharyngitis.

Infections with *Mycoplasma pneumoniae* are infrequently recognized in infants, but the organism is responsible for most pneumonias in school-aged children and adolescents. **Headache, fever, and a conspicuous cough usually overshadow pharyngitis, although complaints of sore throat are common.** The spectrum of disease manifestations, however, tests the mettle of clinicians. Signs and symptoms may resemble varicella skin eruptions, Stevens-Johnson syndrome, Guillain-Barré syndrome, and Coombs'-positive erythrocyte hemolysis. The organism is quite sensitive to the tetracyclines and erythromycin, both of which are thought to shorten the duration of disease (usually 3–4 weeks) in children. **Tetracycline, of course, should not be used in the first 8 years of life because of dental staining.**

SUGGESTED READING

1. Bisno AL: Group A streptococcal infections and acute rheumatic fever. N Engl J Med 325:783–793, 1991.
2. Dobson SRM: Group A streptococci revisited. Arch Dis Child 64:977–980, 1989.
3. Karpathios T, Drakonaki S, Zervoudaki A, et al: *Arcanobacterium haemolyticum* in children with presumed streptococcal pharyngotonsillitis or scarlet fever. J Pediatr 121:735–737, 1992.
4. Klein JO: Group A streptococcal infections: An era of growing concern. Pediatr Infect Dis J 10(Suppl), 1991.
5. Stevens DL, Tanner MH, Windship J, et al: Severe group A streptococcal infections associated with a toxic shock-like syndrome. N Engl J Med 321:1–7, 1989.

7

HOARSENESS

David S. Smith, M.D.

Hoarseness is a common complaint resulting from various disorders that mask the distinctive tone and quality of the voice. The length, mass, and tension of the vibratory segment of the cords, as well as the shape of their margins, relate to pitch and timbre of the infant's cry, which may be altered by congenital and acquired lesions. Most infants and children with hoarseness have self-limited complaints; for others the problem may be accompanied by airway obstruction or progressive symptoms of local or systemic disease.

DIFFERENTIAL DIAGNOSIS (Table 1)

Newborn Infant

Congenital anomalies of the larynx include laryngocele or cysts that arise from the laryngeal ventricle. Although usually filled with air, the laryngocele may become infected. The mass effect often produces obstructive symptoms in addition to hoarseness. **Webs** represent adhesions between the anterior ends of the false cords or the true cords. Webs of the false cords produce primarily obstruction, whereas webs of the true cords not only may impede air flow but also shorten the vibrating length of the vocal cord and thus alter pitch. Web formation may follow trauma as well as infection, occurring most often after intubation. **Injury to the arytenoid cartilage** may also occur with intubation. Fissures or clefts representing incomplete closure of the posterior larynx are uncommon; about 20% are associated with tracheoesophageal fistula. The accompanying hoarseness may be secondary to secretions and contamination of the airway, because aspiration is a continuing problem. The cry is weak.

Unilateral cord paralysis usually results in hoarseness; obstructive symptoms are minimal or absent, unless the airway is further compromised by inflammatory disease. Choking and coughing due to aspiration, however, may accompany the vagal paresis with dysfunction of the cricopharyngeal muscle and loss of sensation to the superior half of the larynx from the superior laryngeal nerve. Stridor, if present, may be worse when the infant is awake and may be positional. Sleeping on the side of the paralyzed cord may allow the cord to fall away from the midline. Cord paralysis may improve with time or with compensatory movement of the opposite side. Bilateral palsy does not appear to alter the quality of the voice but is associated with a weak cry, dyspnea, and stridor. Neonatal **mysathenia gravis** and lesions that are either **supranuclear** (bulbar palsy, hydrocephalus, subdural hematoma) or **nuclear** (brainstem compression, Dandy-Walker cysts, Arnold-Chiari malformation) are among the neurogenic causes of hoarseness secondary to vagal nerve dysfunction. Infants born to and breast fed by **thiamine-deficient** mothers may have hoarseness as well as aphonia.

Infants, Children, and Adolescents

Routine screening of the newborn infant has virtually eliminated the clinical diagnosis of **congenital hypothyroidism**. In addition to prolonged unconjugated hyperbilirubinemia, hypothermia, and constipation, hoarseness and

TABLE 1. Differential Diagnosis of Hoarseness

Age group	Category	Condition	Features
Newborn infant	Congenital anomalies of larynx	Web	Stridor and weak cry; look for ventricular septal defect
		Cyst or laryngocele	May become infected, but usually filled with air
		Fissure or cleft	20% have tracheoesophageal fistula
	Miscellaneous	Arytenoid cartilage dislocation	After intubation
		Hypothyroidism	Prolonged unconjugated hyperbilirubinemia, constipation, vocal-facial cry asynchrony
		Hypocalcemic tetany	Hoarseness and stridor; look for anomalies of the aortic arch and thymus
		DeLange syndrome	Growling and coarse cry, hirsutism, distinctive facies
		Cri-du-chat syndrome	Partial deletion of short arm of chromosome 5
Infants, children, and adolescents	Infectious or inflammatory causes	Croup syndromes	
		Common cold, sinus disease, postnasal drip	Impaired nasal breathing; hoarse on arising
		Congenital syphilis	
		Acquired immunodeficiency syndrome, neutropenia	Patients with AIDS usually have hepatomegaly, adenopathy, and oral candida
		Tuberculosis, histoplasmosis	
		Corticosteroid inhalation therapy	Prolonged use in patients with asthma
	Noninfectious inflammatory causes	Respiratory allergies	Seasonal pollenosis
		Gastroesophageal reflux	
		Angioneurotic edema	Hoarseness with oropharyngeal edema
		Cricoarytenoid arthritis	Juvenile rheumatoid arthritis
Infants, children, and adolescents *(cont.)*	Traumatic causes	Vocal cord nodules	Fibrous nodules preceded by small hemorrhages in vocal cords
		Foreign body	Preceded by sudden episode of choking
		Laryngeal fracture	Clothesline injuries from snowmobiles, bicycles, minibikes, strangulation attempts
		After intubation	Common and usually transient, except with granulomas
	Tumors	Papillomas	Most common sexually transmitted disease in U.S.; hoarseness may be followed by obstructive symptoms
		Hemangiomas	Skin involvement in 50%
		Rhabdomyosarcoma	Painful hoarseness
		Leukemic infiltration	
	Neurogenic	Supranuclear	Bulbar palsy, hydrocephalus, subdural hematoma
		Nuclear	Brainstem compression (Dandy-Walker cyst, Guillain-Barré syndrome)
		Peripheral	Myasthenia gravis, sarcoid, vincristine toxicity, enlarged left pulmonary artery or left atrium, thiamine deficiency, mediastinal tumor
		Allergic reactions	Angioneurotic edema
	Miscellaneous	Amyloidosis	Deposition of amyloid in vocal cords
		Farber disease	Hepatomegaly, painful swelling in multiple joints
		Infantile Gaucher disease	Hepatomegaly, pseudobulbar palsy, opisthotonos
		Mucolipidosis II	I-cell disease
		Lipoid proteinosis	Deposition of lipid and mucopolysaccharide substance in skin, tongue, and airway
		Smoking	
		Sicca syndrome	Ectodermal dysplasia, cystic fibrosis, antihistamine therapy
		Pubertal voice changes	

a gravelly voice gradually became apparent in the untreated infant. **If one flicks the toes of infants with congenital hypothyroidism, there is usually a delay of several seconds between facial grimacing and onset of an audible hoarse cry, whereas in a normal infant vocalization and facial grimace are synchronized when a painful stimulus is applied. Hypocalcemic tetany** may be accompanied by stridor and hoarseness.

Respiratory human papillomavirus infection transmitted to the infant at delivery may result in recurrent **papillomatosis** of the airway. Symptoms begin in the early months of infancy, and hoarseness is common. Over 60 varieties of human papillomavirus have been identified by DNA probes. Of these varieties, which represent the most commonly sexually transmitted disease in the United States, type 11 has been associated with papillomatosis of the airway in the newborn infant. The estimated risk of acquiring respiratory papillomatosis from a clinically infected mother ranges from 1:80 to 1:15,000. **Routine cesarean sections in infected mothers are not recommended; infants born to such women should be observed carefully for hoarseness and stridor.** Surgical laser excision is the therapy of choice; use of interferon has had mixed reviews. Tracheotomy should be done only if other therapies fail, because it may speed progression of the disease to more distal portions of the respiratory tree.

Most children and adolescents develop hoarseness in association with **upper respiratory tract infections**, particularly with impaired nasal breathing. Symptoms are usually transitory and most obvious on arising after a night of mouth-breathing. This pattern is common in children with seasonal pollenosis or perennial allergic rhinitis; sinus disease and postnasal drip often contribute to the problem. Symptoms may be more dramatic and associated with airway obstruction in many of the croup syndromes (see chapter 8). Parainfluenza virus type 1 is responsible for most cases of acute laryngotracheitis, but many other organisms should be considered, including *Hemophilus influenzae* type b and, on rare occasions, *Corynebacterium diphtheriae*. A muffled voice rather than hoarseness usually accompanies acute epiglottitis in association with dysphagia, drooling, a characteristic posture, insistence on sitting, and stridor.

Hoarseness from mycotic infections due to *Candida* and *Aspergillus* species has been observed as an early sign in infants infected with the **human immunodeficiency virus**. Fungal overgrowth in the airway also may be seen with other immunologic disorders, such as defective neutrophil motility and neutropenia induced by chemotherapy. Overgrowth of *Candida* may complicate the prolonged use of inhaled corticosteroids.

Noninfectious causes of hoarseness include rheumatoid arthritis, sarcoidosis, leukemic infiltration, and tumor. **Vocal cord nodules** or "screamer's nodules" due to vocal abuse are often found at the junction of the anterior and middle third of the membranous cords in hoarse preschoolers. These well-organized fibrotic nodules rarely require treatment. In older children who ride bicycles, minibikes, or snowmobiles, as well as in children involved in sports, **external trauma** may result in injury to the larynx and/or trachea. Gross subcutaneous emphysema, hemoptysis, and stridor may present the physician with a life-threatening emergency. Hoarseness and cough are evident immediately after injury. **Diagnostic interventions, including lateral neck roentgenograms and laryngoscopy, should be considered in patients with the following clinical conditions associated with hoarseness:**

1. Congenital hoarseness
2. Laryngeal trauma
3. Symptoms that persist longer than 2–3 weeks
4. Hoarseness and stridor of unknown cause
5. Progressive hoarseness of unknown cause
6. Suspicion of foreign body
7. Cutaneous hemangiomata or lymphangioma of head and neck

SUGGESTED READING

1. Cotton RT, Richardson MA: Congenital laryngeal anomalies. Otolaryngol Clin North Am 14:203, 1981.
2. Filter MD, Poyner RE: A descriptive study of children with chronic hoarseness. J Community Disord 15:461, 1982.
3. Passy V: Hoarseness: Evaluation and treatment. Prim Care 9:337, 1982.

8

STRIDOR AND UPPER AIRWAY OBSTRUCTION

Daniel V. Schidlow, M.D.
David S. Smith, M.D.

Stridor is a rough, crowing sound caused by the passage of air through a narrowed upper airway. The upper airway, defined as the portion of the respiratory tree proximal to the thoracic inlet, includes the pharynx, larynx, and extrathoracic trachea.

Stridor occurs or worsens during inspiration. The extrathoracic airway normally narrows during the inspiratory phase of respiration because the pressure outside the airway exceeds slightly the pressure inside. Conditions causing further decrease in the lumen of the airway will generate an obstruction to airflow and stridor.

The characteristics of sound may vary according to the underlying pathology. For instance, the noise associated with laryngomalacia has a characteristic low-pitched, vibratory quality, whereas the sound of congenital subglottic stenosis may be faint, higher-pitched, and fixed. With severe narrowing of the air passage, **stridor may be audible both in inspiration and expiration, but it always tends to be worse during inspiration.**

Some authors categorize stridor as laryngeal, tracheal, and even upper airway (as opposed to laryngeal). This separation, in our view, is confusing. Serious narrowing of the intrathoracic trachea due to a vascular ring, for instance, can cause a loud noise heard in both phases of respiration. Acoustically, it may be difficult to determine whether the noise is a loud wheeze or stridor. The important point is to determine in what phase it worsens: if it worsens or becomes louder on expiration, then the lesion is intrathoracic; if it worsens on inspiration, the lesion is located above the thoracic inlet. Confusion may arise in instances in which two conditions are present—e.g., a vascular ring and laryngomalacia. In this situation, accurate clinical diagnosis may not be possible, and endoscopic or radiographic examination is required.

Difficulty with intake of air causes prolongation of the inspiratory phase and underaeration of the lungs. These phenomena are distinctly different from the prolongation of expiration and overaeration characteristic of intrathoracic airways obstruction. Although children with stridor can be tachypneic, the respiratory rate never exceeds 40–50 respirations per minute. **If the child is very tachypneic, one should suspect a concomitant lower respiratory disease.**

Voice changes may occur in association with upper airway obstruction. For instance, paralysis of the vocal cords results in dysphonia, whereas subglottic stenosis results in decreased volume of the voice as well as stridor, because a much smaller air column is making the vocal cords vibrate. Involvement of the supraglottic area, proximal to the vocal cords, can result in a hyponasal or muffled voice, which is characteristic of children with severe tonsillitis and epiglottitis. Other signs and symptoms associated with upper airway obstruction and stridor include abnormalities in swallowing and cough, particularly in patients with severe inflammatory involvement of the hypopharynx, as seen in epiglottitis, or obstructions of the esophagus, as seen in tight vascular rings. Extreme compression or inflammation of the esophagus also may result in swallowing dysfunction.

A barking cough (or "barking seal" cough) is characteristically heard with viral croup and laryngeal foreign bodies as well as in many children with psychogenic cough.

Stridor and upper airway obstruction may be categorized in many ways. Probably most useful is a separation of symptoms into acute and chronic or recurrent categories, because patients present in one of these patterns to the practitioner. The common causes of acute stridor are viral laryngotracheitis (croup), epiglottitis, bacterial tracheitis, foreign body aspiration, spasmodic croup and angioedema, and peritonsillar or retropharyngeal abscess. Chronic stridor is usually due to anatomic causes, which may be intrinsic or extrinsic, congenital or acquired (Table 1). Below is a brief description of conditions that cause stridor.

ACUTE STRIDOR

Laryngotracheitis

Laryngotracheitis occurs most commonly between the ages of 3 months and 1 year. It rarely occurs in the first few months of life, but if it does, **congenital compromise of the airway** must be looked for. A host of infective agents are associated with the disease, usually parainfluenza viruses. Parainfluenza type 1 accounts for at least one-half of the cases during the fall and winter months. Parainfluenza type 2 is less frequent and causes a milder form of the disease. Influenza type A often produces a more severe illness that may progress to lower airway involvement. Measles is commonly complicated by laryngotracheitis (Table 2).

TABLE 1. Most Common Causes of Stridor

Acute
Infectious
Viral tracheobronchitis (croup)
Bacterial tracheitis
Epiglottitis
Mechanical
Foreign body aspiration
Chronic
Congenital
Laryngomalacia
Vocal cord paralysis
Subglottic stenosis
Hemangiomas
Vascular rings
Acquired
Postintubation scarring
Foreign body aspiration
Mediastinal masses
Cardiovascular causes (congenital heart disease—postsurgical nerve damage)
Tumors (papillomas)

The onset is usually gradual. Symptoms, which include a croupy cough, hoarseness, and sore throat, vary greatly but are usually accompanied by fever. Seasonal patterns, both nationally and locally, soon become apparent. Most children recover after a few days regardless of therapy; in small numbers of patients, the airway is seriously threatened. The most urgent challenge to the physician is to differentiate laryngotracheitis from acute epiglottitis. Clinical skills are taxed in assessing the severity of upper airway obstruction. A lateral neck radiograph may be of great value in identifying the child with deteriorating clinical status who is in need of an artificial airway. The use of aerosol racemic epinephrine (2.25%-1:8 dilution) may provide transient relief but commits the child to hospitalization because of concerns about rebound and recurrence of obstruction. Improvement does not differentiate among other causes of upper airway obstruction, including epiglottitis. More reliable information for determining the need for intervention is obtained from blood gas values; hypoxemia and hypercapnia underscore the urgency of the situation. Mild hypoxemia may accompany upper airway obstruction in children until muscle exhaustion results in hypoventilation with severe hypoxemia and hypercapnia.

Although much controversy surrounds the use of corticosteroids in laryngotracheitis, in large measure because of the difficulties in designing clinical studies and the great clinical variations in the syndrome, many clinicians use a single injection of dexamethasone in a dose of 0.6 mg/kg on diagnosis. Disagreement also persists about the benefits of a cool mist therapy. Many physicians use this therapy in the home or hospital despite the relative lack of scientific support for it. Antibiotics have no benefit in what is almost universally a viral syndrome. **Sedation should be avoided**; orotracheal intubation and tracheotomy are usually not necessary but may be indicated in children who quickly deteriorate.

Acute Spasmodic Laryngitis

Acute spasmodic laryngitis (or "midnight croup") is a distinct entity that is well known to physicians but still defies definition of pathogenesis. It is often seen in the winter months, cases cluster in families, and recurrences are common. The patient is frequently 1–3 years of age (although the disease can occur in school-aged children), has a preceding upper respiratory infection, and goes to bed without cough but often with nasal obstruction. Sudden onset of a croupy cough and marked inspiratory stridor occur a few hours into sleep, awakening the parents as well as the family doctor. It is reassuring to know that this sudden and dramatic onset of symptoms occurs in the absence of fever. Improvement has been credited to hot steam in bathroom showers, but children appear to be equally improved by exposure to cold and dry night air. Use of corticosteroids should be unnecessary, and no data support this therapy. Recurrence on the following night or with subsequent respiratory infections is not uncommon. Spontaneous recovery is expected. Often children are asymptomatic the following morning. Whether this entity represents a form of airway reactivity is unclear. Treatment with bronchodilators does not appear reasonable unless the symptoms recur with some frequency.

Bacterial Tracheitis

Bacterial tracheitis appears to be a secondary complication of a primary laryngotracheitis; most commonly it is related to superinfection with *Staphylococcus aureus.* Typically the child appears to be recovering from the original episode and develops fever, increasing stridor, and toxicity. Neutrophilia may accompany the illness. Prompt recognition and attention to the patency of the airway are very important. Antibiotic therapy should include adequate coverage for staphylococcus. The lateral neck radiograph may show subglottic narrowing and proximal distension indistinguishable from viral croup. Endoscopy with adequate cultures of infected materials confirms the diagnosis.

TABLE 2. Etiologic Agents in Laryngotracheitis

Agent	Frequency
Parainfluenza virus type 1	Most common
Parainfluenza virus type 2	Common
Parainfluenza virus type 3	Common
Influenza virus A	Very common
Influenza virus B	Rare
Other viruses: measles, respiratory syncytial virus, adenoviruses, rhinoviruses, enteroviruses, herpes simplex virus	Rare
Bacterial agents	
Mycoplasma pneumoniae	Rare
Corynebacterium diphtheriae	Rare

Epiglottitis

Epiglottitis was once among the most serious life-threatening emergencies in children. It appears to be decreasing in incidence, probably as a result of widespread immunization with the *Hemophilus influenzae* type B vaccine. Children from 1–5 years of age are most commonly affected, although on rare occasions adults have developed the disease. Abrupt onset and early toxicity, together with a painful sore throat, fever, drooling, and anxiety, are common. Children insist on sitting with a characteristic protrusion of the chin and limited neck mobility. Minimal tachypnea accompanies increasing respiratory stridor. Within hours, some children progress to shock, cyanosis, prostration, and death.

Manipulation of the oropharynx to visualize the airway should be scrupulously avoided, because such maneuvers may precipitate airway obstruction and respiratory arrest. Total control of the airway, preferably in the operating suite, should precede or accompany any attempt at visual diagnosis. Likewise, it is hazardous to place children with epiglottitis in a supine position, because gravity-associated alterations in the position of the epiglottis also may increase airway obstruction. Children also are at risk during transportation and preferably should be intubated before intrainstitutional transport.

Diagnosis is made under direct visualization of the upper airway in the operating suite. Many centers use the lateral neck radiograph to visualize the typical "swollen thumb" appearance of the epiglottis. Proper precautions must be taken (see below). The primary therapy in the child with epiglottitis is establishment of an airway, preferably by nasotracheal or orotracheal intubation. Bacteremia is usually present, and appropriate antibiotic coverage for *H. influenzae* (usually with cefuroxime) should be instituted after successful intubation. Extubation is usually possible after 36–72 hours. Progress of the patient is followed by direct laryngoscopy while the patient is intubated. Metastatic disease in the meninges is uncommon. Antibiotic prophylaxis may be indicated for family contacts. In contrast to children who develop meningitis, high titers of antibodies to *H. influenzae* type b usually develop after epiglottitis.

Foreign Body Aspiration

Lodging of foreign bodies in the upper airway, particularly the larynx, may cause acute and violent stridor and respiratory distress in a previously healthy child. The onset of symptoms is rather acute and violent. The condition is most common in preschool and school children who may be playing or putting small objects in their mouth. It also should be suspected in children with older siblings who may have introduced small objects into the younger child's mouth. The presence of an upper respiratory tract infection with nasal obstruction may enhance the likelihood of aspiration.

General Rules of Management

1. **Patients tend for unknown reasons to worsen at night.** This fact should be taken into consideration when treatment is prescribed, particularly if the child is seen during daytime hours.
2. **Severe obstruction with cyanosis and respiratory insufficiency is *always* a potential occurrence in children with acute-onset stridor.** The patient must be kept under observation, and the parents or personnel in charge of the child must receive precise instructions.
3. **Periodic evaluation of the degree of obstruction is important.** Whether general clinical observation or semiquantitative scoring methods are used, the important point is to detect signs of worsening of obstruction or early respiratory failure.
4. **The most useful noninvasive laboratory tests in the management of acute stridor are lateral neck radiographs.** In the case of suspected foreign body aspiration, endoscopy of the airway is mandatory. In cases of epiglottitis, the supraglottic tissues appear edematous ("swollen thumb" sign), and edema of the hypopharyngeal and laryngeal tissues is present. Subglottic obstructions cause dilatation of the airway proximal to the obstruction ("ballooning" of the hypopharynx). For further clues to the radiographic evaluation of patency of the upper airway, the reader is referred to chapter 37.
5. **It is very important that an individual with experience in airway management and resuscitation be with the patient at all times during diagnostic examinations.** Most institutions require that a physician accompany the patient at all times during the process of obtaining lateral neck radiographs. Factors such as manipulation of the patient's airway and anxiety may trigger acute obstruction and respiratory arrest.
6. **Attempts to dislodge a suspected foreign body in the larynx or lower airway by means of physical therapy and postural drainage are highly dangerous and unnecessary.** If a foreign body is floating in the airway, maneuvers such as a back blow may cause it to impact in the vocal cords, obstructing the glottis with catastrophic results.
7. **Endoscopic evaluation of the airway *must* be done by an endoscopist with experience in the treatment of children.** If at all possible, the patient should be transferred to a facility at which a pediatric endoscopist and pediatric equipment are available.
8. **Sedation of patients with upper airway obstruction is usually contraindicated.** Sedation may cause obtundation or loss of reflexes with an increased risk of airways obstruction and aspiration.
9. **Although administration of humidified cold air is popular, there are no scientific data to indicate that this therapy is more useful than leaving the child in room air.** The confinement to a mist tent creates extreme anxiety in some children to the point that symptoms are aggravated; such children may be better off in room air.

CHRONIC STRIDOR

The causes of chronic stridor are usually anatomic abnormalities, which may be congenital or acquired.

Laryngomalacia

Laryngomalacia is the most common congenital laryngeal abnormality causing stridor. Symptoms may be present at birth but frequently are delayed until the first or second month of life, when the infant starts making more vigorous respiratory efforts and becomes more active. Stridor usually worsens in the supine position and with agitation or feeding. The typical quality of the stridor is vibratory and quite loud. There are no changes in the quality of the voice, and cough is usually absent. The etiology is unclear but is probably related to immaturity and excessive softness of the cartilaginous and muscular support of the supraglottis. Indrawing of the epiglottis and prolapse of the arytenoids and aryepiglottic folds can be observed during inspiration (Fig. 1). Most infants improve spontaneously before 18 months of age. On rare occasions, surgical intervention such as resection of the arytenoid cartilages is indicated when airway obstruction results in obstructive apnea or severe feeding difficulty.

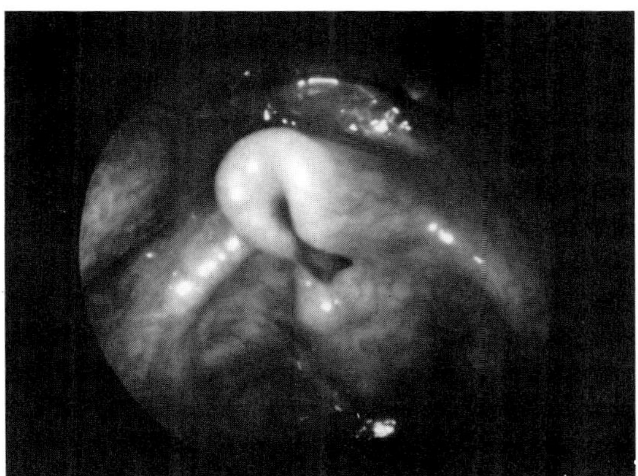

FIGURE 1. Indrawing of the epiglottis and prolapse of the arytenoids and aryepiglottic folds during inspiration.

Vocal Cord Paralysis

Vocal cord paralysis is the second most common cause of airway obstruction in the neonate. Bilateral cord paralysis usually results in severe acute airway obstruction that requires intubation and tracheotomy. The vocal folds fail to abduct on inspiration, although the cry may be relatively normal. High-pitched inspiratory stridor is usually heard. Congenital abnormalities of the central nervous system with herniation of the brainstem may accompany bilateral cord paralysis, although often the pathogenesis is unclear. Spontaneous improvement may occur in some infants in the first few years of life.

Unilateral cord paralysis, which is more common than bilateral involvement, requires a search for pathology involving the recurrent laryngeal nerve. Stridor may be minimal, occurring only with agitation or upper respiratory tract infection. Placing the infant in the lateral decubitus position on the involved side may result in disappearance of the stridor as the paralyzed cord falls away from a paramedian position. A weak and often hoarse cry is usually present, and infants with bilateral cord paralysis are at risk for aspiration. Clinicians should exclude associated abnormalities of the cardiovascular system (the "cardiovocal syndrome"—see chapter 30).

Subglottic Stenosis

Although subglottic stenosis is a rare condition, it is the third most frequent lesion causing stridor in the first months of life. Stridulous breathing is often present in both inspiration and expiration. Obstruction is usually most marked 2–3 mm below the true vocal folds and consists of thickening of the soft tissues of the subglottic trachea. Symptoms vary from severe distress with cyanosis to the more frequent occurrence of minimal stridor, unless the airway is further compromised by acute infection. One should exclude congenital subglottic stenosis in the infant with Down syndrome and noisy breathing. Congenital subglottic stenosis tends to be cylindrical (Fig. 2), whereas acquired lesions are caused by irregular wedges of granulation or cicatricial tissue (Fig. 3). Acquired subglottic stenosis is commonly the result of injury caused by the tip of an endotracheal tube or excessive, vigorous suctioning. Prolonged intubation also may result in the development of paralysis or granulation tissue in the vocal folds, both of which may lead to stridor. **There is no clear relationship between the length of time that the newborn infant is intubated and the development of the lesion.**

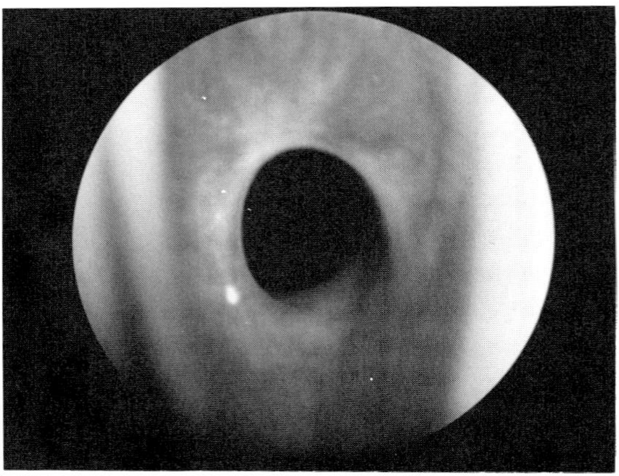

FIGURE 2. Congenital subglottic stenosis is generally cylindrical.

Thus, children with a history of a very short intubation time may develop subglottic scarring.

Most infants with congenital stenosis improve spontaneously with growth of the laryngeal structures. More aggressive therapy, such as surgical tracheal remodeling or laser resection of redundant tissue, may be indicated in cases of severe lesions.

Subglottic Hemangioma

Subglottic hemangioma presents usually in the first 5 or 6 months of life. Two-thirds of cases occur in girls. Hoarseness is commonly associated with stridor; symptoms are worsened with crying and colds. Fifty percent of all patients have associated skin hemangioma. **Hemangioma of the face or neck in a stridulous child should raise the suspicion of a similar lesion in the airway.** Most improve spontaneously, particularly when the growth of the lesion abates before 1 year of age. About one-third of the lesions appear to respond to corticosteroid therapy, whereas others necessitate treatment with endoscopic laser surgery. Radiation should be avoided because of risk of thyroid carcinoma. Other angiomatous diseases that are biologically aggressive and life-threatening have responded to antiproliferative agents, such as interferon alpha-2A, in limited trials. These agents may have promise for selected patients. The reader is advised to consult chapter 7 for a more complete listing of congenital anomalies and acquired lesions of the larynx, including noninfectious inflammatory diseases, neoplasms, trauma, and metabolic conditions that often cause stridor as well as changes in the quality of the voice.

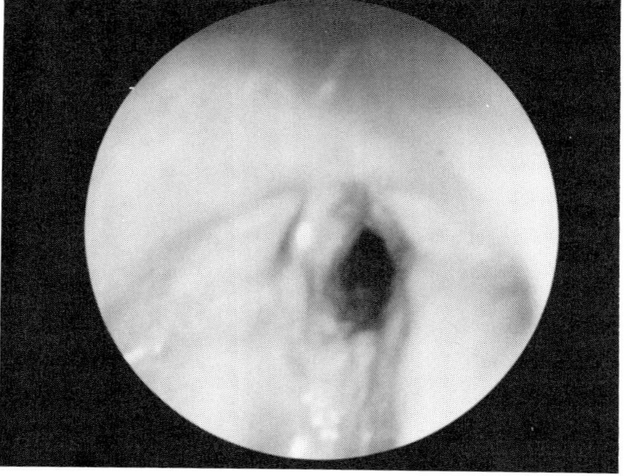

FIGURE 3. Acquired subglottic stenosis is caused by granulation or cicatricial tissue.

Vascular Compression Syndromes

There are several types of vascular compression of the airway. The most severe result in an encircling of both the trachea and the esophagus by vascular structures (the true vascular ring). During the fourth week of intrauterine life, with the development of the bronchial arches, six bursts of aortic arches develop, albeit not simultaneously. Derivatives of the fourth arch on the right become the proximal right subclavian artery, whereas the left fourth aortic arch forms part of the arch of the aorta. On rare occasions, a vascular ring around the trachea and esophagus results from failure of the *distal* portion of the dorsal aorta to disappear. As a result, both the right and left arches arise from the ascending aorta. In most instances, the right arch of the aorta is larger and passes in a retroesophageal position, causing varying degrees of compression of the airway and esophagus. Thus, depending on the relative tightness of the ring, infants may display symptoms of stridor and dysphagia from the first hours of life or remain relatively symptom-free except when stressed. Flexion of the head and neck may worsen symptoms. Diagnosis is usually made by barium esophagogram or other radiographic techniques (see chapter 38). Surgery involves division of the smaller arch, usually the anterior one. The ligamentum or ductus is usually divided with attention to the proximity of the recurrent larygneal nerve.

Almost equal in frequency to a double aortic arch is the presence of a right arch of the aorta with a retroesophageal component. A normal left ductus arteriosus or ligamentum arteriosum attaches to the descending aorta and forms a vascular ring that may produce symptoms identical to those seen with a double aortic arch. Symptoms are usually exacerbated with feeding, crying, and concomitant infections of the upper respiratory tract. Symptoms typically seem to worsen with time since the mediastinal structures become increasingly compressed by the vascular structures.

Another cause of stridor and dysphonia is gastroesophageal reflux, which causes acute and chronic inflammatory changes in the larynx (a popular diagnosis with otolaryngologists).

General Principles of Diagnosis

1. **The most efficient method of diagnosis of chronic stridor is endoscopy of the airway.** Flexible laryngoscopy and bronchoscopy are especially useful in the observation of dynamic changes of the airway while the patient is lightly sedated. The endoscopist can compress the chest, flex the neck, and, in short, duplicate situations that may cause or aggravate obstruction. This type of examination helps the diagnosis of laryngomalacia and tracheomalacia, which are dynamic conditions. During endoscopy in patients with laryngomalacia, the epiglottis can be visualized folding up on itself, and arytenoid cartilages and aryepiglottic folds tend to collapse into the lumen. The ultimate choice of instrument, of course, is up to the specialist.

2. **The most useful noninvasive method that can be done at any center is the barium esophagogram.** This examination, which includes a lateral radiograph of the neck as well as a chest radiograph in the esophagogram itself, is particularly useful in the diagnosis of extrinsic compressions of the airway, including vascular rings. The reader is referred to chapter 38 for further details.

3. **In older patients, pulmonary function testing, particularly flow volume curves, may demonstrate a fixed extrathoracic obstruction** (see chapter 41). The latest technology also allows such testing to be done on infants. The curves may be flattened due to obstruction of airflow.

SUGGESTED READING

1. Kilham H, Gillis J, Benjamin B: Severe upper airway obstruction. Pediatr Clin North Am 34:1–13, 1987.
2. Smith DS: Corticosteroids in croup: A chink in the ivory tower? J Pediatr 115:256–257, 1989.
3. Wood RE: Spelunking in the pediatric airway: Explorations with the flexible fiberoptic bronchoscope. Pediatr Clin North Am 31:785–799, 1984.

9

WHEEZING AND LOWER AIRWAY OBSTRUCTION

Howard B. Panitch, M.D.

Wheezing is sign of intrathoracic airway obstruction. It is a high-pitched musical sound usually loudest during expiration, but it also may be present during inspiration. Generation of a wheeze depends on (1) narrowing or compression of the airway and (2) sufficient airflow to make the noise. Air does not move quickly enough through peripheral or small airways to generate noise, and velocity decreases further when the airways are swollen or partially obstructed by secretions. Small airway obstruction leads to wheezing when the expiratory pressure required to overcome the obstruction also causes compression of larger, more central airways.

When wheezing is associated with small airway obstruction, the degree of airway narrowing varies from place to place within the lung, because airway compression and mucous plugging are not uniform. The generated sounds also vary in quality and acoustical characteristics according to location and thus are called **heterophonous.** In contrast, when wheezing results from a large or central airway obstruction (e.g., tracheal compression, bronchomalacia), the acoustical quality of the wheeze is constant throughout the thorax, although the loudness diminishes with distance from the site of obstruction. This type of wheeze is called **homophonous**.

Wheezing may be acute, chronic, or recurrent. When infants or young children present with sudden onset of wheezing, the sound is usually heterophonous; the one possible exception is aspiration of a foreign body. **By far, the most common cause of acute wheezing in children under 2 years of age is bronchiolitis. In older children, asthma is responsible for most acute episodes.**

Causes of chronic or recurrent wheezing include (1) reversible or transient conditions, such as inflammation or bronchospasm associated with asthma, cystic fibrosis, bronchopulmonary dysplasia, or gastroesophageal reflux, and (2) anatomic abnormalities, such as intrinsic narrowing, extrinsic compressions, or narrowing of the airway associated with forceful expiratory effort and an abnormally collapsible airway wall (Table 1). Anatomic lesions typically cause homophonous wheezing, because they involve a central airway.

ACUTE WHEEZING

Causes

Bronchiolitis. Bronchiolitis is acute inflammation of the small airways. The term typically refers to a viral lower respiratory illness characterized by tachypnea, dyspnea, and wheezing. The most common infectious agent is respiratory syncytial virus (RSV), although other viruses, such as parainfluenza types 1 and 3, adenovirus, influenza virus, and enterovirus, may cause the disease as well. Rapid techniques of viral detection, such as fluorescent antibody staining of epithelial cells obtained from nasal washings, can confirm the etiology.

The patient usually has an antecedent history of coryza, and fever may be present. The disease

TABLE 1. Causes of Wheezing in Children

Homophonous	Heterophonous
Acute	
Foreign body aspiration	Bronchiolitis Asthma
Persistent or recurrent	
Nonstructural	
Gastroesophageal reflux	Asthma
Retained foreign body	Cystic fibrosis
Chronic bacterial bronchitis	Bronchopulmonary dysplasia
	Immotile cilia syndrome
	Gastroesophageal reflux
Structural	
Tracheomalacia/ bronchomalacia	
Vascular compression/ rings	
Tracheal stenosis/webs	
Cystic lesions/masses	
Tumors	

occurs most commonly between 1 and 6 months of age, although it may occur anytime within the first 2 years of life. The respiratory rate is elevated to 50–60 breaths/minute but may be as high as 80 breaths/minute. Because airway obstruction is acute, the partial pressure of carbon dioxide (PCO_2) in not elevated unless obstruction is severe and the infant becomes fatigued. In contrast, the most common blood gas abnormality is hypoxemia, which is readily corrected by the administration of supplemental oxygen. As a rule of thumb, when the respiratory rate is greater than 60, the PO_2 is less than 60 torr. Dehydration occurs because increased fluid requirements due to tachypena and fever are accompanied by decreased fluid intake due to dyspnea. The illness is usually self-limited, with symptoms resolving in 7–10 days. In children with underlying cardiopulmonary disease, however, the course may be protracted.

Airway obstruction results from mucosal inflammation, necrosis, and sloughing as well as from edema of the airway wall and increased production of secretions. Bronchoconstriction may also contribute to airway narrowing. A subset of patients demonstrates improvement after bronchodilator therapy, although which patients will respond cannot be predicted by symptoms or family history. Thus a therapeutic trial of bronchodilators, administered by aerosol in the office, is the simplest way to determine whether or not such therapy should be prescribed.

Infants who are hypoxemic or too distressed to drink enough fluids to maintain adequate hydration should be hospitalized. Treatment is supportive, involving oxygen supplementation and fluid administration to correct deficits and to supply the increased demands. Bronchodilator aerosols (albuterol, metaproterenol) are routinely administered in the hospital if a beneficial effect is noted. No evidence indicates that corticosteroids alone hasten resolution of symptoms or relieve airway obstruction, although the combined use of bronchodilators and corticosteroids may have an additive effect. Use of corticosteroids should be restricted to infants who demonstrate a significant bronchodilator response.

Antiviral therapy (ribavirin) is reserved for hospitalized infants younger than 6 weeks of age, infants with respiratory failure, or infants with underlying cardiac or pulmonary disease and immunodeficiency. Antibiotics are typically not indicated in otherwise healthy infants, because bacterial superinfection is rare. Recently, passive immunization with RSV-hyperimmune globulin has been shown to decrease both the incidence and the severity of lower respiratory tract illness in high-risk infants. This specially formulated immune globulin is not yet readily available, but its prophylactic use may become an important component in the care of high-risk infants.

Asthma. Acute wheezing may mark the first episode of asthma or reactive ariways disease. **No child is too young to have reversible airway obstruction.** Even preterm airway smooth muscle may respond to bronchoconstrictor and bronchodilator agents, and newborns have been shown to display airway reactivity.

Asthma refers to recurrent episodes of airway obstruction associated with bronchoconstriction and airway inflammation. Thus, it is not possible to confirm the diagnosis during the first acute episode. Improvement in respiratory function after administration of a bronchodilator, however, should be ascertained by noting change in respiratory rate, use of accessory muscles, degree of retractions, wheezing, and air entry in any patient who presents with acute onset of heterophonous wheezing (see chapter 13 for further discussion).

Aspiration of a Foreign Body. Aspiration of a foreign body should be suspected in any child who has unequal breath sounds, localized homophonous wheezes, or localized hyperinflation or atelectasis on chest radiographs, **even without the history of a choking episode.** Infants younger than 6–9 months are unlikely to aspirate a foreign body, because they are not mobile enough to get their hands on one. Older siblings, however, may bring the foreign body to a younger infant.

In adults foreign bodies are more likely to lodge in the right main bronchus, because it is wider than the left and makes less of an angle with the trachea, but this fact does not apply in children, in whom lodging may occur in either bronchus. Occasionally, the foreign body may trigger a generalized irritant response, and diffuse heterophonous wheezes also may be present.

The diagnosis is aided by the demonstration of atelectasis or localized air trapping on chest radiographs obtained during inspiration and expiration. Decubitus views of the chest may show impaired emptying of the affected area when it is dependent (see chapter 37). Absence of radiographic findings does not rule out a foreign body. **If aspiration of a foreign body is suspected, rigid bronchoscopy is mandatory. A retained foreign body may also cause chronic or persistent wheezing when the diagnosis is delayed because there is no history of a choking episode and respiratory compromise is mild.**

General Rules of Management

1. **Hypoxemia should *always* be corrected with administration of supplemental oxygen** in patients with acute-onset wheezing, because they do not depend on an "hypoxic drive" to maintain respirations. Hypoxemia results from areas of ventilation-perfusion inequality. Hypercapnia occurs with severe obstruction and hypoventilation due to respiratory muscle fatigue.

2. Parenteral fluids should be used judiciously to replace deficits and ongoing losses. **Excessive fluid administration may exacerbate airway obstruction by causing interstitial edema.**

3. It is reasonable to administer an aerosolized bronchodilator to any patient with heterophonous wheezing to determine whether or not there is improvement. Aerosolized bronchodilators represent the optimal route of administration for infants. Occasionally, two or three aerosol treatments are required before a discernible improvement is noted. On rare occasions, bronchodilators may worsen wheezing. In such patients, the physician should consider the possibility that the central airways are abnormally collapsible, and further use of bronchodilators must be withheld.

4. A chest radiograph in two views (frontal and lateral) should be obtained in any patient with acute onset of homophonous wheezing, unequal breath sounds, or hypoxemia to rule out obstruction of a central airway.

5. When aspiration of a foreign body is suspected, bronchoscopy is mandatory.

6. Atelectasis during acute episodes of wheezing occurs frequently, because mucus glands are numerous and collateral ventilation is poorly developed in infants and young children. Bronchoscopy should not be performed during the acute phase of wheezing. Most areas of atelectasis will clear slowly with conventional therapy and passage of time. Bronchoscopy should be reserved for patients whose atelectasis fails to resolve after several weeks of therapy or patients in whom an anatomic obstruction of the bronchus is suspected.

PERSISTENT OR RECURRENT WHEEZING

Nonstructural Causes

Asthma or Reactive Airways Disease. Asthma is the most common cause of wheezing among children. As many as 40% of children with reactive airways disease have perennial symptoms. Patients with undiagnosed or poorly controlled asthma may have daily cough and wheeze, with frequent exacerbations following even trivial exertion. The most common triggers of exacerbations of asthma in children include upper respiratory infections and exercise (see chapter 13). Other chronic diseases that cause persistent or recurrent wheezing are discussed elsewhere in this text (e.g., cystic fibrosis, chapter 14; bronchopulmonary dysplasia, chapter 21).

Gastroesophageal Reflux. Gastroesophageal reflux (GER) is defined as the retrogarde passage of stomach contents into the esophagus secondary to relaxation of the lower esophageal sphincter. GER is differentiated from vomiting by the fact that it is passive and not accompanied by reverse peristalsis of the esophagus. GER occurs frequently in most infants without causing medical problems and is self-lmited. A subset of infants, however, develops chronic pulmonary symptoms. GER may occur in older children and also complicate the course of patients with asthma.

Wheezing from GER results either from reflex bronchospasm after esophageal irritation or from aspiration of gastric contents. Massive aspiration is extremely uncommon; instead, small amounts of gastric contents may be aspirated frequently. Wheezing is often homophonous, as lobar and segmental airways become narrowed by inflammation and edema, but heterophonous wheezing also may occur. Although many older patients will not complain of heartburn or brackish taste in their mouths, GER should be considered in patients whose symptoms worsen after meals or when they are supine. A barium swallow should be obtained in any patient in whom GER is considered, principally to evaluate the anatomy of the upper gastrointestinal tract for evidence of esophageal inflammation and stricture, gastric outlet obstruction, or intestinal malrotation. The study is not sensitive for GER, and when reflux is present, a causal relationship to wheezing cannot be assumed. If the history is highly suggestive of GER and no abnormality is seen on the barium swallow, medical therapy may be instituted without further testing.

More sensitive tests for reflux, such as radionuclide scintigraphy (GER scan) or extended pH probe monitoring, should be performed if symptoms persist despite medical therapy or if the history is only mildly suggestive of GER. The GER scan also assesses gastric emptying, whereas pH probe monitoring, together with clinical assessment, allows correlation of reflux events with episodes of wheezing. Occasionally, these studies yield equivocal or contradictory results. In such situations, bronchoscopy with bronchoalveolar lavage can aid in the diagnosis of GER with aspiration. The airways appear edematous or inflamed and friable. Excessive numbers of lipid-laden macrophages from bronchoalveolar lavage specimens provide some indication of aspiration. Similar problems occur in children with swallowing dysfunction, who aspirate directly "from above," without first regurgitating gastric contents.

Treatment of GER entails a stepped approach of increasing intervention. Chalasia precautions, involving the use of small frequent feedings, prone positioning and elevation of the head of the crib, are the least invasive and often resolve GER. If symptoms persist, medications that decrease gastric acid production (ranitidine, 2–4 mg/kg/dose, twice daily, or cimetidine, 20–40 mg/kg/day, given every 6 hr) are used in combination with medications that increase the speed of gastric emptying (metoclopramide, 0.1 mg/kg/dose, given 4 times/day, 20 min before meals and at bedtime) or directly increase the sphincter tone of the lower esophagus (bethanechol, 2.9 mg/m^2/dose, 3 times/day). Surgical treatment, or fundoplication, is reserved for patients with severe life-threatening events or for patients whose symptoms persist despite medical therapy.

Chronic bronchitis. Chronic bronchitis in children is usually associated with lung diseases in which bacterial infection and altered host defenses are common (e.g., cystic fibrosis, bronchopulmonary dysplasia, immotile cilia syndrome). Recently attention has focused on a group of patients who have had prolonged courses of wheezing unresponsive to bronchodilator therapy and no underlying chronic disease. Most of these patients either developed wheezing after an acute illness (often RSV disease) or had conditions that kept the airways irritated (GER with presumptive aspiration). Bronchoscopic evaluation disclosed diffuse airway edema with inflamed, friable mucosa. Quantitative cultures of bronchoalveolar lavage fluid yielded significant amounts of bacteria, the majority of which (*Moraxella* sp., nontypable *Hemophilus influenzae*) were beta-lactamase positive (Alpert BE: personal communication). Thus, in patients with chronic wheezing unresponsive to bronchodilator therapy, it is reasonable to try a 2–4 week course of beta-lactamase-resistant antibiotics.

Structural Causes

Wheezing that results from a structural lesion of the airway is virtually always homophonous. Any patient also may have asthma and heterophonous wheezes, which are heard in addition to the central airway wheeze.

Tracheomalacia or Bronchomalacia. The airways of infants and young children are more deformable and collapsible than those of adults. When exposed to high collapsing pressures, as during coughing or crying, young patients are more likely to develop central airway narrowing. Similarly, young patients with fixed peripheral airway obstruction may develop central airway narrowing because of the increased pleural pressures generated during exhalation. In addition, because the immature airway is so deformable, it is more likely than the adult airway to sustain injury after exposure to positive pressure. **Thus, the incidence of "acquired" tracheomalacia or bronchomalacia is much higher in infants with a history of prematurity and mechanical ventilation.**

Congenital tracheomalacia or bronchomalacia may cause wheezing from birth, but more commonly wheezing becomes apparent in the first 2–3 months of life as the infant becomes more active and generates stronger respiratory efforts. When the intrathoracic airway alone is involved, expiratory homophonous wheezing is present with a quiet inspiratory phase. If extrathoracic tracheomalacia is also present, a high-pitched inspiratory stridor may also be present. **Intrathoracic tracheomalacia or bronchomalacia should be suspected in infants who wheeze loudly during activity but are quiet at rest.** Because the degree of airway narrowing depends on the amount of collapsing pressure applied, wheezing is loudest during periods of increased expiratory effort (crying, agitation). In contrast, wheezing may disappear during sleep when expiration is unlabored. Similarly, respiratory infections may worsen airway collapse by causing the infant to exert an increased effort during breathing.

The diagnosis of tracheomalacia or bronchomalacia is made clinically and may be confirmed endoscopically. The ideal study employs flexible bronchoscopy with light sedation so dynamic events can be seen. During spontaneous expiration, the trachea or bronchi narrow by more than 50% of their resting caliber. When bronchoscopy is not available, fluoroscopy of the airway can demonstrate collapse during exhalation.

When central airway collapse is severe, the patient should be referred to a pulmonologist or otolaryngologist. Treatment options include bronchoconstrictor therapy, placement of a tracheostomy tube to bypass the collapsible segment, prolonged use of continuous positive airway pressure (CPAP) to stent the airway, or aortopexy to suspend the anterior trachea and widen the airway as the aorta is suspended. Most infants, however, require no specific therapy. Symptoms slowly resolve over the first 2 years of life.

Congenital Heart Disease and Vascular Rings. Other patients at risk for central airway collapse are those with congenital heart disease or vascular rings (see chapter 30). Many experts believe that prolonged compression of the airways during fetal development results in a permanent defect in cartilage, because after surgical repair, many patients have persistent tracheo- or bronchomalacia at the site of compression and so continue to wheeze.

Other structural lesions that cause wheezing are considerably less common. Tracheal stenosis, tracheal webs, and complete cartilaginous rings with absence of the pars membranacea are congenital lesions that may cause critical narrowing of the airway. Acquired tracheal stenosis may result from repeated local trauma in patients with artificial airways. Because these lesions do not allow airway caliber to change during inspiration or expiration, they usually cause biphasic noises; they can be distinguished only by endoscopy. Wheezing in patients with congenital lobar emphysema may arise from airflow through a narrowed bronchus of the involved lobe or from a bronchus compressed by the overexpanded lobe. Mediastinal masses likewise may compress airways and cause complete or partial obstruction. The chest radiograph may demonstrate a hyperlucent lobe or narrowing of the air column by a mass. Computerized tomography is the best study for evaluating mediastinal structures or masses arising from the mediastinum. Finally, although rare in childhood, endobronchial tumors may cause wheezing. The most likely benign lesions are bronchial adenoma and carcinoid.

General Principles of Diagnosis

1. Symptoms that start early in life are suggestive of congenital lesions, tend to intensify with age, and may become acutely worse during upper respiratory infections. Chronic wheezing that is loudest when the child is active but disappears during quiet breathing or changes

with the child's position suggests a structural lesion of the central airway.

2. The single best noninvasive study in the diagnosis of both wheezing and stridor is the barium esophagogram. The barium-filled esophagus can disclose vascular rings or compressions or cardiac chamber englargement.

3. The most efficient method of evaluating the child with persistent wheezing is pediatric flexible bronchoscopy. Direct visualization of the airway will disclose compression, dynamic narrowing, endobronchial lesions, or mucosal inflammation. Examination of bronchoalveolar lavage fluid may confirm the diagnosis of viral infection, hemosiderosis, or aspiration.

4. Bronchodilator responsiveness or airway hyperreactivity may be objectively assessed in older children by spirometry and airway challenges with cold air, exercise, or methacholine; in infants, by specialized pulmonary function testing equipment. If such equipment is unavailable, **bronchodilator responsiveness can be assessed clinically by observing respiratory rate, severity of retractions and work of breathing, air entry, and wheezing.**

SUGGESTED READING

1. Mair EA, Parsons DS: Pediatric tracheobronchomalacia and major airway collapse. Ann Otol Rhinol Laryngol 101:300–309, 1992.
2. Orenstein SR, Orenstein DM: Gastroesophageal reflux and respiratory disease in children. J Pediatr 112:847–858, 1988.
3. Panitch HB, Callahan CW Jr, Schidlow DV: Bronchiolitis in children. Clin Chest Med 14:715–731, 1993.
4. Prendiville A, Green S, Silverman M: Airway responsiveness in wheezy infants: Evidence for functional β adrenergic receptors. Thorax 42:100–104, 1987.

COMMENTARY

by Daniel V. Schidlow, M.D.

The intrathoracic airway in children is particularly susceptible to insult. Wheezing is a common feature of many diseases. "All that wheezes is not asthma," goes the axiom, but certainly a lot of what wheezes is. The difficulties in elucidating the differential diagnosis and occasionally in determining the site of airways obstrution have been well described in this chapter.

A condition that continues to puzzle physicians is gastroesophageal reflux (GER). Although this condition indisputably causes wheezing and other respiratory complications either by reflex mechanisms or by direct aspiration, in my opinion it is blamed for too many ills. GER has become somewhat of a diagnostic wastebasket in the last few years, into which many unexplained respiratory symptoms, especially wheezing, are thrown.

Gastroesophageal reflux is very prevalent, particularly in infants. Aggressive study would reveal such reflux in asymptomatic infants from time to time. Thus, the finding of GER in a child with respiratory symptoms must be evaluated critically before a cause-effect relationship is assigned. In my view, GER as a cause of respiratory symptoms must be approached almost as a diagnosis of exclusion, in the absence of obvious signs and only after all efforts have been made to rule out other causes of respiratory disease. In my experience, reflux is most often identifiable as the cause of recurrent or chronic lung disease in patients who have basically no gastrointestinal symptoms. Another clinical observation (not scientifically collaborated with controlled studies) is that GER appears to be more prevalant in children who are slightly hypotonic and/or very obese. Clearly, reflux is very prevalent and a relatively common cause of respiratory symptoms in children with neurologic and muscular deficits. GER also should be suspected in patients whose symptoms occur particularly at night, while recumbent, or after meals.

Some clinicians place great stock in the finding of lipid-laden macrophages in bronchoalveolar lavage fluid. Two caveats, however, seem appropriate: (1) this procedure should be performed only after all other avenues for diagnosis have been exhausted, and (2) lipid-laden macrophages are also present in children who have chronic small airway obstruction for other causes. Some authors have proposed semi-quantitative methods, involving determination of relative numbers of lipid-laden macrophages or amounts of fat, as indicators for aspiration. Because there is no gold standard for the diagnosis of aspiration, the data correlating GER with aspiration, using lipid-laden macarophages as indicators, must be critically examined.

We ought to be rather circumspect in diagnosing GER as the cause of respiratory symptoms. When everything is said and done, the diagnosis boils down to good clinical judgment.

10

HEMOPTYSIS

Howard B. Panitch, M.D.

It is uncommon for a child to cough up blood. When it occurs, however, hemoptysis can be terrifying for the patient, the family, and the treating physician. In the majority of cases, with the aid of a thorough history and physical examination and a few simple laboratory tests, the cause of bleeding can be determined and appropriate therapy instituted.

DIAGNOSIS

The first step in the evaluation is to determine that bleeding originated from the lower airways. Bleeding from the nose, nasopharynx, or oropharynx often can be detected by simple inspection. An older child may be able to tell whether the blood was produced with coughing or vomiting, but this differentiation may be impossible in an infant. **When hemoptysis cannot be differentiated from hematemesis by history, a description of the material produced may help to distinguish the site of bleeding.** Blood that emanates from the gastrointestinal tract is typically dark red or brown and may be mixed with food; its pH is acidic. In contrast, blood that originates from the respiratory tract is usually bright red, foamy, and frequently mixed with sputum; its pH is typically alkaline. Some patients complain of a localized area of chest pain or of warmth or gurgling in the chest that correlates with the bleeding site.

Once a pulmonary source has been confirmed, the amount and rate of bleeding must be quantitated. This can be difficult because the blood may be mixed with sputum or saliva, and the anxiety produced by the child's coughing up of blood may result in an exaggerated perception of bleeding by family members. To help the patient to establish the amount of bleeding, one can relate the size of the clot of blood coughed up to different-sized coins (i.e., dime, quarter, half dollar) or estimate how much of a teacup would be filled.

The severity of hemoptysis is determined by both the quantity and the rate of elimination of blood. Mild hemoptysis refers to production of less than 60 ml of blood per day. Expectoration of 200–600 ml of blood in a 24-hour period is considered serious (massive). Smaller quantities of expectorated blood denote severe hemoptysis when bleeding occurs for several days. Losses of 125 ml or more per hour are life-threatening.

Factors that can worsen the prognosis of a patient with hemoptysis include (1) preexisting pulmonary disease; (2) inability to clear secretions because of altered mental status or ineffective cough; (3) coagulation defects; and (4) the rate of bleeding. **In cases of massive hemoptysis, death occurs by asphyxiation, not by exsanguination.**

Once the site and approximate quantity of bleeding have been established, attempts should be made to determine the actual cause of bleeding. It is helpful to consider patients with no known medical history separately from those with a chronic underlying disorder (Table 1). Although many causes of hemoptysis in children have been identified, information concerning their relative frequency is limited.

BLEEDING IN APPARENTLY HEALTHY CHILDREN

In children with no medical history, the most common causes of hemoptysis are acute

TABLE 1. Conditions Associated with Hemoptysis in Children

Children with No Previous Medical History
Tracheobronchitis
Retained foreign body
Congenital malformations
Arteriovenous malformations
Lung parasites
Nonspecific endothelial damage (toxin exposure)
Trauma
Tumors
Thromboembolism
Children with Preexisting Medical Conditions
Cystic fibrosis
Congenital heart disease
Sickle-cell anemia
Autoimmune disorders
Familial telangiectasia (Osler-Weber-Rendu syndrome)
Tuberculosis (old)
Idiopathic pulmonary hemosiderosis

infectious tracheobronchitis and an inflammatory bronchial reaction due to a retained foreign body. Although hemoptysis in adults often suggests the presence of a neoplastic lesion, in a previously well child it does not carry a grim prognosis.

The bleeding associated with bronchitis or tracheitis is usually mild and self-limited. There may be a flulike prodrome before streaks of blood appear in the sputum. Bleeding is caused by friability of airway mucosa, which resolves when the acute infection subsides.

TABLE 2. Clues to the Etiology of Hemoptysis

Diagnosis	Clues
Bronchiectasis	Purulent sputum Digital clubbing Weight loss
Retained foreign body	Lobar or unilateral hyperlucency or atelectasis on plain chest radiograph Asymmetry on lateral decubitus view
Arteriovenous malformation	Bruit Cyanosis, dyspnea on exertion Digital clubbing Cutaneous or mucosal telangiectasia
Connective tissue disorders	Vague constitutional signs Saddle-bridge nasal deformity Malar rash

Bleeding from a retained foreign body can be massive, especially when the aspirated substance is organic material that creates an intense inflammatory reaction. In as many as one-third of patients, a history of a choking episode cannot be elicited. Often the foreign body remains in the respiratory tree for weeks to months before hemoptysis occurs. Organic foreign bodies are radiolucent and cannot be detected on a chest radiograph. If the foreign body allows passage of air around it, air-trapping on decubitus radiographic views or atelectasis may be absent. **In summary, an abnormal radiograph can confirm the presence of a foreign body, but a normal study does not rule it out. Thus, the physician must maintain a high index of suspicion for a retained foreign body in an otherwise healthy child with hemoptysis.**

Other causes of hemoptysis in previously healthy children, all of which are considerably less common, include congenital abnormalities such as enteric cysts or arteriovenous malformations (Table 2). Approximately one-half of the patients with arteriovenous malformations have Osler-Weber-Rendu syndrome, an autosomal dominant condition. Recurrent epistaxis, positive family history, or findings of widespread telangiectasia confirm the diagnosis. Parasitic infections and lung abscesses may erode pulmonary vessels and result in hemoptysis. Worldwide, paragonimiasis and echinococcosis are important causes of hemoptysis in children. Thus, travel and dietary histories are important in determining the etiology of bleeding.

Hemoptysis may be the first manifestation of a systemic immunologic disorder, such as Goodpasture syndrome, systemic lupus erythematosus, polyarteritis nodosa, or Wegener granulomatosis. Malaise, recent weight loss, unexplained fever, hypertension, amenorrhea, or hematuria in an adolescent should prompt further investigation for one of these entities. Although most connective tissue diseases occur more frequently in females, Goodpasture syndrome is seen more commonly in males. Hemoptysis in an infant or young child may represent the onset of idiopathic pulmonary hemosiderosis. Although no single immune response can be demonstrated in patients with this disorder, a subset of patients with specific cow milk precipitins in their serum may show symptomatic improvement with avoidance of cow milk products.

Miscellaneous causes of hemoptysis in previously well children include inhalation of toxic substances that disrupt the endothelial integrity of pulmonary capillaries, such as carbon monoxide, nitrogen dioxide, or crack cocaine. Finally, although rare in children, benign adenomas, malignant primary tumors, or metastatic tumors can cause hemoptysis by erosion into airway mucosa, by postobstructive infection of airways, or by autonecrosis of richly vascularized neoplastic lesions.

BLEEDING IN CHILDREN WITH UNDERLYING CONDITIONS

The most common underlying condition associated with hemoptysis in children is cystic fibrosis. Severity of hemoptysis ranges from blood streaks in sputum to massive bleeding. Chronic inflammation associated with bronchiectasis induces formation of anastomoses between pulmonary and bronchial systemic arteries, causing brisk bleeding in some cases.

Patients with congenital heart disease may experience hemoptysis when the lesions cause either pulmonary venous obstruction or a marked reduction in pulmonary artery blood flow. When pulmonary venous pressures are chronically elevated, as with mitral stenosis, dilation or angiomatoid changes of small pulmonary arteries may result in subsequent bleeding. Severe reduction in pulmonary artery blood flow may result in thrombosis of small pulmonary arteries, weakness of pulmonary artery walls, and a marked increase in bronchial artery circulation. These vascular changes occur over long periods of time; thus, bleeding occurs in the adolescent or young adult.

Patients with sickle-cell anemia or other hemoglobinopathies develop thrombosis in situ, which causes pulmonary infarction and occasionally hemoptysis. As previously mentioned, patients with known connective tissue disease may develop pulmonary bleeding as a result of direct injury to the pulmonary vascular bed. In addition, side effects of medications may include abnormalities of coagulation. Finally, patients with pulmonary hemosiderosis develop recurrent pneumonias and anemia. They also may have a history of recurrent wheezing, but unlike children with asthma, they appear ill between exacerbations.

EVALUATION

Mild hemoptysis can be evaluated in the office. In contrast, the child with massive hemoptysis should be admitted to a facility with anesthesiologists who are expert in pediatric airway management. **Bronchoscopy and interventional radiology should be available for the patient with life-threatening hemoptysis.**

Adequate ventilation and oxygenation are the first priorities when bleeding is severe. Pulse oximetry detects oxyhemoglobin desaturation as long as perfusion is adequate. If oxyhemoglobin desaturation is significant (i.e., SaO_2 $<94\%$), an arterial or capillary blood gas sample should be obtained.

After adequate ventilation and oxygenation have been ensured, the intravascular volume status must be determined. Changes in baseline and orthostatic measurements of pulse and blood pressure, which may be the earliest signs of serious hypovolemia, signal the need for urgent fluid replacement.

All patients with massive bleeding should have a complete blood count, platelet count, and type and cross-match in expectation of transfusion. Anemia may be absent if adequate time has not passed to allow equilibration of the intra- and extravascular spaces. The white blood cell count may be elevated in patients with chronic infection, whereas eosinophilia is suggestive of parasitic infections or exposure to toxic substances such as crack cocaine. Assessment of platelet number and coagulation profiles can rule out a bleeding diathesis.

Once ventilation and circulatory status are stabilized, efforts must be directed toward determining the site and the cause of bleeding. The nose and mouth must be examined to identify bleeding from the upper airway. Telangiectasia in the nose or under the tongue confirms the diagnosis of Osler-Weber-Rendu syndrome. Auscultation of the chest may disclose a bruit associated with an arteriovenous malformation: when the patient is asked to inspire against a closed glottis, pulmonary blood flow increases and the bruit becomes louder. Digital clubbing points to bronchiectasis or significant shunting through an arteriovenous malformation. Cutaneous telangiectasia or a malar rash is suggestive of connective tissue disease.

A chest radiograph should be obtained in all patients. It may be normal in as many as one-half of all cases, or it may show a discrete mass, an infiltrate, or unilateral hyperinflation (suggestive of an aspirated foreign body). In patients with chronic lung disease, a prominent pulmonary blood vessel may point to the bleeding site. Computerized tomography (CT) with contrast or angiography can confirm the diagnosis of congenital malformations in patients with suspicious radiographs (see chapter 38).

Rigid or flexible bronchoscopy may be useful in visualizing blood emerging from a particular lobar bronchus, especially if the bleeding has not completely subsided. Rigid bronchoscopy is preferred when bleeding is active, because the instrument has a larger suction channel and the patient's airway can be controlled during the procedure. In addition, if a foreign body is present, it can be extracted. We have used flexible bronchoscopy and bronchoalveolar lavage instead of gastric washings and lung biopsy to detect hemosiderin-laden macrophages for the diagnosis of pulmonary hemosiderosis. Angiography is not a useful procedure to localize active bleeding, although the presence of dilated or tortuous vessels in a particular area correlates closely with bronchoscopic visualization of blood emanating from the corresponding bronchus.

MANAGEMENT

In patients who are bleeding briskly or who have signs of respiratory compromise (hypoxemia, hypercapnia, increasing dyspnea), the first step is to secure the airway by endotracheal intubation. Endoctracheal intubation also should be performed in any patient unable to cough to protect the airway. If the bleeding site can be identified, keeping the ipsilateral side dependent helps to avoid soiling the better-functioning lung.

Adequate intravenous access must be established, with catheters large enough to push fluids quickly. Crystalloid can be used as the initial volume expander until blood type and cross-match studies allow replacement of appropriate blood products. Packed red blood cells should be given if signs of hypovolemia ensue.

Further management of hemoptysis is dictated by the etiology of bleeding. For instance, in a patient with cystic fibrosis who experiences hemoptysis during a pulmonary exacerbation, aggressive antibiotic treatment and pulmonary drainage techniques are important modalities for treating infection and decreasing inflammation.

Most episodes of hemoptysis subside within a few days without specific therapy. If, however, bleeding continues unabated or the patient becomes further compromised, specific therapies are necessary to slow or stop the bleeding. Options include intravenous infusions of premarin or pitressin, embolization of bronchial arteries, or balloon catheter tamponade of the bronchus from which blood is emanating. If bleeding persists despite such interventions, lung resection should be considered. Lobectomy should be performed only as a last resort in patients who have a reasonably good chance of postoperative recovery and reasonably good pulmonary functions.

In summary, hemoptysis is an uncommon event in children, but its presence demands prompt attention. Every effort should be made to quantitate the amount of bleeding and to determine the bleeding site. In approximately 20% of cases, despite exhaustive investigation, no etiology for hemoptysis will be found. The prognosis for patients with essential hemoptysis is excellent, and the likelihood of recurrence is low.

SUGGESTED READING

1. Conlan AA: Massive hemoptysis—Diagnostic and therapeutic implications. Surg Annu 17:337–354, 1985.
2. Haroutunian LM, Neill CA: Pulmonary complications of congenital heart disease: Hemoptysis. Am Heart J 4:540–559, 1972.
3. Levine BW: Case records of the Massachusetts General Hospital. N Engl J Med 309:1374–1381, 1983.
4. Winter SM, Ingbar DH: Massive hemoptysis: Pathogenesis and management. J Intens Care Med 3:171–188, 1988.

11

COUGH

Daniel V. Schidlow, M.D.

Cough is a reflex defense mechanism of the respiratory tree. Its main objective is to rid the tracheobronchial tree of foreign particles and mucus. Effective cough mechanism is necessary to maintain clean airways, particularly when mucociliary clearance is damaged.

The cough reflex involves three main sites: (1) the cough receptors located in the nose, sinuses, pharynx, trachea, ear canal, and pleura, among other areas; (2) the cough center located in the brainstem, to which efferent stimuli arise and are processed; and (3) effectors, such as the diaphragm and intercostal muscles, that participate in the active mechanism of cough after efferent impulses are received from the cough center.

The actual mechanism of cough consists of a short inspiration and inflation of the lungs with air, followed by closure of the glottis, compression of the air, and contraction of chest, abdominal, and perineal muscles. This preparatory stage, during which increased airway pressure is created, is followed by a sudden opening of the glottis and the generation of high-velocity airflow during exhalation. **Cough can be caused by one or all of the following mechanisms: (1) airway inflammation and production of excessive mucus, (2) spasm of bronchial smooth muscle, and (3) direct stimulation of cough receptors.**

COUGH IN THE FIRST MONTH OF LIFE

Cough in the neonatal period is always abnormal and a cause for concern. It is a reflection of disease, usually of some severity. Although it is common for newborn infants to sneeze, it is abnormal for them to cough. The cough reflex is not well developed early in life and is totally absent in premature babies. As the child gets older, the cough reflex rapidly develops. Causes of cough in the neonatal period are listed in the mnemonic **CRADLE** (Table 1). Of the conditions listed, heart failure is the least common as a cause of cough. The incidence of respiratory infections seems to be increasing as rates of immunization against pertussis infection decrease, and HIV infection, among others, rises. Bronchiolitis due to respiratory syncytial virus (RSV) in the winter months causes cough and apnea in this age group.

COUGH IN INFANTS

In infants beyond the neonatal period, cough secondary to acute viral infections is quite common. When cough persists beyond the expected time of resolution of the disease, physicians must think of other possible diagnoses. **The most common cause of chronic or persistent cough in infants is reactive airway disease.** The cough has a brassy quality, and the child may sound congested with increased transmission of breath sounds that have a "wet" quality, characteristic of increased secretions in the respiratory tract. The examiner must try to differentiate between upper airway (i.e., nose and hypopharynx) congestion, which is characteristic of rhinitis and postnasal drip, and lower airway noises caused by mucosal edema, increased secretions, and bronchospasm.

TABLE 1. Causes of Cough in the Neonatal Period

C	**C**ystic fibrosis
R	**R**espiratory infections
A	**A**spiration (swallowing dysfunction, gastroesophageal reflux, tracheoesophageal fistula)
D	**D**yskinesia of cilia
L	**L**ung, airway, and vascular malformations
E	**E**dema (heart failure)

Expiratory wheezing and prolonged exhalation are associated with lower airway noises. Cough associated with postnasal drip tends to be worse in the recumbent position, usually when the child is put to bed and when the child awakens in the morning.

Infection with *Bordetella pertusis* may cause cough that persists for up to 6 months. Whereas some children present with the characteristic "whoop" of varying intensity, others do not. Children with cystic fibrosis, with a foreign body retained in the airway, or with pulmonary staphylococcal infection may have a cough with pertussoid characteristics. Children infected with *Chlamydia trachomatis* have a staccato cough, characterized—as the musical term suggests—by bursts of short, brassy cough. Infection with RSV and other viruses may present with cough that persists for a few months after the initial episode.

Other causes of cough in this age group include extrinsic compression of the airways by enlarged vessels in patients with congenital cardiac disease; edema and increased respiratory secretions due to heart failure; and aspiration due to swallowing dysfuncion. Gastroesophageal reflux conceivably causes cough by direct stimulation of cough receptors with acid or by inflammation due to aspiration of stomach contents into the airway.

COUGH IN SCHOOL-AGE CHILDREN AND ADOLESCENTS

The most common cause of cough in school-age children and adolescents—by far—is asthma, followed in frequency by postnasal drip. Cystic fibrosis, as well as other less common causes of pulmonary inflammation, must be kept in mind. Tuberculosis is not a common cause of chronic cough in otherwise healthy children, but it occurs more often in settings such as immune deficiency.

Psychogenic cough or "cough tic syndrome" is a puzzling and relatively frequent cause of persistent cough in this age group, particularly in adolescents. The cough, which is dry, vibratory, and throaty, has been described by several authors as similar to a barking seal or as having a honking quality. It ranges in severity from mild throat-clearing to fits of uncontrollable, violent cough, occasionally associated with subsequent vomiting and exhaustion. The symptom may appear spontaneously or follow a respiratory infection; it has no clear pattern other than absence during sleep or when the patient is deeply distracted. Patients usually go from specialist to specialist in search of a physical diagnosis; family life and school attendance are disrupted, and a vicious cycle is established. In our experience, children with psychogenic cough tend to be good students, compulsive and eager to please. They suffer from other somatic symptoms, such as abdominal pain and headaches, and come from families in which somatization, talk about symptoms, or actual diseases are common. Approach to treatment ranges from benign neglect (shifting the focus of attention to everyday concerns and away from the symptom) to self-hypnosis and family therapy. In many cases, the cough is a manifestation of underlying stress and conflict. Although therapies such as wrapping the child in a tight-fitting sheet may occasionally work, **such maneuvers basically have a placebo or aversive effect and do not address the underlying conflict or personality characteristics that make the patient prone to other psychosomatic ailments.**

PHYSICAL EXAMINATION

The physical examination is important. In examining the child, one must look for allergic shiners, nasal crease, hypertrophy of the turbinates, polyps, enlarged tonsils, retractions, wheezing, and clubbing of the digits. Wheezing commonly is not heard during normal breathing, and one needs to help the patient to generate a forceful exhalation to create dynamic compression of the airways ("to squeeze the wheeze") (see chapter 9). If pulmonary function testing is not available, one may administer an inhaled bronchodilator and then listen again after 10–15 minutes to see whether the cough has been relieved or wheezing has disappeared. This procedure helps to confirm the diagnosis of airway reactivity.

The most useful laboratory test is measurement of pulmonary function. Evidence of airway reactivity with decrease of airflows and reversibility by bronchodilators confirms the diagnosis of reversible airway obstruction. Provocation with exercise (running up and down stairs) or exposure to cold air may elicit some wheezing and an abnormality in the pulmonary function test. A sweat test should be obtained in any child with chronic cough, particularly if purulent sputum is expectorated, if weight gain is poor, or if other signs of cystic fibrosis are present. A culture may help to determine the etiology of the cough if purulent secretions are produced, because the presence of *Staphylococcus aureus* or *Pseudomonas* sp. will steer the physician in the direction of a chronic disease of the airways, such as cystic fibrosis.

In general, laboratory studies for patients with chronic cough in the absence of recurrent pulmonary infiltration and fever do not yield very helpful results. We believe that the laboratory work-up should be highly focused and basically should confirm clinical suspicions rather than serve as a screening device. Our primary work-up of patients with chronic cough includes a chest radiograph, a sweat test, and evaluation of pulmonary function. In other patients, we also may obtain a complete blood cell count to detect eosinophilia, lymphopenia, or leukocytosis, which point to an allergic, immunologic, or infectious etiology. Measurement of serum immunoglobulins has a very low yield, particularly in the absence of recurrent severe infections. Determination of serum levels of immunoglobulin E (IgE) is of limited usefulness. Elevated serum concentrations may point to an allergic diathesis, but a normal level does not rule out allergy.

The management of cough is obviously directed to its cause. Statistically, airway reactivity is the most common cause of chronic cough, and we recommend **a trial of bronchodilator therapy either by aerosol or orally.** Cough suppressants and decongestants are usually quite ineffective, because the doses necessary to relieve or suppress cough are often associated with undesired symptoms. Preparations containing dextromethorphan or codeine may be more useful in the relief of acute cough caused by viral or respiratory infections, allowing sleep for weary children and parents. One must remember that the administration of such preparations is treatment of the symptom, not of the underlying condition.

SUGGESTED READING

1. Cloutier GM, Loughlin CM: Chronic cough in children: A manifestation of airway hyperreactivity. Pediatrics 67:6–12, 1981.
2. Konig P: Hidden asthma in children. Am J Dis Child 135:1053–1055, 1981.
3. Lavigna JV, Davis AT, Fauber R: Behavioral management of psychogenic cough: Alternative to the "bedsheet" and other aversive techniques. Pediatrics 87:532–537, 1991.
4. Taylor JA, Novack AH, Almquist JR, Rogers JE: Efficacy of cough suppressants in children. J Pediatr 122:799–802, 1993.

12

CHEST PAIN

Richard J. Scarfone, M.D.

Chest pain is a common complaint among children, exceeded only by headache and abdominal pain as a reason for outpatient visits. The mean age of children presenting with chest pain is 12 years; it is found with equal frequency in males and females.

Chest pain in children is rarely associated with serious organic disease, yet the evaluation of such patients can be challenging. Pain may arise from one of several different organ systems, and prognosis is almost always favorable. Laboratory assessment often is not helpful, and the many cases in which an etiology is not found produce anxiety for patients, parents, and physicians. This chapter serves as a practical approach to the evaluation of the child with chest pain, with emphasis on the most common causes.

HISTORY

A detailed history is essential in assessing the child with chest pain. It is always helpful if the child is old enough to describe the pain in his or her own words. It should be ascertained when the child first experienced the symptom. In one series, children presenting to an emergency department with chest pain of more than 6 months' duration had a significantly higher incidence of nonorganic illness than children with less chronic pain. In a study of children diagnosed with idiopathic chest pain, not a single patient was subsequently diagnosed with an organic illness after a 3-year follow-up. Chronic chest pain, therefore, is usually not associated with serious underlying pathology.

The location of the pain is important. Pain that is localized and superficial is likely to originate from the chest wall; pain localized to the breast of an adolescent male may simply represent gynecomastia. The clinician should ask about the severity of the child's pain. Is it interfering with daily activities? Does it prevent the child from participating in enjoyable activities, or is a component of secondary gain involved? The frequency of the pain may help to establish the diagnosis. Pain that is present all the time may be pleuritic or originate in the chest wall. Pain that is intermittent, on the other hand, may have one of many different etiologies, including psychogenic, asthma, hyperventilation, or esophagitis. Is trauma to the chest wall a possible cause? Is the child involved in sporting activities or vigorous exercising such as push-ups? Has the child had a recent fall in which the chest may have been injured?

What are some of the factors that precipitate the pain? Pain with exertion raises concern for a cardiac etiology. Pain that occurs most commonly after a meal may represent esophagitis. If coughing or deep breathing exacerbates the pain, it may be pleuritic in origin.

Many studies have shown that psychogenic chest pain is among the most common types in children, especially adolescents. Questions about school performance, emotional stress, separations (e.g., divorce), or recent death of a loved one need to be asked. Is the child frequently anxious or bothered by other complaints, such as difficulty sleeping, headaches, or abdominal pain? Psychogenic pain is not a diagnosis of exclusion; it is based on the responses to questions such as these. If emotional stressors are associated with the pain, especially in the absence of constitutional signs or symptoms such as fever or weight loss, psychogenic pain should be suspected.

A family history is important. Of interest, among children presenting to an emergency department with chest pain, those diagnosed with a nonorganic etiology were more likely to have a family history of heart disease or chest pain than those with an organic etiology. Children are suggestible and may harbor fears about their own health when a loved one is ill. Conversely, hypertrophic obstructive cardiomyopathy has an autosomal dominant transmission in some cases, and mitral valve prolapse is familial. Both, however, are relatively uncommon causes of chest pain in children.

Past medical history should focus on chronic diseases that may produce chest pain. Examples include asthma, sickle-cell anemia, and congenital heart disease. Review of systems should include questions about constitutional symptoms such as cough or fever. Children with fever are more likely to have organic disease than children who are afebrile.

PHYSICAL EXAMINATION

Although a complete physical examination should be performed for every child with chest pain, examination of the chest and heart is most likely to help in establishing a diagnosis. Children with an abnormal physical examination are 12 times more likley to have organic disease than children with no abnormalities.

Inspection of the chest is important. A patient with bronchospasm may have substernal or intercostal retractions, whereas a patient who is hyperventilating will appear hyperpneic and may have carpal pedal spasm. Trauma may be marked by contusions or abrasions. An adolescent with gynecomastia will typically have enlarged breasts and tender nipples.

Auscultation of the lungs should be performed carefully. Examination may reveal a focal area of decreased breath sounds suggestive of pneumonia or a pleural effusion. The presence of rales or rhonchi also suggests pneumonia; wheezing, poor aeration, and a prolonged expiratory phase indicate bronchospasm.

Careful palpation of the chest wall often reveals the diagnosis. Chest pain that is easily reproducible by palpation is musculoskeletal in origin. The pectoral muscles are commonly strained during exercise and will be tender to palpation. Reproducible tenderness at the costochondral junctions indicates costochondritis, and reproducible tenderness elsewhere may represent a region of microtrauma. Less commonly, palpation may reveal the presence of subcutaneous emphysema, suggesting pneumothorax or pneumomediastinum.

Although cardiac etiologies for chest pain are uncommon in children, examination of the heart is obviously important. Physical findings with mitral valve prolapse may be subtle, such as a midsystolic click and late systolic murmur. The patient should be examined in the upright, supine, and standing positions to increase the possibility of eliciting such findings. Supraventricular tachycardia is the most common significant dysrhythmia in children. The patient may feel heart palpitations, and the examiner discovers a regular, rapid rhythm. Heart rates are above 220 beats/minute in infants and above 150 in older children. A less common cause of chest pain in children is pericarditis. A friction rub may be heard, and the heart sounds are often muffled. Patients usually assume an upright posture, leaning forward to decrease the degree of pain.

DIFFERENTIAL DIAGNOSIS

The differential diagnosis for chest pain in children is broad, encompassing a number of organ systems and diseases. After the history and physical examination, the physician should be able to narrow the possibilities. This section presents some of the causes of chest pain in children with an emphasis on the most common (Table 1).

Many studies have found that musculoskeletal and psychogenic factors are among the most common causes of chest pain in children. In a large prospective study of children presenting to an urban pediatric emergency department with chest pain, about 25% were diagnosed with idiopathic chest pain and 25% were found to have musculoskeletal etiologies, including costochondritis. About 10% of the children were diagnosed with psychogenic chest pain, whereas less than 5% had cardiac disease. The incidence of cardiac disease was low despite the fact that every patient initially diagnosed with idiopathic, psychogenic, musculoskeletal, or gastrointestinal pain or costochondritis received an electrocardiogram (EKG) and echocardiogram as part of the study. Adolescents were more likely than younger children to have a psychogenic cause for pain, whereas children less than 12 years of age were twice as likely to have a cardiorespiratory etiology.

Idiopathic chest pain was the most common diagnosis, even though each patient received a complete evaluation. Other studies also demonstrate that one-fourth to one-half of children with chest pain are undiagnosed after an initial outpatient evaluation. The natural history of such patients is resolution of symptoms without complications. In a study that followed children initially diagnosed with idiopathic chest pain, none was subsequently diagnosed with organic disease.

TABLE 1. Differential Diagnosis of Pediatric Chest Pain

	Common Causes	Uncommon Causes
Idiopathic		
Psychogenic		
Musculoskeletal	Trauma Costochondritis	Tietze syndrome Precordial catch
Tracheobronchial	Asthma Cough Pneumonia	Pleural effusion Pneumothroax Pneumomediastinum
Gastrointestinal	Esophagitis	Esophageal foreign body
Cardiac	Mitral valve prolapse Supraventricular tachycardia	Hypertrophic obstructive cardiomyopathy Myocarditis Pericarditis Aortic stenosis
Other	Hyperventilation Gynecomastia Sickle-cell anemia	

Psychogenic Chest Pain

Idiopathic chest pain is clearly a diagnosis of exclusion; the diagnosis of psychogenic chest pain, on the other hand, is based on positive historical information in conjunction with exclusion of other etiologies. Unlike a malingerer, the child with psychogenic chest pain experiences real pain, but it has no organic basis. A profile of the child with psychogenic chest pain has emerged from a number of studies. Psychogenic pain is more frequent in adolescents, particularly females. Moreover, in the large majority of such children, the pain lasts for more than 1 week. Sleep disturbances and other somatic complaints, such as headache and abdominal pain, are common. A positive family history of chest pain is also quite common.

Children who have recovered from acute life-threatening illnesses or accidents are at risk for experiencing psychogenic pain. The parents of the so-called vulnerable child, fearing that the child will die prematurely, are overprotective and highly sensitive even to mild complaints.

About one-third of children with psychogenic pain report a recent stressful event in their lives. Because the history establishes the diagnosis, it is imperative to inquire about a recent death or separation, problems at school, aggression, depression, anxiety, physical illness, or disability. When a definite emotional origin can be identified for the pain and no organic factors can be found, the diagnosis of psychogenic pain is established.

Musculoskeletal Chest Pain

Common

Trauma. Musculoskeletal chest pain includes any pain originating from the pectoral or intercostal muscles, ribs, sternum, or overlying skin. It is the most common specific cause of chest pain and often results from muscle strain, as with exercising or after minor trauma. The patient typically experiences sharp localized pain that is exacerbated by movement. The physical examination is diagnostic. Pain that is well localized and reproducible with palpation has its origin in the chest wall. No further diagnostic tests are needed unless the patient has other findings.

When the child has experienced significant trauma to the chest wall (e.g., pedestrian vs. motor vehicle), chest pain may result from a rib fracture, pneumothorax, hemothorax, or pulmonary or cardiac contusions. The physician must evaluate the patient for the presence of a flail chest, diminished breath sounds, or distant heart sounds. The level of intervention (e.g., thoracentesis) is dictated by the patient's clinical state. All such patients should be stabilized and transfered to a tertiary care center.

Costochondritis. Costochondritis, an inflammation of rib cartilage in the region adjacent to the sternum, is diagnosed in 10–20% of all children with chest pain. As with other musculoskeletal pain, the child usually experiences sharp anterior pain that may radiate to the chest. Costochondritis may result from trauma to the chest wall or follow a viral illness. The pain is usually unilateral; bending, twisting, or other stretching motions may aggravate it. As with other musculoskeletal pain, costochondritis is diagnosed by eliciting tenderness while palpating the affected rib cartilage.

Uncommon

Tietze Syndrome. The diagnosis of Tietze syndrome is made on the basis of a characteristic swelling of the chest wall: a single, nonsuppurative, spindle-shaped swelling usually at the right sternoclavicular junction. This condition is most likely due to microtrauma; biopsy specimens show only increased cartilage without inflammatory changes. The pain, which is localized, usually lasts days to weeks, although the swelling may last longer.

Precordial Catch. Precordial catch or "Texidor twinge" is marked by the sudden onset of pain localized to the left sternal border or cardiac apex. The pain typically lasts less than 5 minutes but may recur frequently for a few hours or remain absent for months. It may not be easily distinguished from angina except by its short-lived nature and lack of radiation. This innocuous condition is not well understood, but some believe that it results from pressure on an intercostal nerve, which produces pain from the parietal pleura.

Tracheobronchial Causes of Chest Pain

Common

Asthma. Asthma is one of the most common reasons for children to visit a physician, and a small percentage of patients complain of chest pain at the time of an acute exacerbation. The most common etiology for such pain is a straining of chest wall muscles due to tachypnea, coughing, or retracting. Anxiety also may be a factor. Less common but potentially more serious causes of chest pain in an acutely wheezing child, such as pneumothorax or pneumomediastinum, need to be considered. Ventilation/perfusion mismatching may lead to hypoxemia and angina. In addition, medications used to treat asthma, such as beta-adrenergic agents or theophylline, can cause dysrhythmias, including supraventricular tachycardia, which in turn can cause ischemic chest pain. Therefore, the child with acute asthma and chest pain needs to be evaluated carefully. Oxygen saturation should be determined, and a chest radiograph should be obtained. If an irregular rhythm or extreme tachycardia is present, an EKG is warranted.

Cough. Chest pain secondary to cough accounts for about 10% of cases of chest pain in children and is most likely related to a straining of chest wall muscles. The physician must determine whether the cough is producing chest wall pain or whether an underlying condition, such as pneumonia or aspirated foreign body, is causing both the cough and pain. A chest radiograph is often helpful in this setting.

Pneumonia. Children with pneumonia may experience irritation of the parietal pleura by microorganisms and inflammatory cells that cause pleuritis. In addition, chest pain secondary to coughing may produce chest wall strain. Clinical clues to the diagnosis include fever, tachypnea, retractions, rales, or localized diminished breath sounds.

Uncommon

Pleural Effusion. Among the causes of pleural effusions in children are infections, collagen vascular diseases, and trauma. The patient with a pleural effusion typically has a vague history of poorly localized, unilateral chest pain. Clues to the diagnosis include decreased or absent breath sounds, orthopnea, or fever. Breathing deeply may increase the pain (see chapter 19 for a more detailed discussion).

Pneumothorax and Pneumomediastinum. Pneumothorax (see chapter 23) is a rare cause of chest pain in children. The pain is usually described as sharp, especially with deep inspiration, and may radiate to the shoulders or neck. Other clinical manifestations depend on how large the pneumothorax is. Most patients have dyspnea and tachycardia.

A pneumomediastinum can result from trauma and may be seen in patients with an acute exacerbation of asthma. The hallmark is sharp substernal chest pain that may mimic angina. A large leak may result in subcutaneous air in the neck, shoulder, or chest. Subcutaneous air, which can be easily palpated, helps to establish the diagnosis.

Gastrointestinal Causes of Chest Pain

Common

Esophagitis. Esophagitis may manifest as chest pain, especially in children with gastroesophageal reflux. In classic cases, the pain occurs soon after a meal and is worse in the supine position. This condition may be overdiagnosed. In a retrospective study it was found to be the cause of chest pain in 7% of children, but when stricter definitions were used in a prospective series of adolescents with chest pain, esophagitis was diagnosed with much less frequency.

Uncommon

Esophageal Foreign Bodies. Foreign bodies such as coins can be lodged in the proximal esophagus and produce chest pain. This is seen most frequently in toddlers, usually with a history of severe coughing or choking. All foreign bodies in the esophagus need to be removed endoscopically to avoid complications such as strictures or perforation. Alternatively, a child with achalasia, an inability of the lower esophageal sphincter to relax, may have food matter lodged in the esophagus. Lodged food can lead to the sensation of a foreign body, vomiting, dysphagia, and referred chest pain.

Cardiac Causes of Chest Pain

Common

Mitral Valve Prolapse. Although mitral valve prolapse is believed to be one of the more common cardiac causes of chest pain, the incidence and significance of such pain are unclear. In one series, 18% of children with mitral valve prolapse reported chest pain. In another series, however, chest pain occurred no more frequently in children and adolescents with mitral valve prolapse than in those without the disorder. Thus, the relationship may be an association rather than cause and effect.

Patients with mitral valve prolapse presumably have pain secondary to ischemia of the papillary muscle and/or left ventricular endocardium, although this is not well established. A midsystolic click or late systolic murmur is characteristic. Such findings may be difficult to elicit, and the patient should be examined in the supine, sitting, and standing positions. Some patients with mitral valve prolapse have normal cardiac examinations, leaving the physician to ponder whether to refer all undiagnosed patients to a cardiologist for exclusion of mitral valve prolapse. Given the benign nature of the disorder, most patients do not need to be referred for an echocardiogram, unless clinical findings suggest mitral valve prolapse or another cardiac disorder or unless the pain recurs frequently or interferes with daily activities.

Supraventricular Tachycardia. Supraventricular tachycardia (SVT) is the most common significant dysrhythmia in children. Precipitating factors include congenital heart disease, fever, and medications, especially sympathomimetics and beta-adrenergic agents. Older children with SVT often complain of palpitations and chest pain due to decreased diastolic filling, myocardial hypoperfusion, and ischemia.

The pediatrician must distinguish SVT from sinus or ventricular tachycardia. The rate in SVT is usually more rapid than in sinus tachycardia—typically 150–250 beats/minute, and unlike ventricular tachycardia, the EKG reveals a narrow QRS complex with atypical or absent P waves. The RR interval is very regular and does not vary with the respiratory pattern of the patient. If vagal maneuvers are unsuccessful in terminating the dysrhythmia, the child should be transfered to a tertiary care center for more definitive treatment.

Uncommon

Aortic Stenosis. Aortic stenosis accounts for about 5% of all congenital cardiac lesions in childhood. Most children with aortic stenosis are asymptomatic at the time of diagnosis, which usually is based on the presence of a systolic murmur heard best at the upper right sternal border. A thrill may be palpable, and diastolic murmurs occur frequently. Left ventricular outflow obstruction can lead to myocardial ischemia. The resultant substernal chest pain is anginal in quality and may radiate to the neck, back, abdomen, or upper extremities. In addition, many patients have fatigue, dyspnea, syncope, and signs of congestive heart failure. The diagnosis is suspected on the basis of the findings on cardiac examination, EKG findings of left ventricular hypertrophy, and cardiomegaly on chest roentgenogram. Such patients should be referred for echocardiography.

Myocarditis. Most commonly caused by viruses, myocarditis may result in chest pain due to ischemia or dysrhythmia. Patients may have fever, dyspnea, and evidence of congestive heart failure. Heart murmurs or friction rubs may be heard. Chest radiographs most frequently show cardiomegaly; S-T depression and T-wave inversion may be seen on EKG.

Pericarditis. Disease processes that may involve the pericardium in children include infections and autoimmune disorders such as systemic lupus erythematosus and juvenile rheumatoid arthritis. Clinical signs and symptoms vary according to the amount of fluid in the pericardial space. Typically, however, the first symptom is a sharp, stabbing pain over the precordium or left shoulder. This pain is aggravated by coughing or deep breathing and may be relieved somewhat by sitting and leaning forward. A friction rub, narrow pulses, distant heart sounds, and pulsus paradoxicus may be present. The pediatrician must have a high index of suspicion to establish the diagnosis, because laboratory findings are nonspecific.

Cardiomyopathy. Hypertrophic obstructive cardiomyopathy, formerly known as idiopathic hypertrophic subaortic stenosis, is a disorder characterized by massive ventricular hypertrophy with decreased distensibility and impaired filling. In some families, the disease is transmitted in an autosomal dominant pattern. Clinical features range from no symptoms to chest pain, dyspnea with exertion, and syncope. A systolic murmur heard best at the left sternal edge and apex is usually present. EKG findings of left ventricular hypertrophy and cardiomegaly on chest radiograph suggest the diagnosis, which is confirmed after myocardial biopsy.

Miscellaneous Causes of Chest Pain

Hyperventilation. In one prospective series 23% of adolescents seen in an outpatient clinic for chest pain were diagnosed with hyperventilation. Most patients who hyperventilate do so as a direct result of stress or emotional upset. However, organic causes of hyperventilation should be kept in mind during evaluation, including diabetic ketoacidosis, aspirin overdose, and severe pain. Hyperventilation produces chest pain as a result of hypercapneic alkalosis or coronary artery vasoconstriction. Breathing into a closed space such as a paper bag usually is enough to abort an attack; patients do not require further evaluation unless an organic etiology is suspected.

Gynecomastia. Gynecomastia, an enlargement of one or both breasts, occurs commonly in adolescent boys. The nipples are often tender to light touch; even clothing may cause discomfort. Gynecomastia typically lasts about 2 years, and patients need reassurance only.

Sickle-cell Anemia. Children with sickle-cell anemia frequently experience chest pain as part of a vasoocclusive crisis. Sickled red blood cells occlude arterioles, leading to ischemia and pulmonary microinfarcts. It is difficult to distinguish between children with pulmonary infarcts and children with pneumonia, either clinically or radiographically. Many of these children require intravenous fluids and narcotics for pain relief.

EVALUATION AND MANAGEMENT

"Is this pain likely to be of cardiac origin?" is the first question that the clinician must ask when evaluating a child with chest pain. Pain worsened by exertion or associated with syncope, palpitations, a friction rub, muffled heart sounds, or a pathologic murmur is suggestive of cardiac disease. For such patients, electrocardiograms and chest radiographs should be obtained. More sophisticated testing, such as Holter monitoring or echocardiography, may be needed for patients in whom cardiac disease is suspected but who remain undiagnosed after the intitial evaluation.

For children in whom cardiac disease is not suspected, the indiscriminate use of laboratory studies is of limited value. In a large prospective study in an urban pediatric emergency department, EKGs were obtained for all patients with either suspected cardiac chest pain or no clear diagnosis after history and physical examination. Ony 1 of 191 EKGs revealed an abnormality that was not suspected after physical examination. In a retrospective study of children presenting to an emergency department with chest pain, over 90% of chest radiographs were normal, and all abnormal findings were suspected before the radiograph was obtained.

Clearly, when a diagnosis has been made after a history and physical examination, further studies need not be obtained. In addition, when the initial assessment fails to ėstablish a diagnosis and neither cardiac nor pulmonary disease is suspected, EKGs and chest radiographs are generally not indicated. The natural history of patients with idiopathic chest pain is resolution without complications.

SUMMARY

Although chest pain is a prevalent problem among children, **cardiac causes of chest pain are uncommon. Younger children with chest pain are more likely to have cardiorespiratory disorders, whereas children older than 12 years are more likely to have psychogenic chest pain. Children with chronic chest pain are less likely to have an organic etiology.** In evaluating children with chest pain, it is not unusual to fail to establish a diagnosis after an initial assessment. The natural history of children with idiopathic chest pain is resolution without complications. In many cases, the diagnosis is established by history and physical examination, and further testing is unwarranted. If a cardiac etiology is suspected, then a chest radiograph and EKG should be obtained. In other cases, however, laboratory tests are generally not helpful in establishing a specific diagnosis; often, abnormal studies are not significant or reveal only previously known or clinically suspected problems.

SUGGESTED READING

1. Asnes RS, Santulli R, Bemporad JR: Psychogenic chest pain in children. Clin Pediatr 20:788–791, 1981.
2. Brown RT: Recurrent chest pain in adolescents. Pediatr Ann 20(4):194–199, 1991.
3. Coleman WL: Recurrent chest pain in children. Symposium on Recurrent Pain in Children, 1984.
4. Driscoll DJ, Glicklich LB, Gallen WJ: Chest pain in children: A prospective study. Pediatrics 57:648–651, 1976.
5. Epstein SE, Gerber LH, Borer JS: Chest wall syndrome. JAMA 241:2793–2797, 1979.
6. Feinstein RA, Daniel WA: Chronic chest pain in children and adolescents. Pediatr Ann 15(10):685–694, 1986.
7. Pantell RH, Goodman BW: Adolescent chest pain: A prospective study. Pediatrics 71:881–886, 1983.
8. Perry LW: Pinpointing the cause of pediatric chest pain. Contemp Pediatr 2:71–96, 1985.
9. Rowland TW, Richards MM: The natural history of idiopathic chest pain in children. Clin Pediatr 25:612–614, 1986.
10. Selbst SM: Evaluation of chest pain in children. Pediatr Rev 8(2):56–62, 1986.
11. Selbst SM: Chest pain in children. Pediatrics 75:1068–1070, 1985.
12. Selbst SM, Ruddy RN, Clark BJ, et al: Pediatric chest pain: A prospective study. Pediatrics 82:319–323, 1988.

COMMENTARY

by David S. Smith, M.D.

The clinical profile of the child with recurrent abdominal pain and other somatic complaints is less apt to be present in the patient with chest pain. The incidence of organic disease appears to be higher with chest pain than with recurrent abdominal pain. One is impressed, however, that the patient is often an adolescent who comes from a "painful" family in which stress is poorly handled.

As with recurrent abdominal pain, certain clinical associations increase the risk of organic disease. Fever, weight loss, sleep disruption, and young age demand a more aggressive approach to diagnosis, and clearly pain of rapid onset is more commonly associated with an organic disease.

Pain of cardiac origin is uncommon, and one cannot help but speculate that the pain of mitral valve prolapse is more common after the diagnosis has been established. There is no clear pathophysiologic mechanism whereby mitral valve prolapse would cause chest pain.

Musculoskeletal problems are among the most common causes of chest pain; the presence of tenderness in the chest wall is usually reassuring. With increasing numbers of young adolescents, male and female, engaged in vigorous sporting activities, including weightlifting, the symptom of chest pain has become a common cause of office and emergency department visits. As with any complaint of pain, however, one must be cautious; the first steps are a complete history and a careful physical examination.

13

ASTHMA

David G. Tinkelman, M.D.

Despite scientific advances regarding allergy, asthma, and immunology, the morbidity and mortality associated with asthma have increased steadily in the last decade. Among children asthma remains the number-one chronic medical illness that requires physician visits and hospitalization. Overall, more than 6 billion dollars are spent annually on the care of asthma in the United States. This chapter deals with specific issues related to the diagnosis and management of asthma in children as well as general pathophysiology of the disease.

DIAGNOSIS

In 1991 the National Heart, Lung, and Blood Institute (NHLBI) issued a report entitled *Guidelines for the Diagnosis and Management of Asthma.* In this report asthma is defined as "a lung disease with the following characteristics: **(1) airway obstruction that is reversible (but not completely so in some patients) spontaneously or with treatment; (2) airway inflammation; and (3) increased airway responsiveness to a variety of stimuli.**" This definition is rather complex and actually describes the pathophysiologic events that characterize the disease. Airway hyperresponsiveness is the hallmark of asthma; increased reactivity of the airways differentiates the asthmatic from the nonasthmatic child. Although it is not clear that a single mechanism is responsible for this state, airway inflammation is thought to be the major underlying pathophysiologic state that increases airway reactivity (Fig. 1). Other mechanisms thought to play a role are alterations in the bronchial epithelium, dysfunction of the autonomic nervous system, and alterations in the smooth muscle lining the airways of the lung. Signs of inflammation can be found in the airways of mild, asymptomatic asthmatic patients as well as in the severe asthmatic child in respiratory distress. Several studies have demonstrated a direct correlation between the levels of inflammatory cells (eosinophils and neutrophils) and mediators and the development of airway hyperresponsiveness and asthma symptoms. It appears that **control of airway inflammation leads to control of the disease.**

The level of airway hyperresponsiveness varies considerably in the asthmatic child, depending on various conditions, including but not limited to the allergic state, exposure to pollutants, and presence of infection. The level of reactivity determines the potential sensitivity of the asthmatic child to acute exacerbations of asthma. The events leading to symptoms vary somewhat with the child, the exposure, and the degree of inflammation already present. The most common reactions start with alterations in the level of obstruction in the airway and the increased production of mucus in the airways. The severity of airway obstruction depends on the degree of spasm of bronchial smooth muscle, mucosal edema, and mucosal secretion. Obstruction causes a musical wheeze as air is transported through a narrowed airway. As the degree of obstruction increases, hyperinflation of the lungs occurs and the patient increases his or her respiratory rate to improve gas exchange. Hypersecretion of mucus usually leads to coughing.

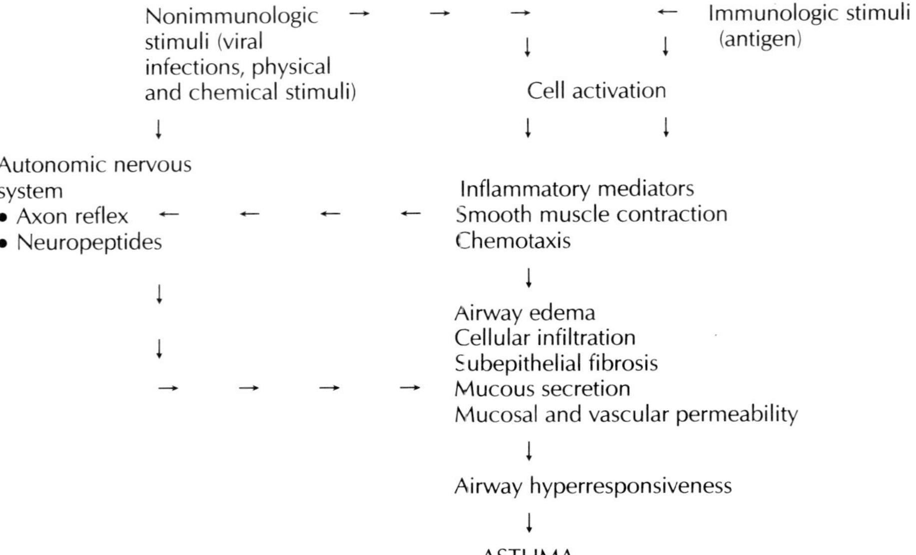

FIGURE 1. Proposed pathways in the pathogenesis of bronchial inflammation and airway hyperresponsiveness.

The presentation of asthma varies greatly from child to child and from attack to attack. Levels of bronchial hyperreactivity (BHR) can be assessed in different ways. A nonexact measurement can be made simply by history. Once the level of inflammation increases, symptoms subsequently increase. Questions regarding coughing with sleep, activity, or laughing may give some indication of changes in BHR. BHR also can be measured by comparing the variability in twice-daily peak flow measurements. As the degree of inflammation increases, the difference between morning and evening values also increases.

The best measurement of BHR is with chemical bronchial challenges. Measurement of methacholine sensitivity is an accurate, reproducible means of measuring BHR in older children and adults. It is more difficult in the small child, but possible.

Triggers of Asthma

Many different events can trigger an exacerbation of asthma. Many asthmatic children have allergies, and exposure to the allergen leads to the release of mediators, mobilization of cells, and onset of symptoms. A similar reaction can occur after a viral infection, exposure to pollutants, exercise, and emotional stress. As indicated above, the level of preexisting airway inflammation dictates the type and severity of response. In the typical asthmatic patient with an ongoing inflammatory reaction, exposure to allergen is associated not only with an acute reaction, resulting in bronchospasm, but also with a delayed reaction, consisting of mobilization of inflammatory cells. This leads to occurrence of a second or late-phase reaction from 6–24 hours after the immediate or early reaction. Persistent exposure is followed by a chronic inflammatory state and chronic symptoms of asthma.

EVALUATION OF THE CHILD IN THE OFFICE SETTING

History

The history of the child who has or is suspected of having asthma must include the following:

1. A complete description of the symptoms:
   (a) Presenting symptoms such as coughing, wheezing, dyspnea, chest discomfort (tightness or pain), or sputum production
   (b) Pattern of symptoms, including onset, severity, duration, character, diurnal variation, and effect on sleep and activity

(c) Precipitating events such as allergic factors, nonspecific exposures, presence of infection, emotional factors, weather changes, and exercise and their relationship to symptoms

2. History of associated illnesses, including symptoms of rhinitis, sinusitis, polyps, or eczema

3. Previous evaluations and medications and any other illnesses or medications

4. Environmental history, including the immediate environs of the child, with special attention to the bedroom and other areas where the child spends a lot of time (day care or school), the presence of animals, pollutants (smoke), and type of heating and air-conditioning

5. Impact of the disease on the child and family, including previous hospitalizations, days missed from school, and the effect on growth, behavior, and school performance

6. Family history of allergy, asthma, or other medical problems

Physical Examination

The basic physical examination of the child with asthma should always include examination of the upper airways, lower airways, and extremities.

Upper Airways. The examination of the upper airways includes the ears, nose, and throat. Attention should be paid to any indication of rhinitis or sinusitis that may be important in the complex of presenting symptoms.

Lower Airways. The examination of the lower airways should begin with attention to the manner in which the child is breathing and the respiratory rate. Is the child in distress, using accessory muscles, or retracting? Is there a difference in the inspiratory and expiratory phases of respiration? Are breath sounds audible in all lung fields? What is the quality of the lung sounds? Is there wheezing? Is it in all lung fields? Is it with inspiration or expiration or both? Are there other adventitious sounds? Is there any alteration in the chest configuration?

Extremities. Examination of the extremities should begin with the skin. Does the child have indications of active or recent atopic dermatitis or urticaria? Is there any evidence of clubbing of the fingers? (It is rare for a child with asthma to have digital clubbing.)

Laboratory Studies

The single most important laboratory study in evaluating the child who has or is suspected of having asthma is spirometry. It is the only method of qualifying airway obstruction. Spirometry measurements help to evaluate the severity of obstruction, limitation of airflow in the large and small airways, and degree of reversibility of the obstruction (see chapter 41).

Other tests may be of help in the diagnosis and in ruling out other problems, including chest and sinus radiographs, a complete blood cell count, and in some patients a bronchial provocation test. Selection of specific tests should be individualized.

MANAGEMENT (Fig. 2)

Regardless of the severity of asthma in the child or adult, efforts should be made to establish the best possible control over environmental precipitating factors. Both parents and physicians often overlook the importance of this aspect of therapy and almost totally disregard it. More time should be spent on control of environmental precipitating factors than on any other aspect of the total management plan. The initial focus of the physician should be to reduce or eliminate exposure to pollutants, irritants, and allergens in the child's bedroom, where the child often spends the majority of the day, where the child stays when sick, and where the parent can effect change. For instance, keeping the windows closed is an important way of reducing nighttime exposure to pollens and molds. Exposure to both of these allergens usually follows a particular seasonal pattern, depending on geographic area. Careful attention to such exposures should be stressed to the parents.

The most common and important indoor allergen for many children with allergic asthma is the house dust mite, which thrives in high humidity and feeds on human skin. Therefore, their highest concentrations are found in pillows, mattresses, upholstered furniture, stuffed toys, and carpet. The house dust mite is relatively big and is not found in still air. High concentrations can be found after vacuuming and after playing in a room with carpet and furniture. Studies have demonstrated that

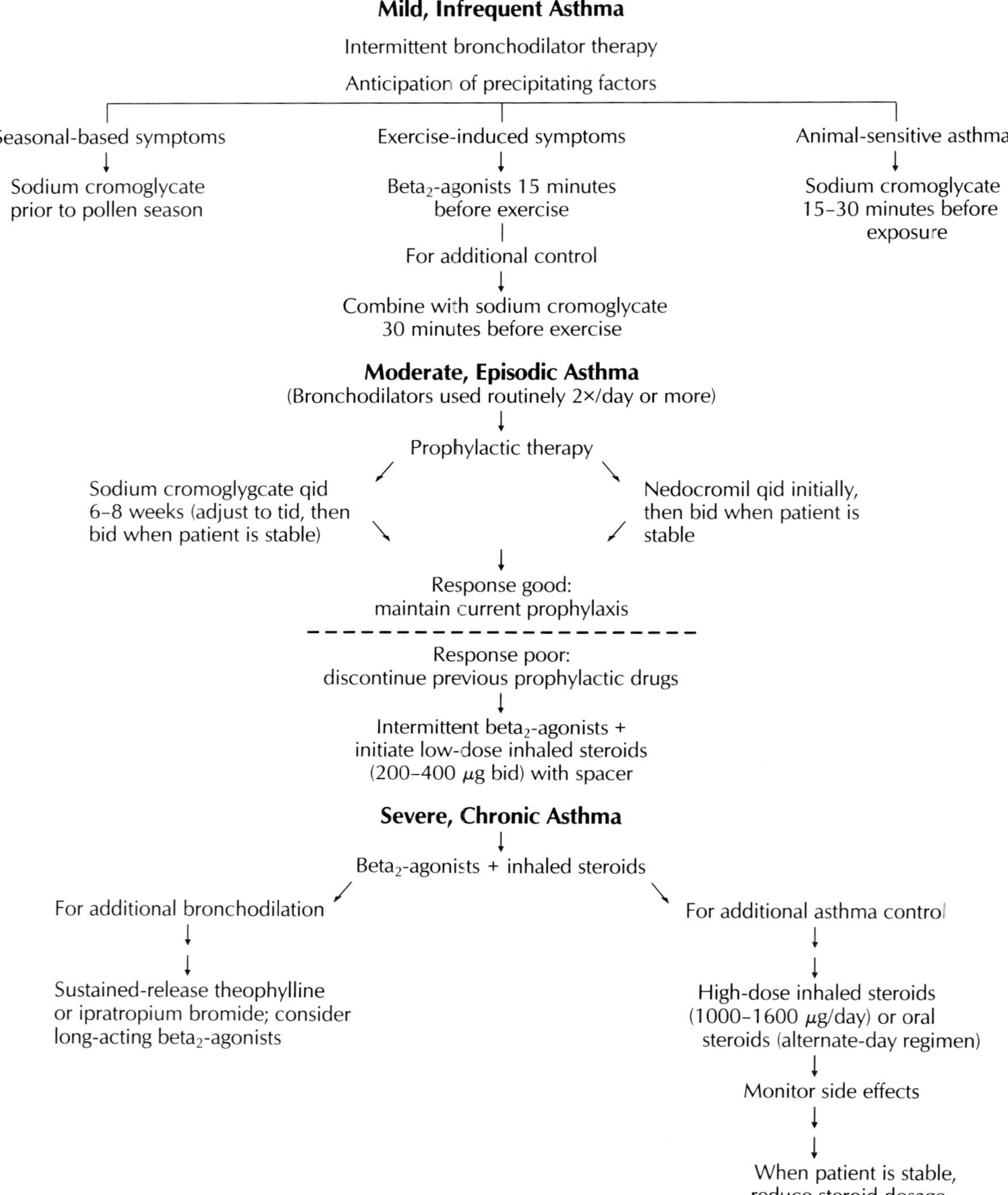

FIGURE 2. Therapeutic approach to the treatment of asthma.

reduction of levels of the dust mite is directly associated with reduction in BHR and symptoms. Essential measures to reduce exposure to the house dust mite in the bedroom include the following:

1. Encasing the box spring, mattress, and pillow in airtight covers with a zipper with overlying tape;
2. Washing the bedding in water at a temperature of 130°F weekly;

3. Removing carpet that is laid on concrete;
4. Using double-layered vacuum cleaner bags and added exhaust filters to make vacuums more efficient;
5. Removing or washing stuffed toys in water (130°F) weekly or placing them in a plastic bag and freezing overnight weekly; and
6. Keeping the bedroom free of clutter.

Probably the item of environmental control associated with the greatest emotional turmoil for the child is the removal of pets from the bedroom area and from the house. Because children develop strong emotional bonds with their pets, this difficult and delicate issue must be addressed by the physician to establish control over BHR. Frequent (weekly) washing of cats and dogs has been shown to reduce significantly the levels of dander.

Another item of environmental control that is fraught with emotional issues is the presence of cigarette smoke in the house. Without question, tobacco smoke is an irritant that can precipitate increased reactivity and inflammation of the airways. **The environment of the asthmatic child should be free of cigarette smoke.** Tobacco smoke is made up of very fine particles that remain airborne for long periods and also penetrate furniture and draperies. Therefore, smoking should not occur in the home.

The NHLBI guidelines have classified asthma into three stages: mild, moderate, and severe. It is possible, and indeed likely, that these stages overlap and that a child with asthma can go from one stage to another quite easily and frequently. The degree of inflamation leading to airway hyperreactivity and airway obstruction determines the type and severity of asthma symptoms.

Mild Asthma

The child with mild athma has minimal disability. Mild cough or wheezing one or two times a week is easily controlled with inhaled or oral bronchodilator therapy. Children rarely wake up at night or early in the morning because of asthma; usually they can play with their peers and experience exercise-induced coughing or bronchospasm only with extended or vigorous exercise. When spirometry is performed, lung volumes and flows are normal, and peak flow meter readings vary little from day to day.

Moderate Asthma

Children with moderate asthma have symptoms more than 2 days a week, with coughing or wheezing. They may have had infrequent but more severe attacks that required urgent physician care. They are on the edge of having persistent symptoms (coughing or wheezing). They cough or wheeze easily with exercise, wake up wheezing or coughing at least once a week, and, in general, have persistent problems with asthma. Observable changes in pulmonary function show evidence of airflow obstruction and variability in diurnal peak flow measurements of more than 20%. Such children have reached a level of airway inflammation that requires antiinflammatory therapy. The inflammation has produced airway obstruction and a level of airway irritability that predisposes the child to frequent, acute exacerbations of symptoms. Athough the need for beta-agonist therapy persists and even increases, the children require specific antiinflammatory therapy on a long-term basis. Present options for treatment in children are limited because of licensing as well as available formulations.

The first choices for antiinflammatory therapy are cromolyn or the newly released nedocromil, which has properties and activity similar to cromolyn. Presently nedocromil is available only in a metered-dose inhaler (MDI) of 2 mg/dose and is approved only for children over 12 years of age. The initial dosage of 4 mg four times a day can be reduced to twice daily after control has been established (usually 4 weeks at least). Long-term studies of nedocromil are not available.

The most potent method of reducing the inflammatory process is the administration of corticosteroids. Oral corticosteroids quickly control the inflammatory reaction and allow normal activity to resume. Unfortunately, oral corticosteroids have the potential for inducing many side effects, even in small doses of short duration. The development of inhaled corticosteroid preparations has significantly reduced the potential for side effects because of the reduced amount of systemic steroid administered.

Presently, inhaled corticosteroids are available only for administration through MDIs. Three preparations are currently marketed in the United States: beclomethasone dipropionate (BDP), flunisolide, and triamcinolone. Although some studies have compared these agents clinically, few data suggest that one is superior to another for children, milligram for milligram. The agent most studied in children in the United States is BDP. The currently recommended dosage is 100 μg (two puffs) four times daily; however, the actual dose administered is 42 μg per puff. Studies indicate that this dosage is effective in reducing airway reactivity and in establishing good control over moderate asthma. One recent study suggests that some children, especially boys in the growing years, may have growth retardation with this dosage. Therefore, as soon as the asthma is well under control, the dosage should be decreased to 100 μg three times a day or twice daily if possible. Weight gain, cataract formation, and some metabolic disorders have been reported with inhaled corticosteroids. It is unclear, however, whether such complications have been associated with higher doses of inhaled corticosteroids or with the administration of systemic corticosteroids before or during the periods of observation.

The effect of inhaled corticosteroids on the hypothalamic-pituitary-adrenal (HPA) axis is also unclear; reports in the literature are conflicting. The discrepancy may be related to the method of testing. Measurement of morning levels of serum cortisol is clearly the least sensitive method of testing for HPA suppression. Stress tests with insulin or Cortrosyn are more sensitive measurements, as is measurement of cortisol either hourly or in 24-hour urine collections. There is no clearly documented relationship, however, between suppression of the HPA axis and development of side effects. Sensitivity to corticosteroids varies widely in adults, and this is probably true in children as well.

Topical side effects in children, although less frequent than in adults, are also fairly common, including cough, hoarseness, and pharyngeal discomfort. Dysphonia due to vocal cord paresis is far less common.

Spacing devices are probably indicated for all children who need to receive their medication from an MDI (Fig. 3). With corticosteroids, they are even more important. Many different commercially available spacers enhance delivery of medication to the lung, avoid coordination problems between actuation and inhalation, and also significantly decrease the incidence of topical side effects from corticosteroid use. Devices are even available for administration of inhaled medication to very small children. Such devices have not been studied with inhaled corticosteroids, but their effectiveness has been demonstrated with inhaled bronchodilators in young children.

Children who have bronchospastic events despite the use of prophylactic medication may be approached in several ways. The most effective means to control acute bronchospasm is the use of inhaled beta-agonists, as discussed above. For the young child, in whom inhaled formulations may be difficult to deliver effectively, oral formulations may be required. For the child who has early morning increases in symptoms, another approach may be to add a single bedtime dose of sustained-release theophylline (8 mg/kg). This single dose may cover the early morning dip in pulmonary function that awakens the child.

Another approach is to consider that increasing bronchospasm represents an increase in the inflammatory state. Therefore, inhaled corticosteroids may be highly effective. The dose can be increased for several days as the symptoms and peak flow measurements are monitored. When the child is again under control, enjoying normal activity and sleeping through the night, the dose can be reduced to the established prophylactic level. Improvement of symptoms with this approach takes longer than with oral corticosteroids, but it is safer and often meets with less resistance from parents who are reticent about corticosteroid use.

Severe Asthma

The child with severe asthma is relatively easy to recognize. He or she is not able to maintain a normal life. The level of inflammation is such that pulmonary function is reduced on a chronic basis, with daily symptoms of airway obstruction. The child coughs with any activity and may wheeze regularly. The child has difficulty sleeping and gets up during the night or wakes up with chest tightness almost daily. The child with severe asthma requires daily attention and continuous medication to

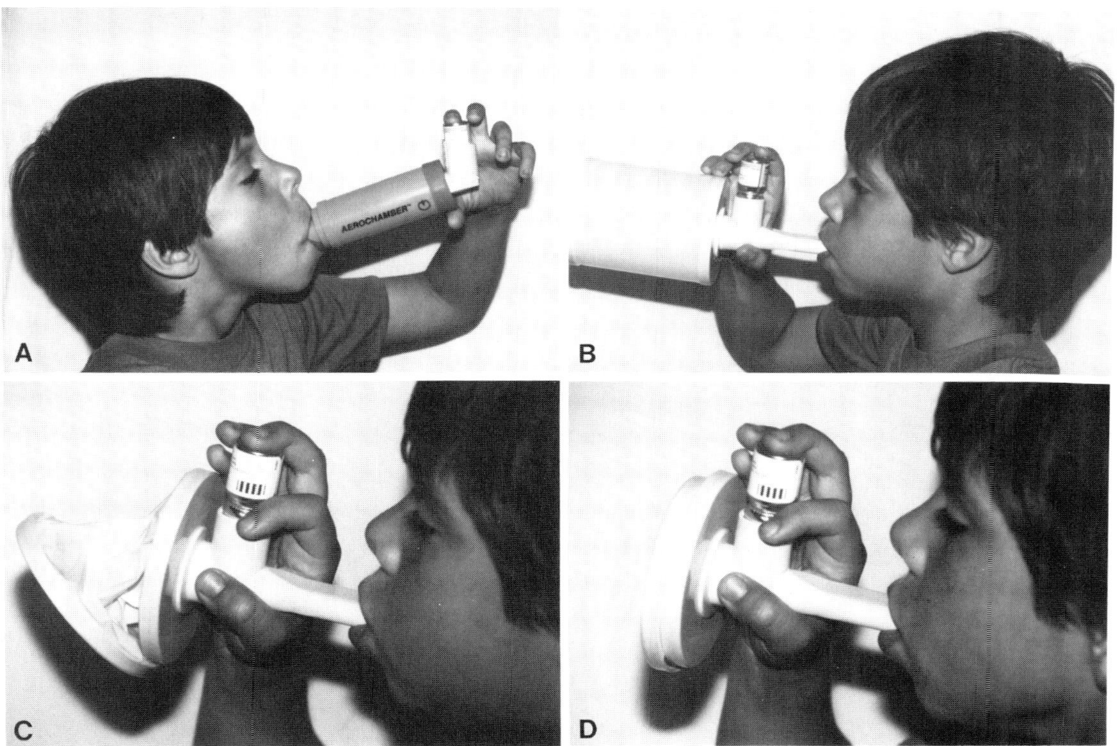

FIGURE 3. Two of the most widely used spacer devices. No coordination between the activation of the inhaler and inhalation is necessary. *A,* Rigid tube, available in several sizes. The patient activates the inhaler, propelling the medication into the spacer, and subsequently inhales slowly. *B–D,* Collapsible chamber. After full exhalation and expansion of the spacer, the patient activates the inhaler and then inhales slowly. Too fast an inspiration results in a whistling sound. The device collapses flat for storage. (Photo courtesy of M.S.) Various devices are available. Some are produced by pharmaceutical companies to be used specifically with their products.

control the inflammatory state and the level of bronchial obstruction.

The approach to the child with severe asthma must be more aggressive (Fig. 4). Both the parents and the child must recognize the severity of the problem and accept a more strenuous medical regimen. A higher level of corticosteroid therapy is required. If the child has been taking cromolyn or nedocromil, it obviously does not control the level of inflammation and may be discontinued. If the child has or has not been receiving inhaled corticosteroids, a relatively high dose administered through a spacing device is necessary. Often a dose of 1000–1600 μg is required for a short period to control the symptoms. If the child is in distress or is already taking a higher dose of inhaled corticosteroids, oral corticosteroids must be started for a short period. For the nonemergency state, a dosage of 2 mg/kg/day of prednisone or prednisolone is usually sufficient to control symptoms in the first 3–5 days. Once the symptoms are better controlled, the dose of the oral corticosteroids can be reduced, whereas the higher dose of inhaled corticosteroids is continued. The physician must take sufficient time to instruct the parents on the potential side effects of the corticosteroids and to describe the process that is taking place and the approach to control it. Parents can judge the effectiveness of the therapy by observation of peak flow measurements at home and should report the child's progress to the office daily.

For additional bronchodilation, sustained-release theophylline (once daily at bedtime), long-acting inhaled or oral beta-2 receptor agonists, and inhaled ipratropium bromide may be considered in addition to the inhaled beta-agonists.

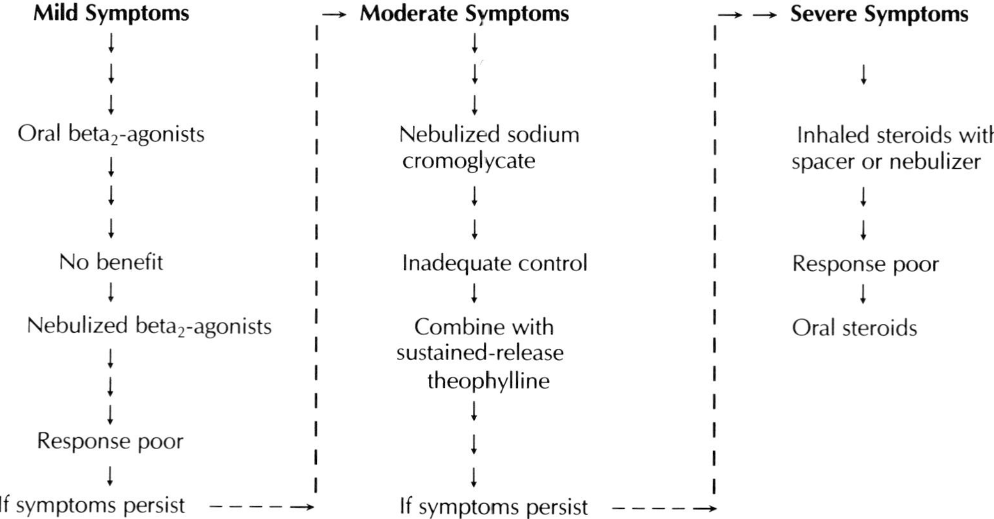

FIGURE 4. Therapeutic approach to treatment of asthma in infants and young children. (Adapted from Tinkelman D, Naspitz C (eds): Childhood Asthma, 2nd ed. New York, Marcel Dekker, 1992.)

SPECIAL PROBLEMS IN TREATING ASTHMA IN THE CHILD YOUNGER THAN FIVE YEARS

Chronic asthma in the child younger than 5 years presents several problems with respect to both diagnosis and management. The hampered ability of the physician to gather historical information, specific objective data, and reproducible physical findings presents a significant hindrance to making the diagnosis and to determining severity. Many problems in treatment relate to availability of specific formulations, lack of data in this age group about drug efficacy and safety, and limitations in measuring the outcome of therapy in small children.

Sources of Descriptive History

The child younger than 5 years can give a limited amount of information to the physician. The parents or guardians, therefore, become the primary source of information. The many limitations in this source of information must be recognized:

1. Parents must be aware that something has occurred in order to report it. A child's coughing during the night or wheezing during the early hours of the morning may go unrecognized because it is not heard by the parents. Another important symptom that may go unrecognized is the sensation of tightness in the chest. The young child is unable to recognize the feeling as an abnormal exercise-induced symptom when playing, and it resolves after the child goes home.

2. The observer often has a bias with respect to severity or even occurrence of symptoms. Quite often parents do not agree on the presence, timing, severity, or type of symptoms present. The perspectives of a grandparent, an estranged parent, and a child-care person may be very different. Naturally they will have different opinions with different assessments of the child's problems.

3. There is no way for an observer to assess the severity of subjective symptoms.

4. The onset of symptoms is often not appreciated. As indicated above, a symptom is often perceived when it impacts negatively on the observer. A night cough "begins" when the parent is first awakened. Wheezing is first appreciated when the day-care worker calls because it has progressed to the point of being obvious.

Dealing with this problem is not easy. The physician needs to instruct parents about what to look for and when to look. Parents need to be taught to look and listen for coughing with activity, laughing, and crying; to record respiratory rates; and to differentiate wheezing from upper airway sounds. It is important for parents to recognize when their child is having difficulty with breathing. Physicians should recognize the lack of complete information and act accordingly. Physicians need to respect the judgment of the mother who observes a subtle change in her child's well-being. **An increase in irritability or a change in feeding may be the first indicator that asthma has become a problem for the child.**

Difficulties of the Physical Examination

The physical examination in a small child is often difficult under any condition and may provide few clues to the diagnosis of asthma. Care must be taken to look for associated signs of respiratory or skin conditions. The child with atopic dermatitis is at a higher risk for asthma. The child with frequent purulent nasal discharge may have acute or chronic rhinitis or sinusitis and, therefore, bronchospastic disease.

Different techniques may be needed to encourage the toddler to take a deep breath and blow out hard. Special toys with lights, pinwheels, or party favors may be useful for such encouragement. Exercise challenges may need to be created to evaluate exercise-induced bronchospasm in the office setting. Care must be taken to make such challenges safe and meaningful. **Bronchial challenges with methacholine or histamine are difficult and should be reserved for the most experienced clinicians in carefully monitored settings.**

Lack of Objective Measurements

Pulmonary function testing in children younger than 5 years is almost impossible in the usual office setting. Some 4-year-old children can generate reproducible peak flow measurements, but the number is relatively small, and the results give no information about the small airways of the lung. This is a major obstacle to optimal care of children younger than 5 years. Infant pulmonary testing is available but requires highly sophisticated equipment and costly procedures; moreover, the reproducibility of such measurements is questionable in children who must be sedated. Certainly, no reliable technique goes home with the parent or can be used in the office. It is almost impossible to judge the degree of obstruction in both the large and small airways on the basis of physical examination, even in the best settings with the best diagnosticians. Thus, a good history, which includes information about symptoms with crying, laughing, and playing, is even more critical in children under 5 years of age. Questions about possible alterations in diurnal activity level may be helpful.

Chronic sinusitis may be missed in this population. The upper airway symptoms may be unnoticed by parents or ignored as unimportant. Affected children may have repeated episodes of respiratory problems, often with intervals of improvement related to antibiotic therapy, and may require further investigation, including radiographic evaluation of the paranasal sinuses.

Avoidance Measures Specific to the Preschool-Age Child

Children under the age of 5 years have several unique features that need to be considered in establishing appropriate environmental avoidance measures:

1. They spend a great deal of time on the floor or ground, whether they are crawling or just learning to walk.
2. For 8–10 hours a day, 5 days a week, they may be in a day-care environment, which is difficult, if not impossible, to control. They may be exposed to smoke, pets, and a carpet full of household mites for most of the day—as well as to viral infections from other children.
3. Finally, when they sleep, they often are surrounded by stuffed animals and dolls that may contain mites.

Observation of the effects of such environmental exposures is usually very limited, and often parents have no choice as to day-care arrangements. Because the children cannot express negative experiences, questioning about day care is very important. The physician also should make positive suggestions about the child's environment, which may take more time and effort than explaining medications.

Availability of Medications

1. Pharmacologic therapy for asthma in young children presents several problems. The pharmaceutical industry has no suitable guidelines for safe testing of medications in the very young child.

2. There are few long-term safety data for children under the age of 5 years, and few consistent studies look at the many parameters of the growing child, both physical and psychological.

3. Children are a poor source for reporting side effects. They are not able to understand such side effects as lethargy, behavioral changes, and nausea. Therefore, data concerning medications rely totally on observable side effects or poorly trained observers (i.e., parents and guardians).

4. The data about the effect of diet on most medications administered to small children are poor. Such studies require multiple blood samples from many children of different sizes and ages who are on different types of diets.

5. It is costly and difficult to develop formulations for children of this age. Solutions of medications are unstable or present difficulties with bioavailability.

ESTIMATION OF SEVERITY OF ASTHMA IN THE PRESCHOOL-AGE CHILD

The need to establish criteria for estimating the severity of both acute and chronic asthma is just as important in the very young child as in older populations. The same categories of mild, moderate, and severe apply, although the boundaries are more nebulous and based primarily on subjective measurements. The first persons to make such estimations are the parents or caregivers. Proper written instructions in appropriate language are critical to any management program if parents and caregivers are to assess their children with confidence. Instructions for action, particularly in the labile asthmatic child, are equally essential.

Acute Asthma

Normal. The child is happy and able to sleep, eat, and play as usual.

Mild. The first sign of change or trouble may be subtle, such as an increase in respiratory rate with activity. The child may or may not become irritable, but feeding may become more difficult. Coughing associated with activity, lying down, crying, or laughing may be the first sign of trouble. The child may choose to watch television or read rather than to run or to ride a bicycle with friends. Wheezing may not be audible to the parent but usually can be heard with the end of a deep inspiratory or expiratory effort, such as crying or peak flow effort.

Moderate. The respiratory rate is increased, even at rest. The child may start to look anxious to the parent, a sign not obvious to casual observers such as day-care workers and physicians. There is usually more coughing with activity and lying down. The child may awaken from sleep with coughing. Wheezing is heard more easily by the parent. In most cases, the child cannot eat, sleep, or play without some increased work of breathing and coughing but is not in distress at rest. The child is usually still happy and alert. This level of severity rarely makes the child look ill to the casual observer and may be noticed first by parental intuition, which should not be dismissed. A plan of action is needed to keep the child from deteriorating rapidly.

Severe. The child is in trouble. Wheezes are easily heard by caregivers. The child has retractions. Talking is an effort, as is eating, sleeping, and any activity. The child appears anxious, pale, and possibly cyanotic. The respiratory rate may be significantly increased. In some older children, however, the rate may not be so high because of the time spent in the expiratory phase and the depth of the inspiratory effort. Severe asthma is an emergency for the child and needs immediate medical care. In severe obstruction, wheezing in fact may be diminished or absent because of insufficient airflow to produce sound. This grave, life-threatening situation can be misinterpreted by the caregiver or novice in medical practice.

Chronic Asthma

Normal. The child is happy and performs all age-related activities without problems on a daily basis.

Mild. The child has infrequent difficulty with asthma. There may be isolated, easily controlled episodes with respiratory tract infections that do not require physician or hospital visits for treatment. Usually such children do well for most of the year and have only two or three episodes during the winter months. They are easily recognized and treated at home with proper brochodilator therapy.

Moderate. The child has fairly frequent episodes of wheezing, although the episodes may be confined to the fall and winter months. Night coughing may be present with some frequency. Such children require nebulization therapy for increased symptoms more than once a month, usually during the fall and winter months and often for several days at a time. They need an urgent care visit to a medical facility more than once a year and may have 1-3 short courses of systemic corticosteroids annually. One hospitalization a year may be needed. They do well between episodes and may have normal growth and development.

Severe. The child definitely needs frequent care, is very labile, and advances from a normal appearance to respiratory difficulty in a short period, usually three or four times a year. Such children are in the urgent care facility on a monthly basis in the winter and require short bursts of corticosteroid therapy more than two or three times a year. They usually are admitted to the hospital more than once a year.

THERAPY FOR THE PRESCHOOL-AGE CHILD WITH CHRONIC ASTHMA

Administration of medication is a problem because of the many factors surrounding this "simple" task that are unique to preschool-age children. Factors such as type of formulation, taste, time to administer nebulization, cross-reactivity with other common medications such as erythromycin, and feeding schedules must be considered in recommending medication for the small child.

Prophylaxis

Cromolyn. **Without question, cromolyn should be the first prophylactic agent tried in preschool-age children.** Use of the MDI may be difficult, but it is worth a try in all age groups, including the very young, for the following reasons: (1) parents do not want to be "tied" to a machine; (2) personnel at some day-care centers will not administer nebulization or will do it less effectively; and (3) children do not like to be still for the time necessary for administration of the nebulization.

Therefore, administration of cromolyn with a spacing device may be an appropriate way to begin. The dosage may be 2 or 3 inhalations through a spacing device 3 or 4 times a day. If this is impossible or totally ineffective, a nebulized formulation will be necessary. Adequate instruction must be given to the parent on the various ways the nebulizer can be used so that the best way of giving the child adequate medication can be found. Because few controlled studies have examined the effectiveness of cromolyn therapy in the very young, it should be assumed that the percentage of children who will respond is the same as in older children or adults (approximately 65%). However, because the dose is so variable, the success rate may be lower.

Inhaled Corticosteroids. The child who fails cromolyn therapy and continues to require long-term treatment is a candidate for inhaled corticosteroids. The choices of formulation are limited. Data pertaining to effective as well as potentially toxic doses in preschool-age children are unavailable. The physician must be an excellent observer and recordkeeper to avoid the potential side effects associated with corticosteroids. Because the only form available is the MDI, a spacing device must be used. Care must be taken to choose a spacing device that can be accepted by the child without too much difficulty, or therapy surely will fail. Parents need to be instructed in the use of several different devices and should choose the one that appears most effective. Monitoring for side effects, particularly growth-related ones, is essential. Neither the relationship between dose and effectiveness nor the effects on the HPA axis or growth suppression have been established for the small child. **Growth suppression is possible, especially in the years of rapid growth. Accurate growth measurements must be taken routinely.** Children requiring more prolonged therapy also should have periodic eye examinations to look for cataract formation.

Bronchodilator Therapy

Inhaled Beta-Agonists. Although studies of all the specific agonists have not been performed, sufficient data suggest that inhaled beta-agonists are effective in the management of acute asthma in small children. The specific dose recommendations must be tempered with the knowledge that it is difficult to judge the amount of medication that reaches the lungs in this (or any) age group. Inhaled beta-agonists are best suited for treatment of acute exacerbations of bronchospasm, or assumed bronchospasm, in small children.

When beta-agonists are administered from an MDI, the use of a spacing device facilitates drug administration and delivery. In the smaller child, studies have shown a bronchodilator effect from drugs administered with a device attached to a face mask. Administration is often difficult, and the exact dose is usually much less than expected; therefore, a third or fourth puff may be needed to achieve clinical benefit in the small child with wheezing. More medication is thought to be administered with a nebulizer because the dose is much greater than with the MDI. The customary dose of albuterol solution is 0.25 ml with 2 or 3 ml of saline for the child younger than 2 years or 0.5 ml in the same saline solution for the older child.

Parents may use various techniques for administering medication with a nebulizer. One technique is a face mask. More than 75% of the drug usually ends up on the outside of the mouth with this technique, but a sufficient dose is administered to have some clinical benefit. A less common technique is to hold a mouthpiece in the child's mouth. This technique, when done effectively in the cooperative older child, results in the administration of a much higher dose of medication into the mouth; therefore, a smaller dose may be needed. The most commonly used technique, especially in the smaller child, is to hold the mouthpiece, updraft nebulizer, or tubing 2 or 3 inches from the child's nose and mouth and to have the child inhale the mist. In this technique, the vast majority of the medication is lost; to achieve clinical benefit, the dose should be increased to 0.5 ml of albuterol with 3 ml of saline solution.

Oral Beta-Agonists. Oral beta-agonists probably have little if any use in adults and older children. However, in the small child, in whom it is difficult to administer sufficient quantities of inhaled medication to control symptoms, especially at bedtime, oral beta-agonists are indicated. It should be stressed that oral formulations may have significant adverse effects on the small child, including insomnia, irritability, and alterations in feeding patterns. The dose may need to be titrated not only on the basis of clinical effect but also on the degree of behavior change. For the small child, a starting dose of 0.5 mg of albuterol may be increased as tolerated, whereas in the 4-year-old child a starting dose of 2 mg is often tolerated. Proper instructions about the possible adverse effects must be given to all parents because the profile of adverse effects varies greatly among children. Parents who understand the possible side effects and the recommended adjustments in dosage are less likely to discontinue the therapy.

Theophylline. The numerous formulations of theophylline facilitate its administration in small children. Theophylline has the same well-described side effects in preschool as in school-age children and adolescents. However, it is hard for the child to describe headaches and nausea, and such effects may be interpreted only after extremes of irritability and vomiting. Because children older than 1 year metabolize theophylline quite rapidly, the advantage of once-daily dosing is probably lost in this age group. Night dosing may give several hours of bronchodilator efficacy and may be used in the same way in small children as in older patients to alleviate the early morning declines in pulmonary function.

Parents should be advised about the effects of fever, viral infections, and concomitant medications on the metabolism of theophylline as well as about proper administration techniques of "sprinkle" formulations (i.e., mix sprinkles in cold foods, no chewing allowed, follow with liquids, and administer at regular dosing intervals).

In general, the management of the young child is similar to that of the older child or adult; however, it takes a little more time and care to evaluate the clinical state and to establish proper management. Medications and dosages are summarized in Table 1.

CONCLUSION: GOALS OF THERAPY (NHLBI)

Management of asthma should have the following goals:

- **to maintain normal levels of activity (including exercise);**

TABLE 1. Available Medications and Recommended Doses for Treatment of Chronic Asthma

Drug	Oral Route	Inhaled
Cromolyn		MDI: 1 mg/puff, 2 mg 3–4 times a day Nebulizer solution: 20 mg/ 2cc tid
Nedocromil		MDI: 2 mg/puff, 4 mg 3–4 times a day
Beta$_2$-adrenergic agents		
Metaproterenol	<6 years of age: 1.3–2.6 mg/kg/day 6–9 years: 10 mg 3 or 4 times/day >9 years: 20 mg 3 or 4 times/day	MDI: 650 μ/puff, 2 puffs every 3–4 hr as needed 5% Nebulized solution: 0.2 ml every 4–6 hr as needed
Terbutaline	0.075 mg/kg 3 times/day	MDI: 200 μ/puff, 2 puffs every 4–6 hr as needed
Fenoterol	0.2 mg/kg 3 times/day	MDI: 200 μ/puff, 1–2 puffs every 4–6 hr as needed 0.5% Nebulized solution: 0.01 ml/kg every 4–6 hr as needed
Albuterol	0.15 mg/kg 3 times/day	MDI: 100 μ/puff, 2 puffs every 4–6 hr as needed 0.5% Nebulized solution: 0.02 ml every 4–6 hr as needed
Procaterol	0.5 mg/kg tid	MDI: 10 μ/puff, 1–2 puffs every 6 hr as needed
Pirbuterol		MDI: 200 μ/puff, 2 puffs every 6 hr as needed
Bitolterol		MDI: 370 μ/puff, 2 puffs every 4–6 hr as needed
Salmeterol		MDI: 25 μ/puff, 2 puffs every 12 hr
Inhaled corticosteroids		
Beclomethasone dipropionate	Use with spacer	MDI: 50 μ/puff, 2 puffs 3–4 times/day; increase as necessary
Triamcinolone	Use with spacer	MDI: 100 μ/puff, 2 puffs 3 times/day increase as necessary
Flunisolide	Use with spacer	MDI: 250 μ/puff, 2 puffs bid; increase as necessary
Theophylline	Many formulations available. Dose can be administered initially as 16 mg/kg/day in divided doses. Monitor clinical status and theophylline level and adjust dose.	

MDI = metered-dose inhaler.

- **to maintain near-normal pulmonary function rates;**
- **to prevent chronic and troublesome symptoms (e.g., coughing or breathlessness during the night, during the early morning, or after exertion);**
- **to prevent recurrent exacerbations; and**
- **to avoid adverse effects from medications.**

Physicians are entrusted by parents to accomplish these goals. We should strive to keep the child with mild asthma from having exacerbations of airway inflammation and obstruction and to return the child with moderate or severe asthma to normal daily activity and lifestyle as quickly and as safely as possible.

SUGGESTED READING

1. Becker AB, Nelson NA, Simons FER: Inhaled albuterol vs. injected epinephrine in the treatment of acute asthma in children. J Pediatr 102:465–469, 1983.

1a. Bergsman DA, Cooley JR, Tinkelman DG: Practice parameter: The office management of acute exacerbations of asthma in children. Pediatrics 93:119-126, 1994.
2. Booij-Nord H, DeVries K, Sluiter HR, Oro NGM: Late bronchial obstructive reaction to experimental inhalation of house dust extract. Clin Allergy 2:43-61, 1972.
3. Ellis EF: Theophylline toxicity. J Allergy Clin Immunol 76:297-301, 1985.
4. Godden DJ, Crompton GK: An objective assessment of the tube spacer in patients unable to use conventional pressurized aerosol efficiently. Br J Dis Chest 75:165, 1981.
5. Guidelines for the Diagnosis and Management of Asthma. Washington, DC, National Asthma Education Program. National Heart, Lung, and Blood Institute, National Institutes of Health Publication No. 91-3042, 1991.
6. Hargreave FE, Ryan G, Thomson NC, et al: Bronchial hyperresponsiveness to histamine or methacholine in asthma: Measurement and clinical significance. J Allergy Clin Immunol 68:347-355, 1981.
7. Konig P: Inhaled corticosteroids—their present and future role in the management of asthma. J Allergy Clin Immunol 82:297-306, 1988.
8. Salmeron S, Guerin JC, Godard P, et al: High doses of inhaled corticosteroids in unstable chronic asthma. Am Rev Respir Dis 140:167-171, 1989.
9. Schwartz AL, Lipton JM, Warburton D, et al: Management of acute asthma in childhood: A randomized evaluation of beta adrenergic agents. Am J Dis Child 134:134-138, 1980.
10. Tinkelman DG, Lutz C, Conner B: Methacholine challenges in the management of young children. Ann Allergy 66(3):225-230, 1991.
11. Tinkelman D, Reed CE, Nelson HS, Offord KP: Aerosol beclomethasone dipropionate compared to theophylline as primary treatment of chronic mild to moderately severe asthma in children. Pediatrics 92:1, 1993.
12. Toogood JH: Complications of topical steroid therapy for asthma. Am Rev Respir Dis 14:589-596, 1990.
13. Weiss et al: An economic evaluation of asthma in the United States. N Engl J Med 326:362-368, 1992.

COMMENTARY

by Daniel V. Schidlow, M.D.

There are many approaches to the management of asthma. The basic principles, however, are always the same: (1) bronchial spasm *and* inflammation must be treated in order to successfully control the symptoms. (2) The patient must be given as little medication as possible but as much as necessary to curb symptoms and to allow the child to participate fully in everyday activities. The child's activities should not be curtailed with the aim of reducing dosage or number of medications, but rather the therapy should be adjusted. (3) The environment and psychological makeup of the child should be taken into account in treating and educating patients and families.

The categorization of the severity of asthma into mild, moderate, and severe serves the purpose of reminding practitioners of the pathogenesis of symptoms and helps them to adjust therapy accordingly. As pointed out in the text, patients with asthma may, at different times, "cross" categories. Some authors prefer to classify the symptoms of asthma as sporadic, periodic, and persistent (continuous). These terms reflect the variable nature of symptoms and their behavior over time. A patient can have sporadic but severe symptoms (for instance, patients with severe reactions upon exposure to specific allergens).

The NHLBI guidelines underscore the value of education and environmental control. They provide a source of organized diagnostic and therapeutic approach to asthma. I am somewhat concerned, however, about turning this consensus document into incontrovertible gospel, or having it become the standard of care against which all medical practice is measured. Many physicians (myself included) take issue with the extensive use of peak flow measurements in the management of asthma. Although there may be a role for such measurements in selected patients, it is hazardous to base therapeutic decisions on the most unreliable of all pulmonary function tests. As pointed out by Dr. Tinkelman in this chapter and by Dr. Allen in the chapter on pulmonary function, peak flow measurements are gross assessments of airway patency and do not appropriately reflect changes in small airways, which in some patients are the only manifestation of airway inflammation. Furthermore, in the hands of anxious or compulsive parents and patients, peak flow meters can create a veritable "peak flow obsession." I prefer to educate families and patients in early recognition of symptoms of asthma and their appropriate therapy and rarely resort to the use of peak flow measurements at home. If patients remain symptomatic in spite of what appears to be adequate therapy, five main causes for "treatment failure" must be considered: insufficient dose of medication; need for additional drugs; lack of adherence to treatment recommendations, including technique in the use of inhalers; presence of environmental or psychosocial triggers; and the possibility that the diagnosis of asthma is incorrect (another condition is contributing to or causing the symptoms).

The management of asthma is gratifying because health professionals can make a real difference in the lives of children affected with this disease, prevent serious morbidity and death, and contribute to containing the cost of health care.

14

CYSTIC FIBROSIS

Daniel V. Schidlow, M.D.

Cystic fibrosis (CF) is a genetic disease, inherited in an autosomal recessive manner and characterized by chronic respiratory infection, pancreatic insufficiency, and elevated concentrations of electrolytes in sweat.

The gene for CF is located on the seventh chromosome. Over 240 mutations of the gene associated with clinical forms of CF have been reported. A child with CF inherits two mutations, one from each parent (both are heterozygote carriers). These mutations cause absence or defective production of a transport protein called fibrosis transmembrane conductance regulator (CFTR). This protein is responsible for normal passage of electrolytes through epithelial cell membranes; its absence or deficiency results in defective exit of chloride from cells in epithelial tissues and an increased absorption of sodium from the lumen into the cells and the interstitium. In the respiratory and gastrointestinal tract, as well as in other organs lined with epithelial cells, this defect results in dehydration and increased adhesiveness of mucus. Specific results in the respiratory tree include chronic bacterial colonization, inflammation, and a vicious cycle of cell damage, with release of chemical mediators and proteases, that perpetuates the inflammatory process.

An abnormality in ion transport similar but not identical to that in other epithelia results in the excessive excretion of sodium and chloride through the skin.

The diagnosis of CF is based on clinical presentation in the vast majority of patients and is confirmed by the measurement of elevated concentrations of chloride or sodium (or both) in the sweat. Current technology allows intrauterine detection of mutations of the CF gene as early as the 10th week of gestation by means of chorionic villous sampling and subsequent DNA analysis. In addition, the presence of mutations can be detected by DNA analysis of blood cells, buccal mucosa, or others sources of DNA. Genetic diagnosis should be restricted, however, to families in which there is a known case or to patients in whom the diagnosis of CF cannot be firmly established on the basis of clinical and laboratory data.

Screening of the general population is not recommended at this time. Neonatal screening programs are in place in some states. The finding of elevated immunoreactive trypsinogen in blood (obtained at birth by heel prick onto a filter paper) is highly suggestive of CF.

Cystic fibrosis remains a clinical diagnosis. The most common presenting signs of CF are summarized in the mnemonic CF PANCREAS (Table 1).

COMMENTS AND CAVEATS

Meconium Ileus. About 10% of newborn infants with CF present with meconium ileus and require intervention shortly after birth to relieve the intestinal obstruction. **Children born with meconium ileus have CF until proved otherwise.** The incidence of CF in children with meconium plug syndrome is higher than in the general population; it is prudent to rule out CF in this setting as well.

TABLE 1. Presenting Signs of Cystic Fibrosis

Remember the mnemonic **CF PANCREAS**

C =	**C**hronic cough and wheezing
F =	**F**ailure to thrive
P =	**P**ancreatic insufficiency—signs of malabsorption (bulky, foul stools)
A =	**A**lkalosis and hypotonic dehydration
N =	**N**eonatal intestinal obstruction (meconium ileus) and **N**asal polyps
C =	**C**lubbing of the fingers and **C**hest radiograph with characteristic changes
R =	**R**ectal prolapse
E =	**E**lectrolyte elevation in sweat; salty skin
A =	**A**bsence or congenital atresia of the vas deferens
S =	**S**putum with *Staphylococcus* or *Pseudomonas* (mucoid)

Mild and Atypical Presentations. About 10% of children with CF have normal pancreatic function, are well nourished, and lack the classic signs and symptoms of intestinal malabsorption. Mild or atypical forms of the disease, associated with mutations or combinations of mutations of the CF gene, are reported with increasing frequency. **Basically, no child "looks too good" to have CF.**

Sweat Test. Although DNA testing can unequivocally confirm the diagnosis of CF, the sweat test is still the most important confirmatory laboratory test in most cases. An abnormal sweat test, which is found in the vast majority of patients, confirms abnormality of the sweat glands. This test should be performed by experienced technicians using approved techniques. Siblings of newly diagnosed patients should undergo sweat testing, as should first- and second-degree relatives with suspicious symptoms.

Levels of Care. The care of patients with CF is time-consuming and requires the input of various professionals. Patients are best served by periodic attendance at a center approved by the CF Foundation and ongoing follow-up by a generalist who serves as the frontline caregiver.

Older Patients. CF is no longer exclusively a pediatric disease. Over one-third of patients are 18 years of age or older, and it is predicted that by the year 2000 up to one-half of all patients will be adults. The incidence of complications of CF, such as diabetes mellitus, gallbladder disease, liver disease, and arthritis, is expected to increase as the population of patients ages. In addition, older patients are subject to the general health problems of adults. The need for appropriate services for older patients at CF centers and in the community is an issue of growing importance. CF centers provide access to experimental and new therapeutic modes as well as multidisciplinary care, whereas the generalist can provide ready access to medical care in case of emergencies, early detection of complications or exacerbations of pulmonary disease, and ongoing support for the famliy.

Sinus Disease and Nasal Polyps. The basic defect in ion transport affects all areas of the respiratory epithelium, from the nose to the alveoli. Mucosal thickening of the paranasal sinuses and mucus accumulation are universal in patients with CF. Recurrent exacerbations of sinus disease are also common and are managed in much the same manner as sinusitis of other etiologies. Nasal polyposis is common in patients with CF. The actual reason is not known, but chronic inflammation is believed to be at least a contributing factor. Nasal polyps, which may be one of the presenting signs of the disease, tend to grow back after surgical excision, sometimes very quickly. Unless polyps completely obstruct the nasal passages, cause symptoms such as postnasal drip and cough, or contribute to recurrent sinus disease, most specialists prefer an expectant approach to surgery. Administration of intranasal corticosteroids may help to contain the growth of polyps somewhat.

Pulmonary Disease. The pulmonary disease of CF is characterized by alternating periods of well-being and flare-ups of respiratory infection. Persons with CF may cough and expectorate purulent secretions on a daily basis. Acute and severe exacerbations requiring antimicrobial therapy are easily recognized; many patients, however, experience more subtle deterioration of pulmonary function and increases in symptoms, both of which benefit from aggressive therapy. The aims of therapy are to curb signs and symptoms, to optimize pulmonary function, and, most importantly, to prevent lung damage, thus prolonging life. The most common signs of exacerbation of endobronchial infection in CF again may be summarized by the mnemonic CF PANCREAS (Table 2). Exacerbations of pulmonary infection require treatment with oral or intravenous antibiotics, chest physiotherapy, bronchodilator drugs, and, if necessary, intravenous administration of antimicrobial drugs in the hospital or at home.

Ongoing Therapy. Ongoing therapy of patients with CF must be individualized according to the symptoms and severity of disease. Most patients require some or all of the following: (1) chest physical therapy and postural drainage or alternative methods of lung clearance (e.g., breathing exercises, huffing, special masks, sports); (2) bronchodilators, inhaled sodium cromolyn or corticosteroids; and (3) wetting or mucolytic agents. Patients with exacerbations of reactive airways disease may require periodic administration of prednisone. Oxygen is indicated for patients with hypoxemia. Lung transplantation is now available as the last resort for patients with end-stage lung disease.

Pancreatic enzyme preparations must be administered *with all meals* to patients with intestinal malabsorption. Nutritional, multivitamin, and vitamin E supplements are usually indicated. The doses of enzyme supplements vary greatly from patient to patient. The basic principle is that patients must ingest as much pancreatic enzyme as necessary with each meal to allow weight gain; to avoid flatulence, abdominal distention, and pain; and to facilitate normal or near-normal stool patterns. No dietary restrictions are necessary. Patients must ingest enough calories to allow for normal growth and activity.

TABLE 2. Exacerbation of Pulmonary Infection of Cystic Fibrosis

Remember the mnemonic **CF PANCREAS**

C	=	**C**ough (increase in intensity and frequency, spells)
F	=	**F**ever (usually low grade, unless severe bronchopneumonia is present)
P	=	**P**ulmonary function (deterioration)
A	=	**A**ppetite (decreased)
N	=	**N**utrition (weight loss)
C	=	**C**omplete blood cell count (leukocytosis—left shift)
R	=	**R**adiograph (increased overaeration, peribronchial thickening, and mucus plugging)
E	=	**E**xamination (rales or wheezing in previously clear areas—tachypnea, retractions)
A	=	**A**ctivity (decreased, impaired exercise tolerance, increased absenteeism)
S	=	**S**putum (becomes darker, thicker, and more abundant, forming plugs)

ISSUES OF MANAGEMENT

The practitioner who cares for patients with CF is confronted frequently with several major issues related to management.

When to Prescribe Antibiotics

Aggressive research into prescription of antibiotics continues, because this issue has not been settled satisfactorily to date. The value of ongoing suppressive antistaphylococcal, antimicrobial therapy is currently under study. Most clinicians agree that an increase in cough and sputum production or a change in physical findings is an indication for antibiotics. The choice of antibiotic tends to vary among practitioners, but the most commonly used preparations are cephalosporins. Some clinicians rotate antibiotics at 2-week intervals in an effort to avoid resistance. The quinolones, the only oral antimicrobials proved effective against *Pseudomonas aeruginosa,* are used for more serious exacerbations by some physicians, as intermittent suppressive therapy for sicker patients by others, and as ongoing suppressive therapy by still others (emergence of resistance, albeit reversible, is relatively common). Quinolones have proved quite effective in the control of many exacerbations that in the past would have necessitated intravenous antibiotics.

The use of inhaled antimicrobial drugs for treatment of exacerbation and as suppressive therapy has increased. Aminoglycosides, especially tobramycin, have been shown to be quite effective in high doses (400–600 mg/dose, 3 times a day) with an ultrasonic nebulizer. Such doses require the use of solutions without preservatives; otherwise bronchospasm may supervene. Nebulization of aminoglycosides and other antibiotics has been prevalent for quite a while in Europe, with reasonably good results.

In general, one does what seems to work for the patient; choices are rather empirical. Quite often the choice of antimicrobials does not reflect the sensitivities obtained in antibiograms but rather the observed clinical response. The underlying theory is that the agent may have some suppressive effect in spite of in vitro resistance. Whether some of the observed benefit is due to the killing of undetected sensitive flora or the treatment of unsuspected sinus disease rather than endobronchial infection has not been satisfactorily established.

Intravenous administration of antibiotics is indicated when the severity of deterioration demands aggressive action to curb lung damage. Intravenous therapy may be indicated to arrest slow, progressive deterioration as well as to treat acute exacerbations of lung infection. In patients who respond slowly, oral therapy may prove costly in the long run. If symptoms of acute exacerbation do not improve in about 5 days after initiation of oral therapy or if the patient is very sick, it is best to resort to intravenous treatment. The most commonly used antibiotics are aminoglycosides, especially tobramycin; newer generation cephalosporins, especially ceftazidime; and semisynthetic penicillins, such as ticarcillin or pipericillin. Patients harboring *Staphylococcus aureus* in their sputum should receive an antistaphylococcal drug such as nafcillin or a combination of semisynthetic penicillin and clavulanate. It is best to use the maximal dose of a given antibiotic, with appropriate measurements of serum levels and follow-up for signs of toxicity.

When to Use Bronchodilators

The use of bronchodilators is also a subject of some controversy among practitioners, because it has been observed that in patients with severe lung disease, bronchodilators may cause increased compliance ("floppiness") of large airways and thus increased obstruction. The more practical issue is that in many patients with CF, airway hyperreactivity is ameliorated by bronchodilator drugs. We use inhaled sodium cromolyn to prevent airway reactivity, along with beta$_2$-agonists in patients with reversible obstruction as proved by pulmonary function testing. During wheezing episodes, patients are treated with intravenous theophylline, corticosteroids, inhaled beta$_2$-agonists, or combinations thereof.

What to Do When a Patient Does Not Gain Weight

There are three main reasons for weight loss or lack of weight gain in patients with CF: (1) insufficient caloric intake, (2) excessive fecal loss of calories due to malabsorption, and (3) increased caloric expenditure due to infection. In the absence of severe respiratory problems, one must carefully explore intake of food (with a 3-day calorie count) and pancreatic enzymes (many children and adolescents neglect to take enzyme preparations with all meals). It also may be necessary to measure 72-hour levels of fecal fat or serum levels of vitamin A or E to assess the extent of malabsorption. Psychosocial issues, particularly in toddlers and young children, are particularly important causes of decreased calorie intake and failure to thrive. Good nutrition is of paramount importance in maintaining the welfare of patients with CF. A well-nourished patient fares much better clinically than a patient whose nutritional status is deficient, given similar pulmonary compromise.

Hemoptysis

As pulmonary disease progresses, destruction of bronchial and parenchymal tissue increases. Hemoptysis may range from expectoration of blood-tinged mucus to elimination of large quantities of pure blood. Anastomosis between bronchial and pulmonary circuits, congestion, and erosion of bronchial wall secondary to inflammation contribute to this complication. Expectoration of large amounts (over 1 cup/day) of blood is more characteristic of older, sicker patients, and even in this population it is not common. Expectoration of blood-streaked sputum or small amounts of blood is much more likely. Hemoptysis in young children with CF is exceedingly rare, because collateral circulation needs time to develop.

In most cases, treatment of hemoptysis consists of observation and reassurance. A minimal number of laboratory studies should be done to rule out a disturbance of coagulation. The routine administration of vitamin K, application of ice packs to the chest, discontinuation of physical therapy, and other such measures probably have no effect on the bleeding. It is useful to determine whether the bleeding is associated with an exacerbation of endobronchial infection. Patients with more severe or persistent bleeding should be referred for further therapy (see chapter 10).

Chest Pain

Chest pain is associated with inflammation of the pleural surface, muscular pain from excessive cough, tracheitis, esophagitis, or pneumothorax. It can be quite difficult to distinguish between pneumothorax and pleuritis as the cause of chest pain. The degree of dyspnea is not a good indicator, because a pneumothorax may be small or anxiety over pain may be high and thus exaggerate the degree of breathlessness. In such situations, the approach includes a chest radiograph to detect free air in the thorax or signs of exacerbation of lung disease. Analgesia is always indicated, with care to avoid narcotics, tranquilizers, or drugs that may blunt respiratory efforts.

Abdominal Pain

Abdominal pain is a common cause of telephone calls and office visits. The causes in patients with CF range from school phobia or irritable colon to intussusception or intestinal volvulus, gallbladder disease or pancreatitis. By far, **the most common cause of abdominal pain, particularly in school-age and adolescent patients, is intestinal malabsorption due to inadequate intake of pancreatic enzyme supplements.** A good place to start a work-up is to elicit dietary changes and to determine whether the pain is related to ingestion of meals (particularly fatty ones). Flatulence or changes in stool pattern (bulkier, lighter color, greater frequency) point the physician in the direction of poorly controlled malabsorption. Careful review of enzyme therapy, including changes in doses, preparations, and mode of administration, is essential.

Constipation due to distal intestinal obstruction (meconium ileus equivalent) ranks second in frequency as a cause of abdominal pain. Examination of the abdomen may disclose a fecal mass in the right lower quadrant, abundant stools in the descending colon, and distention. An abdominal radiograph confirms the presence of large amounts of stool in the intestine. The treatment varies from center to center. Some discontinue enzyme therapy in an effort to increase bulk and to soften stools. A good starting point is to administer enough fluids and mineral oil at a dose of at least 60 ml/day. If these measures do not produce relief within 24 hours, enemas with acetyl cysteine may be tried. Another approach involves the use of hyperosmolar solutions such as GoLytely or lactulose. If oral treatment is unsuccessful, enemas of Gastrografin or other hyperosmolar solutions should be attempted under medical supervision. Meconium ileus equivalent frequently occurs during an upper respiratory infection and probably is precipitated by increased dehydration and adhesiveness of mucus. **It is essential not to be contemplative but to act aggressively in the management of such patients.** Occasional patients require surgical intervention because of undue delays in starting therapy or because of the refractory nature of the problem. Patients with previous abdominal surgery (e.g., meconium ileus) should be managed with even more promptness because of the higher potential for mechanical obstruction due to fibrous adhesions.

NEW AND DEVELOPING THERAPIES

The last few years have witnessed a flurry of research in the field of CF. New approaches to the control of the various manifestations of CF are actively pursued by more investigators than ever before.

The most spectacular approach, directed at correction of the genetic defect, is human gene therapy. Investigators have begun to introduce normal genetic material into epithelial cells in an effort to promote production of normal CFTR, thus inducing normal ion transport and effectively correcting the basic defect of the disease. Preliminary trials of human gene therapy directed at the respiratory tree have already started, and data about safety and efficacy should be forthcoming.

Amiloride, a potassium-sparing diuretic, blocks the excessive reabsorption of sodium from the lumen of the respiratory tree. Uridine triphosphate, a nucleotide that induces excretion of chloride from the cell, is also under active investigation. These two drugs, administered as an aerosol, are expected to help in normalizing ion transport in the respiratory tree and to make secretions thinner.

A new preparation, rhDNase (alpha dornase), is entering the market at the time of this writing. This preparation effectively breaks up long strands of DNA liberated by broken neutrophils, present in purulent sputum, and turns the normally viscid mucus into a more fluid, free-flowing liquid that is easier to expectorate.

Other experimental approaches to the control of inflammation and infection include the administration of exogenous, recombinant antiproteases to the lung in an effort to counteract the imbalance created by an excess of neutrophil elastase and other noxious enzymes (individuals with CF produce normal quantities of antiproteases, but the system is overwhelmed by the amount of enzyme present). Other approaches include the administration of antipseudomonas vaccine, monoclonal antibodies, and hyperimmune gammaglobulin along with antiinflammatory drugs. Recent data show that the risks of ongoing, long-term administration of high-dose prednisone outweigh the benefits. Prednisone should be used judiciously in selected patients.

New techniques of chest physiotherapy, choleretic drugs to prevent liver damage (ursodeoxycholic acid), and various other experimental approaches to control the manifestations of CF are constantly under investigation and make the prospects for more definitive therapies very promising in the years to come.

Primary care providers play an important role in the management of patients with CF, as previously indicated. Vaccinations, child advocacy, family support, school health, education about sexuality and prevention of sexually transmitted diseases, along with early detection of complications, planning of home care, and support of research, are important aspects of the role of the primary care provider. Good communication and mutual trust between the CF center and the primary care physician result in the best possible care for patients and their families.

SUGGESTED READING

1. Cystic Fibrosis Foundation Center Committee and Guidelines Subcommittee: Cystic Fibrosis Foundation Guidelines for patient services, evaluation and monitoring in cystic fibrosis centers. Am J Dis Child 144:1311–1312, 1990.
2. Fitzsimmons SC: The changing epidemiology of cystic fibrosis. J Pediatr 122:1–9, 1993.
3. Stern RC: The primary care physician and the patient with cystic fibrosis. J Pediatr 114:31–36, 1989.

COMMENTARY

by Thomas I. Kennedy, M.D.

In this chapter one statement rings frighteningly true: **Basically, no child "looks too good" to have cystic fibrosis.** Because cystic fibrosis is the most common fatal genetic disease in the United States, early detection and treatment are particularly important to limit or delay complications of the disease. This raises the question of who should have a sweat test and when.

Ordering the sweat test can have adverse consequences. Although the test can rule out a chronic, fatal disease, it may raise the anxiety level of parents who are already worried about the child with poor weight gain or recurrent pneumonia. Parents may even show anger and resentment when they are put through such anxiety if test results are normal. When, then, should a sweat test be ordered?

Of course, we think of cystic fibrosis in a child with recurrent pneumonia. In practice, however, it is not always so easy. During a routine examination the mother of a 6-month-old boy mentioned that his skin tasted extra salty to his grandmother. His mother had read that salty sweat may mean cystic fibrosis. Review of the chart revealed that the child was growing and developing normally. He had normal stools. Of note, however, was one episode of bronchiolitis at age 3 months that resolved without incident. Although we attempted to reassure the mother of the unlikelihood of CF, we explained that we could not be 100% certain unless a sweat test was done. In the next month a sweat test confirmed the diagnosis of CF. Even in retrospect I wonder if all physicians would have ordered the test at that time.

Another infant boy was followed for routine care. There was no history of respiratory problems, but he was just beginning to fall off the weight curve. On questioning about stool pattern, the parents admitted that when they change his diaper, family members complain that they have trouble staying in the same room because of the foul odor. Sweat testing confirmed the diagnosis of cystic fibrosis.

In our practice of 15,000 patients, we have very few with cystic fibrosis whom we routinely follow.

Ideally, as primary care physicians, we can play an important role in continuity of care, ready availability, family support, and immunizations. However, this is often not the case. Although the CF center encourages use of the primary physician, after diagnosis the patient and family slowly lose contact with primary caregivers as they become more involved with the center. This puts an additional burden on the specialist, who is expected to be always available as the first and perhaps only caregiver.

The future holds great promise for patients with cystic fibrosis. When and how aggressively to order a sweat test still remains a clinical decision. Perhaps prenatal testing will become routine in the near future, at least for at-risk families. Research into gene therapy may change the face of this disease forever.

15

PNEUMONIA IN YOUNG INFANTS

(Birth through 3 Months)

Sarah S. Long, M.D.

In young infants acute bacterial and nonbacterial respiratory pathogens frequently lead to lower tract disease. Perinatally acquired infection can lead to acute onset of overwhelming pneumonia within hours of birth (e.g., group B streptococci). The pneumonia may be part of disseminated disease (e.g., herpes simplex virus), or its onset may be insidious at 6–12 weeks of age (e.g., *Chlamydia trachomatis*, cytomegalovirus [CMV]). Bacteria are the most frequent causes of pneumonia only in the first few days of life. By the time the infant leaves the nursery, nonbacterial causes are overwhelmingly predominant. In the past, carefully performed prospective studies diagnosed less than 50% of causes of lower respiratory tract infection in young infants. Recent work has uncovered several new pathogens and an improved understanding of the pathogenesis of pneumonia in young infants. Table 1 identifies agents of pneumonia and their relative importance in the young infant; undoubtedly further information will cause shifts within the list.

PNEUMONIA IN THE NURSERY

Bacterial pneumonia in the first few days of life is associated with complications of the peripartum period. Maternal factors, such as premature onset of labor, prolonged rupture of membranes, chorioamnionitis, and systemic disease, as well as infant risk factors, such as prematurity, distress during labor, asphyxia during delivery, and congenital anomalies, increase the likelihood of bacterial infection in the neonate. Most of these events lead to fetal aspiration of material contaminated by maternal vaginal flora. Infection is caused by the most prevalent or virulent pathogens present and spreads systemically from the lower respiratory tract. Groups B and D streptococci and *Escherichia coli* are the most frequent, but *Listeria monocytogenes* cannot be forgotten. Group B streptococci deserve special notation. Although perinatal risks greatly increase the likelihood of disease, a healthy, full-term infant with no risk factors for infection is the usual victim of overwhelming group B streptococcal disease. This anomaly reflects both the special virulence of the bacterium and the susceptibility of the neonate. Whatever the cause of early-onset disease, the pulmonary manifestation may simulate hyaline membrane disease with complete opacification of lungs. Clues to bacterial etiology rather than surfactant deficiency are lack of prematurity, relative ease of ventilation, presence of left shift of the peripheral white blood cell count, acidosis, disseminated intravascular coagulopathy, and shock. Ampicillin plus gentamicin, given intravenously, is appropriate initial therapy for suspected bacterial pneumonia and septicemia in the neonate.

Bacterial pneumonia in the nursery after the first few days of life is almost always a complication of medical intervention. Bacteremia related to intravascular catheters causes systemic illness that may be reflected in deteriorating

TABLE 1. Causes of Pneumonia in Infants Less Than Three Months of Age

	Perinatally Acquired		Community-acquired
	Acute Onset	Insidious Onset	Acute Onset
Bacteria			
Groups B and D streptococci	+ + +	–	+ +
Enteric bacilli	+ +	–	+
*Listeria monocytogenes**	+	–	–
Streptococcus pneumoniae	–	–	+ + +
Hemophilus influenzae B	–	–	+
Staphylococcus aureus	–	–	+
Bordetella pertussis	–	–	+
Treponema pallidum	+	+	–
Viruses			
Herpes simplex	+ +	–	–
Cytomegalovirus	+	+ + +	–
Enterovirus	+	–	+ +
Adenovirus	+	–	+ +
Parainfluenza	–	–	+ +
Influenza	–	–	+ +
Respiratory syncytial virus	–	–	+ + + +
Other			
Chlamydia trachomatis	–	+ + +	–
Ureaplasma urealyticum	–	+ +	–
Pneumocystis carinii	–	+	–

+ + + + = most frequent cause; + + + = frequent cause; – + = less frequent cause; + = occasional cause; — = rare cause; * never to be forgotten.

respiratory function or occasionally actual seeding of the lung. Pneumonia secondary to impaired local defenses related to tracheal intubation or mechanical ventilation is most common. No clinical or radiographic finding differentiates etiologic agents. *Streptococcus* and *E. coli* are causative in the first week, but with increasing duration of nursery stay, use of antibiotics, or parenteral alimentation, *Staphylococcus epidermidis, Staphylococcus aureus,* various gram-negative bacilli, and fungus must be considered. Depending on the above factors and the infant's history of infection and colonization, vancomycin plus either gentamicin or cefotaxime, with or without amphotericin, is an appropriate initial therapeutic choice. Cultures of blood, urine, tracheal secretions, and catheters are helpful in proving a diagnosis and tailoring therapy. Current evidence of efficacy is insufficient to recommend use of intravenous immunoglobulin for therapy or prophylaxis. As the infant approaches 3 weeks of age and continues to have compromising conditions that require intensive care, both community-acquired acute infection and perinatally acquired insidious infections must be considered. Nursery outbreaks of viral disease usually reflect infections in the community. If culture and antigen detection methods fail to aid diagnosis in the infant with severe respiratory deterioration, lung biopsy is sometimes required. Experience with diagnostic mini-bronchoalveolar lavage, which can avert biopsy if the specimen yields a convincing pathogen, is limited but good.

Lower respiratory tract infection in the first week of life may be a manifestation of intrauterine infection with agents such as *Treponema pallidum,* cytomegalovirus, or toxoplasma. Although tachypnea and abnormal radiographs are common in infected infants, pneumonia is usually not the cardinal feature of illness; major clues are growth retardation, jaundice, hepatosplenomegaly, lymphadenopathy, and thrombocytopenia. Perinatally acquired viral infections also must be considered. Onset is acute, frequently with fever. Herpes simplex infection usually begins with fever and appearance of vesicular skin lesions, but pneumonia or signs of visceral dissemination may be prominent and skin lesions may be absent. When the mother is ill in the peripartum period, especially with adenovirus or enterovirus, the neonate may have acute onset of highly morbid or fatal illness in the first week of life with severe involvement of the pulmonary, hepatic, hematologic, cardiac, or central nervous system. Early therapy with intravenously administered acyclovir (10–15 mg/kg every 8 hr) is critical to a good outcome for herpes simplex infection. No therapy has been proved effective for enterovirus or adenovirus disease, although intravenously administered immunoglobulin is sometimes used for neonatal enterovirus infection, and adenoviruses are susceptible to ribavirin in the laboratory.

PNEUMONIA AFTER LEAVING THE NURSERY

After the infant leaves the nursery, bacterial pneumonia accounts for less than 10% of acute lower respiratory tract infections. Viruses acquired from the community cause most acute disease, and some perinatally acquired agents cause insidious disease. The clinical features of pneumonia are not as specific as in older infants. Fever or hypothermia, lethargy, poor feeding, vomiting, and tachypnea are clues. Temperature is sometimes normal. Tachypnea is always present but frequently overlooked. Cough in an infant under 3 months of age is infrequently caused by upper respiratory tract infection and always needs an explanation. It is usually a sign of lower respiratory tract infection, but other important considerations include anomalies of the airway or great vessels, congestive heart failure, and aspiration of gastric contents.

The infant with bacterial pneumonia has lethargy, acidosis, hypotonia, and hypoxemia greatly out of proportion to auscultatory findings in the chest. Both tachypnea with diminished breath sounds and normal auscultatory findings are common. Peripheral white blood cell count is not very helpful, because high counts may be associated with viral infection or stress, and normal and particularly low counts may occur with bacterial pneumonia. Chest radiograph shows hyperinflation with or without patchy infiltrate. Wheezing, interstitial and perihilar infiltrates, or atelectasis suggests a nonbacterial cause of lower respiratory infection. The decision to give antibiotic therapy is based on age, general degree of illness, and reasonable exclusion by clinical assessment of the likelihood of bacterial infection. Table 2 provides guidelines for choosing initial therapy.

Streptococcus pneumoniae is the most common cause of bacterial pneumonia, frequently as a complication of viral respiratory infection. The infant continues to have particular vulnerability to group B streptococci, *E. coli, L. monocytogenes,* and *S. aureus* for the first few months of life. *Hemophilus influenzae* B is a consideration as the infant ages.

For uncomplicated bacterial pneumonia, parenterally administered ampicillin and gentamicin are the therapy of choice for the patient under 2 months; cefuroxime is preferred for the older infant. The infant over 1 month of age with fever and pneumonia as the predominant features of illness and with findings compatible mainly with nonbacterial disease may be given ampicillin alone, because gram-negative bacillary or *Hemophilus pneumoniae* is extremely unlikely. Ampicillin is also a good choice for therapy of pneumonia considered to be due to aspiration of oropharyngeal or gastric contents. The infant who is tachypneic but afebrile and has a preserved sense of well-being, a normal white blood cell count or lymphocytosis, and a diffusely abnormal radiograph, as mentioned above, should not be treated for bacterial pneumonia. If pneumonia is predominant and severe or complicated by pleural fluid or pneumatoceles, nafcillin should be added. For the infant over 2 months of age with complicated

TABLE 2. Therapeutic Considerations for Infants with Pneumonia

Assessment of Pneumonia	Age in Months 0–2	Age in Months 2–3
Probable bacterial	Ampicillin + gentamicin	Cefuroxime
Probable aspiration	Ampicillin + gentamicin	Ampicillin
Fever, possible bacterial	Ampicillin + gentamicin	Ampicillin
Severe or complicated	Nafcillin + ampicillin + gentamicin	Cefuroxime
Afebrile, probable chlamydia, etc.	Erythromycin	Erythromycin
Afebrile, probable viral	None	None

pneumonia, cefuroxime is a good initial choice of therapy. **An infant under 3 months of age with a lung abscess should be investigated for abnormalities such as lobar emphysema, cystic adenomatoid malformation, or pulmonary sequestration.** Third-generation cephalosporins are rarely indicated for pneumonia in previously well infants because they have inferior activity against *S. aureus* and their gram-negative bacillary spectrum is infrequently needed.

A heterogeneous group of perinatally acquired and community-acquired nonbacterial agents are responsible for most lower respiratory tract infections in infants 3 weeks through 3 months of age. These agents account for the steady rate of hospitalization of young infants with lower respiratory disease and superimposed seasonal peaks of community-acquired disease. **The predominant organism overall is respiratory syncytial virus (RSV),** which accounts for one-half of hospitalizations of young infants with lower respiratory disease. Approximately one-half of infants under 3 months of age with RSV and many other acute respiratory virus illnesses are afebrile. The majority of infants with pneumonia due to perinatally acquired CMV, *Chlamydia, Ureaplasma,* and *Pneumocystis* do not have fever. It is useful to consider the clues that differentiate etiologic agents of coughing and wheezing in afebrile infants. Application of facts elicited from the history and findings on examination to the framework of Table 3 usually permits elimination of certain pathogens and focus on a few. *Bordetella pertussis* is included in the scheme because of its importance and certain shared clinical manifestations. ***B. pertussis*, however, is differentiated from other agents because there is no evidence of lower respiratory involvement unless superinfection has occurred.**

Transplacental antibody protection against RSV, influenza, parainfluenza, and other respiratory viruses appears to wane after the first month of life. Viral pneumonia has an acute onset, although disease is heralded by mild upper respiratory signs. Premature infants and infants with previous apnea may have apnea early in the course, especially with RSV and influenza infection. Others have colds or flu at home. Cough and respiratory distress are the cardinal features of illness; prolonged expiration and wheezing are the predominant findings for RSV. Degree of illness is proportional to findings on chest examination. Hypoxemia is out of proportion to both with RSV disease. The chest radiograph is not pathognomonic, but juxtaposed areas of overaeration and atelectasis are typical. Rapid diagnosis of viral respiratory pathogens is possible by examination of respiratory epithelial cells (obtained by nasal wash) stained with fluorescein-labeled specific antibody. **Epidemic disease occurs in previously healthy infants, primarily RSV and influenza in winter and parainfluenza in fall and spring. Infection with *B. pertussis* occurs in any season, although one-half of all cases occur from July through October.**

Improved diagnostic techniques have brought to light only recently the importance of perinatally acquired *C. trachomatis*, cytomegalovirus, *Ureaplasma urealyticum*, and *Pneumocystis carinii* as agents of pneumonia. Except for *P. carinii*, these silent sexually acquired pathogens in the mother are vertically transmitted to the neonate. They share clinical features and together account for at least one-third of lower respiratory disease in the second and third months of life. Pneumonia, which occurs especially in premature infants of low socioeconomic status, is insidious in onset. Cardinal features are cough and minimal respiratory distress in an afebrile infant with poor weight gain. Tachypnea is present but infrequently noticed by the parent. The findings of both diffuse dry rales and diffuse radiographic abnormalities are unexpected, because the infant looks well and has minimal respiratory distress. Hypoxemia is typical only of *Pneumocystis* or severe CMV pneumonia. Pathogens cannot be differentiated by clinical and radiographic features; moreover, many infants have dual infections.

The previously healthy infant with an unremarkable perinatal history who has conjunctivitis, a staccato cough, diffuse rales, eosinophilia, and impressive alveolar and interstitial infiltrates despite minimal distress almost certainly has infection due to *C. trachomatis*. Diagnosis is made by fluorescent antibody staining of scrapings of tarsal conjunctivae, nasopharyngeal, or Leuken's aspirate specimen.

A thin, premature infant who appears chronically ill, has a nonspecific cough, bilateral rales and wheezes, hepatosplenomegaly, diffuse interstitial infiltrate, and hypergammaglobulinemia almost certainly has CMV disease. Diagnosis is

TABLE 3. Clinical Features of Pneumonia in Infants Less Than Three Months of Age

	Respiratory Syncytial Virus	Other Respiratory Viruses	Chlamydia	Cytomegalovirus	Pertussis
Symptoms and signs					
Season	Winter	Unique to each	Any	Any	Any
Onset	Acute, days	Acute, days	Insidious	Insidious	Progressive, days
Others Ill	URI	URI, flu, croup	No	No	Cough
Fever	One-half	Majority	No	Unusual	No
Cough	Yes	Yes	Staccato	Yes	Paroxysmal
Associated features	Apnea, URI	URI, croup, conjunctivitis, rash	Conjunctivitis, failure to thrive	Failure to thrive, hepatosplenomegaly, petechial rash	Apnea, cyanosis posttussive vomiting
General appearance	Ill, not toxic	Ill, not toxic, stridor	Well, tachypnea	Chronically ill	Well between paroxysms
Auscultation	Wheezes, sonorous rales	Rales, wheezes	Diffuse rales	Rales, wheezes	Clear
Cardinal feature	Respiratory distress	Respiratory distress	Cough	Failure to thrive	Cough
Degree of illness	Ill: Findings	Ill: Findings	Findings >Ill	General appearance Ill >respiratory Ill	Ill only a cough
Laboratory tests					
Chest radiograph	Hyperaeration, peribronchial thickening, subsegmental atelectasis	Hyperaeration, ± peribronchial thickening, ± diffuse interstitial infiltrates	Hyperaeration, diffuse alveolar and interstitial infiltrates	Diffuse interstitial infiltrates	Normal or perihilar infiltrate
White blood cell count	Normal or lymphocytosis	Normal or lymphocytosis or neutropenia	Eosinophilia	Normal or eosinophilia or lymphocytosis	Lymphocytosis eosinophilia
Other findings	Hypoxemia		↑ IgG, IgA, IgM	↑ IgG, IgA, IgM, thrombocytopenia	
Diagnostic test	Nasal wash FA, culture	Nasal wash FA, culture, throat culture	Conjunctival scraping FA, Leuken's FA	Leukens, urine culture	NP FA, culture
Treatment	Ribavirin for some	None, ? ribavirin	Erythromycin or sulfisoxazole	None	Erythromycin

URI = upper respiratory infection, Ill = stage Ill disease; FA = fluorescent antibody test; NP = nasopharyngeal.

made by serologic tests and isolation or identification of virus in urine and respiratory specimens.

Pneumocystis pneumonia is much less common, occurring almost exclusively in underweight infants or those infected with the human immunodeficiency virus. Although it can be suspected with few physical findings, profound hypoxemia, and white-out of the chest, some infected infants have a less specific presentation. Diagnosis is made by visualization of protozoa from tracheal or alveolar lavage or lung specimens stained with Gomori silver-methenamine technique.

The high prevalence of *U. urealyticum* in asymptomatic states in women and very young infants makes it difficult to ascribe clinical findings to this agent. The organism is frequently found in dual infections in young infants but has been the sole isolate in afebrile infants with cough and diffuse pulmonary findings. Nasopharyngeal secretions are the best source of specimens for culture. Specimens must be transported and inoculated promptly, because ureaplasms are oxygen-labile.

More than one-half of hospitalized infants with pertussis are under 4 months of age. The clinical illness is identifiable, although the classic whoop is unusual in the young infant. Symptoms begin with ill-defined rhinorrhea and congestion and progress without fever to dramatic, prolonged periods of coughing with red face and bulging eyes. At the conclusion of a paroxysm, when a thick mucous mat is occasionally expelled, the infant may be cyanotic and exhausted. Apnea may occur either after or unrelated to paroxysms. The infant may have more than 20 episodes in 24 hours, set off by sudden noise, light, attempts to feed, or no apparent stimulus. Vomiting, petechiae, subconjunctival hemorrhages, and, on rare occasions, intracranial hemorrhages are associated with coughing. The clue to diagnosis of pertussis is the discrepancy between the appearance of the infant during coughing spells and between paroxysms, when he or she appears well and smiles.

Pertussis infection stops where ciliated respiratory epithelium stops. If pneumonia is present, it is a secondary bacterial complication. The patient then manifests signs and symptoms of bacterial disease. Lymphocytosis in pertussis is related to the ability of the bacterial toxin to modulate margination of cells. Lymphocytes are normal small cells rather than large and atypical, as in viral disease. Profound elevations correlate with severe disease and poor prognosis. Very young infants may have eosinophilia. Diagnosis is made by demonstration of typical coccobacilli on direct fluorescent antibody staining or by culture of nasopharyngeal secretions. Specimens for culture must be put into casamino acid or Regan-Lowe transport medium if they are not inoculated promptly onto specialized agar.

Treatment for bronchiolitis or pneumonia of all etiologies always includes careful supportive therapy (monitoring of oxygenation and adequacy of respiratory function, administration of oxygen and parenteral fluids). Fatigue, metabolic acidosis, and respiratory failure occur rapidly in young infants with lower respiratory disease. An infant requiring oxygen therapy can be monitored frequently by pulse oximetry measurement but should have full blood gas determinations to assess for hypercapnia at least every 24 hours during the acute phase of illness.

Aerosolized ribavirin is used liberally in very young infants with RSV, because their propensity to progress to severe disease and respiratory failure is documented. Infants with history of prematurity, pulmonary or cardiac disease, or immune suppression are treated when diagnosis is confirmed, regardless of degree of illness. Ribavirin is effective in the laboratory against influenza, parainfluenza, adenoviruses, and measles virus. The paucity of clinical information about efficacy limits its use except in special clinical situations.

Amantadine and rimantadine, although effective against influenza A, are not approved for use in infants under 6 months of age. *C. trachomatis, B. pertussis,* and *U. urealyticum* are susceptible to erythromycin in vitro, and clinical data demonstrate its usefulness for the first two (eradication of *B. pertussis* and eradication with clinical benefit in chlamydial disease). Dosage is 40 mg/kg/day divided tid for 14 days for infants 1 month or older. Chlamyidal disease responds to sulfisoxazole (150 mg/kg/day divided tid for 14 days) and *P. carinii* to trimethoprim-sulfamethoxazole (20 mg/kg/day divided q 6 h for 14 days). No therapy has been proved to be efficacious for transplacentally or perinatally acquired CMV infection.

If study of upper respiratory secretions yields no diagnosis and if the patient has progressive respiratory failure or fails to respond to specific therapy over time, a specimen from the lower respiratory tract is required. Lung biopsy affords the opportunity to collect samples for culture as well as to examine the histologic features of disease, sometimes confirming noninfectious etiologies. Bronchoalveolar lavage, which is increasingly common in smaller patients at some centers, allows diagnosis of infectious etiologies, sometimes averting the need for open-lung biopsy.

SUGGESTED READING

1. Abzug MJ, Beam AC, Gyorkos EA, et al: Viral pneumonia in the first month of life. Pediatr Infect Dis J 9:881–885, 1990.
2. Balfour HH Jr, Englund JA: Antiviral drugs in pediatrics. Am J Dis Child 143:1307–1316, 1989.
3. Brasfield DM, Stagno S, Whitley RJ, et al: Infant pneumonitis associated with cytomegalovirus, chlamydia, pneumocystis, and ureaplasma: Follow-up. Pediatrics 79:76–83, 1987.
4. Cassell GH, Crouse DT, Waites KB, et al: Does *Ureaplasma urealyticum* cause respiratory disease in newborns? Pediatr Infect Dis J 7:535–541, 1988.
5. Gan VN, Murphy TV: Pertussis in hospitalized children. Am J Dis Child 144:1130–1134, 1990.
6. La Via WV, Marks MI, Stretman HR: Respiratory syncytial virus puzzle: Clinical features, pathophysiology, treatment, and prevention. J Pediatr 121:503–510, 1992.

16

PNEUMONIA IN OLDER INFANTS, CHILDREN, AND ADOLESCENTS

(4 Months through 18 Years)

Sarah S. Long, M.D.

If one excludes pneumonia secondary to bacteremia or viremia and the rare pneumonia that follows extension from an intraabdominal infection, all pneumonia derives from aspiration of bacteria or contagious spread of viruses or other microorganisms from the upper respiratory tract. The airway is protected at descending levels by anatomic separation from the digestive tract, expulsion by cough, upward sweep of the mucociliary blanket, and phagocytosis by alveolar macrophages. The development of pneumonia depends on the virulence of microorganisms colonizing the upper airways and susceptiblity of the host (i.e., lack of immunity or impairment of natural defenses).

Figure 1 demonstrates examples of impairment of natural defenses. A normal child is susceptible to pneumonia due to *Streptococcus pneumoniae, Hemophilus influenzae,* or respiratory syncytial virus (RSV) because of the intrinsic virulence of the microorganisms and lack of immunity. A child with impaired swallowing or a patient receiving morphine or oxygen therapy is rendered susceptible to pneumonia by indigenous nonvirulent microflora. Double jeopardy occurs when the patient acquires an intrinsically virulent bacterium (e.g., pneumococcus or staphylococcus) during a viral infection that impairs the function of pulmonary macrophages (e.g., influenza, measles). This situation accounts for the excess cases or epidemics of bacterial pneumonia that accompany epidemics of viral diseases such as influenza or measles.

The specific etiologic agent of pneumonia is confirmed in less than one-half of cases, even in prospective studies using multiple microbiologic, serologic, and antigen detection techniques for diagnosis. For purposes of management one can put together the clues of the setting of the patient's illness, the cardinal features of symptomatology, and the physical examination to determine the need for hospitalization, the category of etiologic microorganism and probable specific pathogen(s), and the appropriate therapy. Further investigation by chest radiograph, blood count, or microbiologic testing is reserved for the patient with a confusing clinical picture or degree of illness requiring hospitalization.

MAKING THE DIAGNOSIS OF PNEUMONIA

The diagnosis of pneumonia is a clinical one (Table 1). Noninfectious conditions that share features of pneumonia should be kept in mind, such as congestive heart failure, pulmonary or rib infarction in sickle-cell disease, hydrocarbon aspiration, asthma, autoimmune diseases, congenital anomalies of vascular or pulmonary structure, ketosis, and adult respiratory distress syndrome. General signs of

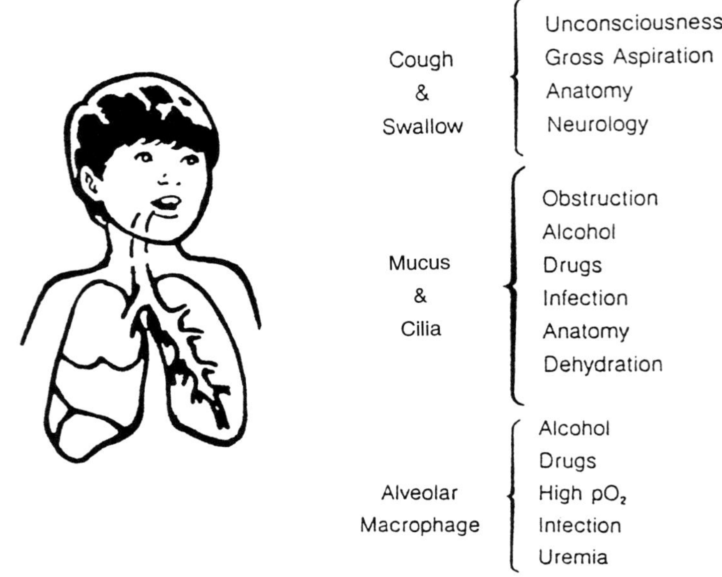

FIGURE 1. Impairments of normal defenses that predispose to lung infection.

infection in patients with pneumonia include fever, malaise, apprehension, chills or rigors, toxicity, and lethargy. **Fever, tachypnea, and cough are the cardinal features of pneumonia. Pneumonia rarely hides behind a normal respiratory rate.** The patient may have trouble getting air in (intercostal retractions) or out (wheezing). Asynchronous chest and abdominal movement or frank cyanosis signifies very severe disease. Abdominal pain and distention, sometimes simulating acute appendicitis, result from swallowing excess air, ileus, or irritation of the diaphragm. Fine end-inspiratory rales are the cardinal auscultatory finding in pneumonia. The young child may not have appreciable auscultatory lung abnormalities or may have only diminished breath sounds, but in the older patient findings by percussion and auscultation usually confirm the diagnosis of pneumonia, suggest the etiology, and predict a complication such as pleural effusion.

TABLE 1. Symptoms and Signs of Pneumonia

Symptoms	Signs	Physical Examination
Fever	Fever	Rales
Rapid breathing	Tachypnea	Wheezes
Cough	Dyspnea	Diminished breath sounds
Vomiting	Retractions	Tubular breath sounds
Poor feeding	Nasal flaring	Dullness to percussion
Irritability	Grunting	Decreased tactile and vocal fremitus
Lethargy	Splinting	Meningismus
Chest pain	Cyanosis	Ileus
Abdominal pain		Pleural friction rub
Shoulder pain		

DIFFERENTIATING ETIOLOGIES OF PNEUMONIA

Table 2 categorizes the features of pneumonia by etiology. No single factor short of direct isolation of the offending agent from lung confirms a diagnosis, but the story usually builds to an accurate conclusion. Virus is by far the most common cause of pneumonia in the infant and preschool-aged child. *Mycoplasma* sp. and probably *Chlamydia pneumoniae* vie with viruses as significant pathogens in the school-aged and adolescent patient.

Bacterial pneumonia, which occurs much less frequently, especially affects infants and toddlers. In the absence of critical illness, low-grade fever suggests nonbacterial etiology. Bacterial pneumonia begins abruptly with high fever and chills and progresses to severe distress in hours, whereas viral pneumonia is characterized by gradual worsening of cough and distress.

TABLE 2. Clues to the Etiology of Acute Pneumonia

	Bacteria	Virus	Mycoplasma
History			
Age	Any, infants	Any	School age
Temperature	Most ≥39°C	Most <39°C	Most <39°C
Onset	Abrupt	Insidious	Worsening cough
Others in home ill	No	Yes, concurrent	Yes, weeks apart
Associated signs, symptoms	Toxicity, rigors	Myalgia, rash, mucous membranes	Headache, sore throat, chills, myalgia
Cough	Productive	Nonproductive	Hacking, usually non-productive
Physical examination			
Pleuritic chest pain	No/yes	No	No
General	Degree illness >findings	Degree illness ≤findings	Degree illness <findings
Auscultation	Confined/no rales, dullness, diminished or tubular sounds	Diffuse, bilateral rales, wheezes	Unilateral rales (≥one lobe), wheezes
Laboratory studies			
Radiograph	Hyperaeration, alveolar patchy or consolidated distribution in lobe or subsegment	Hyperaeration, interstitial infiltrate in diffuse or perihilar distribution, atelectasis	Alveolar and interstitial patchy infiltrate in single or contiguous lobes
Pleural fluid	No/yes → large	No/yes → small	No/yes → small
Peripheral white blood cell count/mm^3	Majority >15,000 granulocytes	Majority <15,000 lymphocytes	Majority <15,000 granulocytes
Sputum	Copious Granulocytes, ingested bacteria	Scant Epithelial cells, mononuclear cells	Scant → copious Mononuclear cells; debris; occasionally granulocytes

Mycoplasma illness begins abruptly with fever, headache, and malaise, but the cough and pneumonia progress gradually over a period of days to a week. The contact setting of the patient's illness is extremely helpful. Bacterial pneumonia is not an epidemic disease. On the other hand, viral respiratory pathogens affect many, and their short incubations mean that others are sick concurrently or quite recently. Mycoplasma affects many family members, but the incubation period is usually 2 weeks; thus contact histories are elicited for the previous 4–6 weeks. Pneumonia is an unusual manifestation of viral or mycloplasma infection. The histories sought in contacts focus on the more common symptoms of myalgia, rash, conjunctivitis, pharyngitis, laryngitis, mouth ulcers, diarrhea, cystitis manifestations of virus or fever, headache, prolonged cough, and the prolonged flu of mycoplasma. One must then examine the patient for such manifestations, remembering that **the more mucous membranes involved (eye, mouth, throat, gut), the more likely the infection is viral. Bacterial pneumonia is special in that the lung is usually the sole affected organ; except for signs of toxicity, findings are confined to the chest.**

Cough is almost universally present, but the young child rarely produces sputum for classification or microscopic examination. The nature of cough is accurately reflected only with adequate hydration. The timbre of the cough in the child with bacterial pneumonia alludes to production and attempted expulsion of thick wet secretions. The irritative dry cough of viral disease produces no mucopurulent secretions and no benefit. The cough of mycoplasma is nine-tenths of the disease. Spasms of nonproductive, hacking, dry, bronchitic, painful cough lead to posttussive vomiting and exhaustion (very much like pertussis infection, except that frequently at the end of paroxysm in pertussis infection a matted cast of denuded mucociliary epithelium is expelled).

Pleuritic chest pain, a sign of bacterial pneumonia, is rarely verbalized by children as pain on inspiration but is manifest as rapid, shallow breathing, immobility, splinting of the affected side of the chest, and expiratory grunting. Pain of pleural irritation is referred to intercostal nerves overlying the pneumonia. If the involved area is the middle third of the diaphragm, pain is referred to the posterolateral neck or shoulder. Pleural irritation over the right upper lobe may elicit meningismus. Grunting expirations in the young child differentiates bacterial from viral pneumonia but also may be a clue to other serious cardiorespiratory problems, such as severe asthma, congestive heart failure, myocardial pain, or purulent pericarditis (see chapters 13 and 30).

The patient's history, setting, and appearance are major clues to the diagnosis of pneumonia, the need for hospitalization, and suspected etiology. The physical examination confirms the diagnosis and aids in differentiating etiologies in two ways:

1. One compares the general degree of illness (distress, toxicity) with the physical findings—in other words, what one sees with what one hears. The child with bacterial pneumonia is toxic, severely distressed, and sometimes cyanotic but has no skin or mucous membrane symptoms and few auscultatory findings. The patient with viral pneumonia appears mildly-to-moderately ill and usually has some skin or mucous membrane manifestations as well as moderate auscultatory findings, most often bilateral rales, occasionally with wheezes. What one sees is what one hears. The school-aged patient with mycoplasma or chlamydia is at the other end of the spectrum. He or she is not ill-appearing and complains mainly of cough, but has rales and rhonchi over half of one lung.

2. One seeks the specific findings that typify pneumonia caused by certain agents. Bacterial pneumonia spreads by the tracheobronchial tree to involve contiguous lung parenchyma. Fine rales, dullness, or tubular breath sounds are anatomically confined, for example, to the right lower posterior chest (right lower lobe), the left mid anterior chest (lingula), or the left superior posterior chest (left upper lobe). Bacterial pneumonia is a consolidative process; tubular or diminished breath sounds, dullness to percussion, and decreased fremitus are clues. Diminished breath sounds suggest bacterial pneumonia complicated by pleural effusion. Viral pneumonia is not anatomically confined and causes bilateral interstitial inflammation; therefore, coarse rales and occasionally wheezes can be heard bilaterally throughout lung fields, with no consolidation and most often without evidence of fluid. The majority of cases of mycoplasma involve only one lung—usually one segment, but sometimes two continguous segments without consolidation. The startling finding is that coarse rales are heard in a patient with no respiratory distress.

LABORATORY CLUES TO THE ETIOLOGY OF PNEUMONIA

The chest radiograph is another way to ask the same questions posed by the physical examination. An overinflated chest denotes acute airway inflammation and is present in all infants with acute pneumonia. Bacterial pneumonia is typified by patchy alveolar, lobular, or, less frequently, lobar parenchymal consolidation, which is anatomically confined. This picture has to be carefully differentiated from the combination of atelectasis and hyperinflation that is the hallmark of viral infection in young children. Radiographic findings in viral pneumonia include perihilar infiltrates and a bilateral interstitial pattern of involvement. The radiographic appearance of mycoplasma is characterized by patchy alveolar and interstitial infiltrates in single or contiguous lobes. Presence of large amounts or rapidly increasing amounts of pleural fluid denotes bacterial disease, as do pneumatocele, abscess, and hydropneumothorax. Small amounts of pleural effusion seen only at the diaphragmatic pleural angle or on lateral decubitus films are not uncommon with any etiologic agent. On rare occasions, large pleural effusions complicate viral pneumonia.

Laboratory tests are divided into two categories: (1) measurements of the nature and degree of inflammatory response and (2) specific pathogen-seeking microbiologic tools. Peripheral white blood cell count is useful in a negative way. **With neither an increase in polymorphonuclear neutrophils nor a shift to immature neutrophils, a bacterial etiology is highly unlikely.** The equation of higher counts with bacterial disease is less accurate, because occasionally viral pneumonia (especially adenovirus and influenza) and mycoplasma cause elevations of the white cell count over 15,000 cells/mm^3.

Thrombocytosis (platelet count >500,000/mm³) is typical of bacterial pneumonia or severe stress. Thrombocytopenia is more typical of viral infection. Sedimentation rate is elevated to variable degrees during pneumonia of any etiology. Extreme elevations (>80 mm/hr) suggest bacterial or noninfectious inflammatory etiologies; extreme depression (<5 mm/hr) is present in early and overwhelming bacterial infections.

Determination of the specific bacteria responsible for pneumonia is usually a statistically based best bet (see below). Gram stain of sputum or an aspirate of the posterior pharynx and trachea (Leuken's aspirate) that shows clumps of neutrophils and a predominant microorganism confirms the diagnosis of bacterial pneumonia and suggests the likely etiologic agent. Viral and mycoplasma pneumonia are characterized by an acellular or mononuclear cell response. In bacterial pneumonia, culture of sputum or upper respiratory or tracheal secretions usually yields the causative pathogen along with noncausative flora. Interpretation of direct Gram stain of the specimen in conjunction with the culture is very useful. Knowledge of upper respiratory flora is also indirectly helpful in choosing antimicrobial agents for the patient with hospital-associated pneumonia. For example, gram-negative bacillary pneumonia does not occur in the absence of colonization of the upper airway. The patient with normal oropharyngeal flora is likely to have a statistically predictable cause of pneumonia (see below). The presence of gram-negative rods in the upper airway is not diagnostic of any disease and does not confirm the etiology of clinically present pneumonia; but it may be a guide to choosing therapy if no more direct specimen is available. Culture of blood and other clinically affected sites (e.g., pleura, cerebrospinal fluid, joint) should be performed for diagnosis and therapy of bacterial disease. Direct rapid tests of sputum and urine for bacterial antigens are available, but they are costly and infrequently positive in cases of pneumonia; in addition, they frequently yield false-positive results and do not include all of the clinically relevant pathogens (see chapter 40).

Specific etiologic agents of viral pneumonia are frequently predictable from the clinical constellation of findings, age of patient, and season (Table 3). Direct fluorescent antibody tests and cultures of nasopharyngeal, tracheal, and bronchoalveolar lavage (BAL) specimens for viral pathogens are rapidly developing techniques in the clinical laboratory. Viral etiology is pursued in patients ill enough for hospitalization and in patients with hospital-acquired disease. Approved or potentially beneficial therapies for RSV, influenza, herpes simplex, and other causative agents make direct testing advantageous. Respiratory epithelial cells are collected by nasal wash or aspiration through endotracheal or tracheostomy tube or with BAL and can be tested directly by specific antibodies or a pooled respiratory panel (Table 4). Tests are expensive and laborious. In a previously healthy infant with a bronchiolitis syndrome in the winter, only the RSV test should be requested initially. In an immunocompromised, severely ill, or older patient the pooled respiratory panel may be more appropriate. Direct antigen detection for cytomegalovirus is reserved for special situations. Culture alone can be performed for

TABLE 3. Prediction of Major Etiologic Agents of Viral Pneumonia

	Relative Frequency by Age			
	4 mo–5 yr	6–19 yr	Peak Season	Associated Findings
Respiratory syncytial viruses (RSVs)	+ + + +	+	Winter → spring	Wheezing, apnea
Parainfluenza viruses	+ + +	+ +	Autumn → fall, spring	Laryngotracheitis, wheezing
Influenza viruses	+ + +	+ + +	Winter	Malaise, pharyngitis, myalgia
Adenoviruses	+ +	+ +	Any, summer	Conjunctivitis, rash, exudative pharyngitis, hemorrhagic cystitis
Enteroviruses	+	+	Summer	Ulcerative enanthem, vesicular and other rashes

+ + + + = most frequent cause; + + + = frequent cause; + + = less frequent cause; + = occasional cause.

TABLE 4. Direct Antigen Detection for Viral Pathogens

Pooled Respiratory Panel	Individual Tests
Respiratory syncytial virus	Respiratory syncytial virus
Influenza A	Rubeola
Influenza B	Herpes simplex
Adenovirus	Varicella-zoster
Parainfluenza	Cytomegalovirus

any of these viruses if a rapid answer is not required. Currently, culture is also performed in many laboratories because it is more sensitive and completely definitive.

Most clinical laboratories do not attempt detection or isolation of *Mycoplasma pneumoniae.* Cold-agglutinating antibodies are present in most children and adolescents when pneumonia is the primary feature of infection. A titer of 1:64 or greater at the time of clinical illness correlates highly with subsequent rise in specific antibodies. Specific antibodies to mycoplasma arise only 3–6 weeks after infection; acute (usually negative) and convalescent serum specimens are necessary.

A newly discovered agent, *Chlamydia pneumoniae,* is probably responsible for almost as much pneumonia in school-aged and young adult patients as mycoplasma. Clinical manifestations are not unique, although patients with chlamydia are more likely to have sore throat, hoarseness, and sinusitis and less likely to have fever. Onset is insidious. Although the organism has been propagated in tissue culture, no rapid diagnostic test is currently available for clinical use. The currently available immunofluorescent test for *Chlamydia trachomatis* antigen does not cross-react with *C. pneumoniae.* The chlamydia complement-fixing antibody test does cross-react, but the result is positive only during convalescence.

CHOOSING THERAPY FOR BACTERIAL PNEUMONIA

If clinical and laboratory clues suggest that the patient has bacterial pneumonia or if it cannot be excluded with a reasonable degree of certainty, one needs to ask the following questions to predict pathogens and to choose therapy:

1. Is the patient otherwise normal? If the answer is yes, only predictable pathogens such as *Streptococcus pneumoniae* or *Hemophilus influenzae b* need to be considered. If the patient is immunologically impaired by disease or drug therapy, etiologic agents cannot be predicted, because less virulent bacteria (such as nontypable *H. influenzae* and *Mycobacterium*), fungi (*Cryptococcus, Aspergillus, Histoplasma*), or protozoa (*Pneumocystis*) may be causative. A swallowing defect, seizure disorder, anatomic defect, or any disorder that causes aspiration may lead to pneumonia caused by bacteria of normal mouth flora.

2. How old is the patient? *H. influenzae b,* a pathogen for the infant and toddler, is unimportant in the immunized and school-aged patient.

3. Is pneumonia complicated by effusion, pneumatocele, abscess, empyema, or empyema necessitans? With uncomplicated bacterial pneumonia, *S. pneumoniae* and *H. influenzae b* account for more than 90% of cases. It is not the nature of *S. pneumoniae* to produce necrotizing pneumonia, effusion, or empyema; it is the nature of Group A streptococci, *Staphylococcus aureus, H. influenzae b,* and anaerobes to do so. For pneumonia complicated by pleural effusion, no organism accounts for more than 20% of cases. A direct specimen of fluid is required for chemical, histologic, and Gram stain examination and for culture.

Table 5 shows the predictable pathogens and appropriate antibiotic therapy for bacterial pneumonia at various ages. Special mention of primary tuberculous pneumonia is necessary. The diagnosis is never suspected early on clinical grounds, because it may present as typical acute bacterial pneumonia or pneumonia complicated by effusion. Primary tuberculous pneumonia has no predilection for any particular area of the lung. One always has to consider the patient's circumstances and to ask pertinent questions of family members. When pneumonia has the radiographic appearance of bacterial disease without the hyperinflation of acute disease, when it has been present for more than a month, or when it is associated with hilar lymphadenopathy or pulmonary calcification, tuberculosis must be excluded (see chapter 18). Mixed-flora anaerobic pneumonia is suspected in any patient who has impaired pulmonary

TABLE 5. Relative Importance of Bacteria in Acute Pneumonia and Initial Therapy

	Uncomplicated Pneumonia		Complicated Pneumonia		Hospital-associated Pneumonia
	3 mo–5 yr	6–19 yr	Pleural Fluid	Lung Abscess	
Agents					
S. pneumoniae	+ + + +	+ + + +	+ +	+	+ +
H. influenzae	+ +	+	+ +	+	+
Group A streptococcus	+	+	+ +	–	–
Mouth flora	+	+	+ + +	+ + + +	+ + +
S. aureus	+	+	+ +	+ +	+ +
Enteric bacilli	–	–	+	+	+ +
*M. tuberculosis**	*	*	*	*	*
Initial therapy					
Outpatient	Amoxicillin Consider erythromycin + sulfisoxazole, amoxicillin + clavulanate, cefuroxime axetil	Penicillin V Consider erythromycin			
Inpatient	Ampicillin Consider cefuroxime, ampicillin + sulbactam	Penicillin G Consider cefuroxime, ampicillin + sulbactam	Cefuroxime or ampicillin + sulbactam	Clindamycin or ampicillin + sulbactam	Clindamycin + aminoglycoside Consider cefoxitin, ampicillin + sulbactam

+ + + + = most frequent cause; + + + = frequent cause; + + = less frequent cause; + = occasional cause; – = rare cause; * never to be forgotten.

defense or who aspirates. Anaerobic bacterial etiology (*Actinomyces* sp. especially) is also suggested by subacute progression to necrotizing pneumonia, lung abscess, or, occasionally, empyema necessitans. With diagnosis of an anaerobic pulmonary infection, the predisposing aspiration event must be sought. If none is apparent, bronchoscopy should be performed in search of a foreign body.

Outpatient therapy for uncomplicated bacterial pneumonia may be amoxicillin for the preschool-age patient and penicillin for the older child. It seems appropriate to overlook possible ampicillin resistance of *H. influenzae* for three reasons: (1) it is an uncommon cause of pneumonia; (2) it infrequently causes disease without systemic illness that leads to hospitalization; and (3) the majority of cases are susceptible to amoxicillin. Alternative therapy, such as amoxicillin-clavulanate, erythromycin-sufisoxazole, or cefuroxime axetil, may be considered if one is more concerned about resistant organisms in the younger age group. Cefixime should not be used because of its poor coverage of pneumococcus. In the older patient, erythromycin is an appropriate alternative, because pneumococcus is susceptible and because mycoplasma and chlamydia are likely, even when bacterial infection is considered as the possible diagnosis.

Inpatient therapy assumes greater importance, because the patient ill enough to require admission is at higher risk for complications of pneumonia, bacteremia, and other foci of infection. In the younger toxic patient, it is difficult to discourage use of cefuroxime because of its added effectiveness against beta-lactamase-producing *H. influenzae b, Moraxella catarrhalis,* and *S. aureus.* If, however, the patient is admitted with history, examination, and laboratory tests suggestive of viral pneumonia but the physician chooses to cover the unlikely possiblity of bacterial pneumonia or if the patient is not very ill, ampicillin is appropriate, safer, and less costly.

If aspiration mouth-flora pneumonia is most likely, the outpatient drug of choice is penicillin G (with instructions to avoid dosing with meals) or clindamycin. Amoxicillin-clavulanate is an attractive choice, especially in preschool-aged patients, because beta-lactamase–producing *Hemophilus* and *Moraxella* as well as penicillin-susceptible anaerobes are effectively covered.

The hospitalized patient with uncomplicated community-acquired aspiration pneumonia usually has failed outpatient therapy. Intravenously administered aqueous penicillin G, clindamycin, ticarcillin-clavulanate, or ampicillin-sulbactam (when approved for use in children) is appropriate; the first is usually very effective as well as cheap and safe.

Therapy for pneumonia complicated by pleural effusion must include agents active against *H. influenzae b* and *S. aureus* as well as pneumococcus and Group A streptococcus. Cefuroxime or ampicillin-sulbactam is a good choice. If anaerobes are likely (because of predisposition or findings on Gram stain of aspirated fluid), clindamycin, ampicillin-sulbactam, or cefuroxime plus metronidazole is appropriate. Therapy is usually altered after microbiologic results.

A major part of therapy for pneumonia complicated by pleural effusion is drainage of the fluid if it is an exudate (protein content fluid:serum = >0.5), if it is purulent (white blood cell count >10,000/mm^3), or if it is present in large amounts. It cannot be overemphasized that the window of opportunity for adequate drainage of pleural empyema closes after 3–4 days when loculation develops, fibrosis and neovascularization begin, and the lung becomes trapped.

Antimicrobial therapy for patients with lung abscess is similar to that for patients with pleural effusion, except that *S. aureus* and anaerobes must be considered as the most likely causative agents. Clindamycin is an excellent choice. Staphylococcal abscesses usually resolve with time, but an aspiration or drainage procedure is sometimes necessary. Anaerobic lung abscesses usually drain spontaneously by the tracheobronchial tree, but bronchoscopy is often required to remove an obstructing foreign body or granulation tissue.

Hospital-associated pneumonia is almost always a form of aspiration pneumonia. The patient's flora, however, may now include enteric gram-negative bacilli or *S. aureus*. A Gram stain and culture of tracheal secretions guide therapy but lead to overtreatment for gram-negative bacillary pneumonia because of frequent colonization of the upper airway in hospitalized patients. Pneumococci, oral streptococci, and anaerobic flora are still preeminent. Ampicillin or broad-spectrum therapy with cefoxitin, ticarcillin-clavulanate, or ampicillin-sulbactam may be chosen initially. If the patient improves rapidly or if the radiographic findings do not progress to a necrotizing pneumonia, the diagnosis of gram-negative bacillary pneumonia is untenable; a penicillin may be substituted. Third-generation cephalosporins are rarely used orally or intravenously, because their gram-negative rod spectrum is not needed, because they have inferior activity against gram-positive pathogens, or both.

Choosing duration of therapy for pneumonia is more a matter of enlightened practice than applied science. For outpatients, 10 days seems appropriate, with extension up to 3 weeks for patients with uncomplicated anaerobic pneumonia. For hospitalized patients with uncomplicated pneumonia, antibiotics are administered intravenously until the presence of bacteremia is excluded and the patient is afebrile for 2–3 days; if bacteremia is present, duration is dictated by the specific pathogen, rapidity of response, and presence of another focus of infection. Therapy for uncomplicated bacteremic pneumococcal pneumonia is usualy 5–7 days of intravenous administration followed by 3–5 days of oral administration. Resolution of radiographic abnormality lags behind clinical response and is not considered in determining duration of therapy. In cases in which it is important to document a normal chest radiograph (e.g., foreign body, anatomic abnormality, cystic fibrosis), film should be obtained 4–6 weeks after occurrence of pneumonia.

Duration of intravenously administered antibiotics for pneumonia complicated by empyema or abscess depends on multiple factors, including the pathogen, adequacy of drainage, and duration of fever. The patient should be afebrile, ambulating, without supplemental oxygen or a chest tube, and without radiographic evidence of reaccumulation of fluid for at least 3–5 days. The best scenario is likely to result from *H. influenzae b* disease, in which the patient presents early because of systemic illness, fluid is drained by the second day, the patient is afebrile by the fifth or sixth day, and intravenous therapy is discontinued by the tenth day. Group A streptococcal or staphylococcal disease is usually the most protracted, with loculated collections or necrotic lung, development of pleural peel, and requirement of multiple drainage procedures before the patient becomes afebrile up to 1 month later. Experience shows that such collections remain infected for weeks, necessitating prolonged intravenous antibiotic therapy and drainage (see chapter 19).

CHOOSING THERAPY FOR NONBACTERIAL PNEUMONIA

For the school-age patient (8 years or older) with signs and symptoms suggestive of infection due to *C. pneumoniae* or *M. pneumoniae,* erythromycin or tetracycline therapy is appropriate, usually for 10–14 days orally, whether on an outpatient or inpatient basis. Erythromycin, clarithromycin or azithromycin would also be expected to be effective. Therapeutic response in the patient with mycoplasma is not dramatic, although prospective studies have shown clinical benefit.

Guidelines for use of antiviral therapy for pneumonia are evolving as experience with efficacy and safety of agents accumulates. Use of ribavirin among the thousands of children hospitalized annually with RSV bronchiolitis and pneumonia is limited by price, inflated concern for toxic environmental effects of the aerosolized form, and a usually good outcome of natural illness. Patients with proved or suspected RSV infection of the lower respiratory tract and underlying conditions that compromise pulmonary or cardiac function or rapidly progressive or severe disease, and infants less than 6 weeks of age with signs of lower respiratory tract involvement or apnea should be treated. Mechanical ventilation, tracheostomy, and endotracheal tube are not contraindications to use of ribavirin, although care must be exercised to maintain patency of the ventilatory equipment. Average duration of therapy in an uncomplicated case is 3 days, but therapy is sometimes extended for longer periods. Adenoviruses, influenza, parainfluenza, and rubeola viruses are sensitive to ribavirin in the laboratory. Limited reports show clinical benefit, but numbers are too small to warrant endorsement of ribavirin except in unusual circumstances.

Ganciclovir is beneficial in compromised patients with pneumonia due to cytomegalovirus. Acyclovir is useful for pneumonia due to herpes simplex virus or varicella virus. Amantadine is highly effective for prophylaxis against influenza A only and, if given early, shortens the course of disease.

SUGGESTED READING

1. Claesson BA, Trollfors B, Brolin I, et al: Etiology of community-acquired pneumonia in children based on antibody responses to bacterial and viral agents. Pediatr Infect Dis J 8:856–862, 1989.
2. Long SS: Treatment of acute pneumonia in infants and children. Pediatr Clin North Am 30:297–321, 1983.
3. Paisley JW, Lauer BA, McIntosh K, et al: Pathogens associated with acute lower respiratory tract infection in young children. Pediatr Infect Dis J 3:14–19, 1984.
4. Peter G: The child with pneumonia: Diagnostic and therapeutic considerations. Pediatr Infect Dis J 7:453–456, 1988.
5. Shann F, Barker J, Poore P: Clinical signs that predict death in children with severe pneumonia. Pediatr Infect Dis J 8:852–855, 1989.
6. Thom DH, Grayston JT, Wang S-P, et al: *Chlamydia pneumoniae* strain TWAR, *Mycoplasma pneumoniae,* and viral infections in acute respiratory disease in a university student health clinic population. Am J Epidemiol 132:248–256, 1990.
7. Tuazon CU, Decker CF: "Atypical" pneumonias: Not so atypical anymore. J Respir Dis 14:1279–1303, 1993.

17

PERSISTENT OR RECURRENT PNEUMONIA

Michael R. Bye, M.D.

In children most episodes of pneumonia are caused by viruses. Because it is often difficult to distinguish a bacterial from a viral pneumonia, most children with pneumonia are treated with antibiotics. Although difficult to prove, the following guidelines are helpful in making the distinction: (1) when the infiltrate is localized to a few segments or lobes and has a dense appearance with air bronchograms, the pneumonia is more likely a bacterial process, and (2) diffuse, patchy interstitial pneumonias are less likely to be bacterial in origin. In the latter cases, the most common infectious agents are viruses, although *Pneumocystis carinii, Chlamydia pneumoniae,* fungi, and *Mycoplasma pneumoniae* need to be considered (see chapters 15 and 16).

The child who has two or more episodes of documented pneumonia may simply have bad luck, but for the child's protection underlying pathology must be considered. In such instances the radiographic pattern of the infiltrates and the history during and between episodes of pneumonia often give clues to an underlying diagnosis. Because the approach to such a child relies heaviliy on the radiographic findings, strong consideration should be given to radiographic confirmation of pneumonia. Although clinical pneumonia may be suspected in the child without preexisting cardiopulmonary disease and with sudden onset of fever, cough, and localized crackles, the radiograph helps to confirm the diagnosis, suggests an etiology, and facilitates follow-up. Because it is impossible to predict who will or will not develop subsequent illnesses of the lower respiratory tract, the radiographic appearance at the first episode may be quite helpful in subsequent evaluations. In addition, if the initial radiograph is abnormal, a subsequent radiograph should be obtained to ensure that the abnormality has cleared. We usually wait 8 weeks before repeating the radiograph. **The abnormality that has not cleared within 8 weeks should be investigated further.**

It is easiest to approach the evaluation of the child with recurrent pneumonia on the basis of radiographic findings. Three patterns of disease merit attention: (1) recurrent pneumonia in the same location; (2) recurrent dense infiltrates in different parts of the lung; and (3) recurrent diffuse and patchy disease.

RECURRENT PNEUMONIA IN THE SAME LOCATION

When the pneumonia recurs in the same location (Table 1), a focal anomaly in the lung or the airway is likely. Poor airway clearance predisposes to pneumonia, and a focal abnormality predisposes to recurrent focal pneumonia. Congenital lesions, especially **sequestration of the lung**, often present as recurrent or persistent pneumonia. Sequestrations are parts of lung, usually in the lower lobes, with abnormal airway connections and abnormal systemic blood supply that result in poor airway clearance. Other congenital lesions, such as **bronchogenic cyst, congenital lobar emphysema,** or **cystic adenomatoid malformation**, may also present as recurrent or persistent pneumonias, although

TABLE 1. Recurrent or Persistent Infiltrates in the Same Area

Proximal airway anomalies
Foreign body
Bronchomalacia/tracheomalacia
Airway stenosis
External compression
Lymph nodes
Vascular rings/slings
Heart, pulmonary arteries
Structural anomalies of the tracheobronchial tree
Distal anomalies
Sequestration
Congenital cystic adenomatoid malformation
Bronchogenic cyst
Congenital lobar emphysema

other clinical presentations of these lesions (such as chronic cysts) are more common.

The most common lesion that practitioners must consider is an **inhaled foreign body**. In one study, almost two-thirds of such foreign bodies were detected within 1 week of aspiration. Thus, one-third of foreign bodies are detected more than 1 week after aspiration. In some instances, the history of aspiration is unavailable. I have seen a plastic toy in the right main bronchus of a developmentally normal 9-year-old boy; neither he nor his family recognized the toy or knew when it got into his airway. In an effort to be "helpful," older siblings and sometimes adults offer infants small items or food that may be aspirated.

Tracheomalacia or **bronchomalacia** may predispose to pneumonia by obstructing the airway, although recurrent or persistent wheezing is a far more common presentation. **Extrinsic compression of the airway** by lymph nodes, aberrant vessels, tumors, enlarged heart, or pulmonary vessels predispose to pneumonia and atelectasis but are more likely to present with noisy breathing. **Structural abnormalities of the tracheobronchial tree**, such as stenosis, atresia, or a localized lack of cartilage (Williams-Campbell syndrome), are rare causes of pneumonia. Localized bronchiectatic changes following an acute episode of pneumonia or repeated injury also may be a source of repeated focal inflammation.

The **diagnostic approach** to the patient with focal persistent or recurrent infiltrates includes a combination of bronchoscopy and computerized tomography (CT) of the chest. Bronchoscopy provides anatomic documentation of the airway and is diagnostic of inhaled foreign body, aspiration syndromes, airway compression, or structural anomalies of the airway. The CT scan also evaluates the more distal airways. If a sequestration is suspected, magnetic resonance imaging (MRI) is a noninvasive method of detecting the anomalous vessel feeding into the sequestered lung. Other diagnostic modalities include aortography, digital subtraction angiography, and noninvasive Doppler-assisted ultrasound (see chapter 38).

If an anatomic abnormality predisposing to pneumonias is found, surgery should be undertaken. If the lesion has already caused two or more episodes of pneumonia, there is no reason to await further episodes. A subsequent pneumonia with a more virulent organism may result in complications.

RECURRENT DENSE INFILTRATES

Recurrent dense infiltrates (Table 2) suggest recurrent bacterial infections, although recurrent atelectasis causes a similar radiographic pattern. The broad categories of possibilities include immune deficiencies, abnormalities in airway secretions, and abnormalities in airway caliber. Although abnormalities in airway caliber may seem the least likely cause of recurrent dense disease, in fact **asthma** is the most common underlying pathology in such patients. The periodic narrowing of the airway, the inflammatory changes, and the abnormal secretions in the airway combine to cause recurrent atelectasis in children with asthma (Fig. 1). This is the

TABLE 2. Recurrent Dense Infilatrates

Asthma
Cystic fibrosis
Ciliary dyskinesia syndrome
Aspiration syndromes
B-cell dysfunction
Acquired immunodeficiency syndrome (AIDS)
Bruton agammaglobulinemia
IgG subclass deficiencies
IgA/secretory IgA deficiencies
White blood cell abnormalities
Chronic granulomatous disease
Phagocytic disorders
Chemotaxis disorders

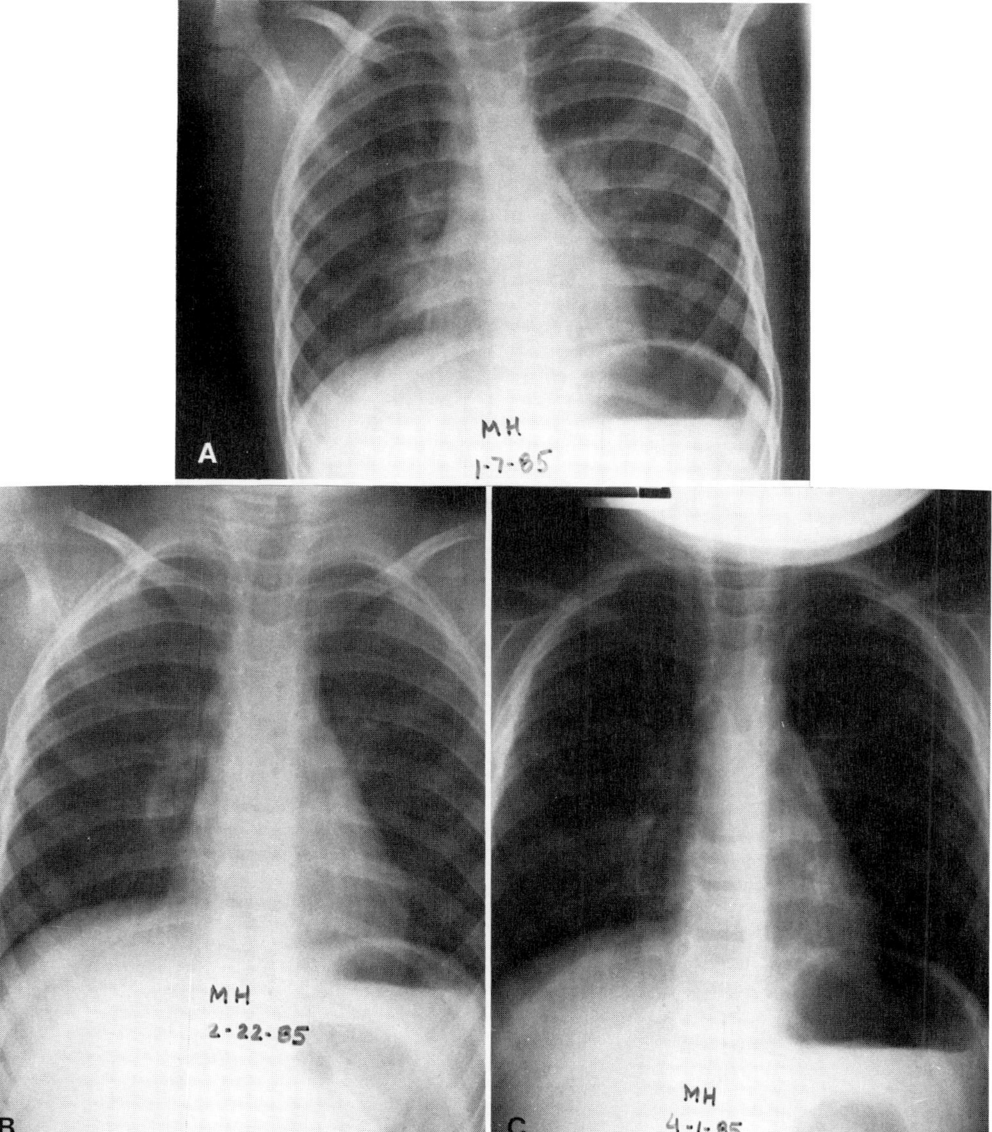

FIGURE 1. This radiograph from a 4-year-old patient with asthma shows right middle lobe and left upper lobe densities *(A)*. *B,* Six weeks later, there is almost total clearing of infiltrations. *C,* Five weeks later, the patient presents with acute wheezing episode and left lower lobe density. Note air bronchogram in the retrocardiac area. Bilateral mild peribronchial thickening and interstitial patterns are seen in all three radiographs.

most common etiology of the dense infiltrates seen in children during an attack of asthma.

Recurrent pneumonia, with or without poor weight gain, must make the practitioner consider **cystic fibrosis** (CF). In CF the secretions are abnormally thick, tenacious, and difficult to cough out. Stasis of secretions predisposes to pneumonia. The organisms commonly found in the airways of children with CF include *Staphylococcus aureus* and *Pseudomonas aeruginosa* (see chapter 14). Poor clearance of secretions is also seen in the **ciliary dyskinesia syndrome** (or immotile cilia syndrome). In this disease, the secretions are normal, but structural abnormalities in the cilia prevent the secretions and debris from being removed adequately. The end result is stasis of secretions, which predisposes to infection and pneumonia. Fifty percent of patients have situs inversus (**Kartagener syndrome**). Patients with ciliary abnormalities usually have involvement of the upper respiratory tract and a history of frequent, recurrent sinusitis and otitis media with sequelae.

Although recurrent diffuse disease is more likely to occur, **recurrent aspiration** may cause the radiographic picture of recurrent focal pneumonia. Aspiration is more common in children who are neurologically impaired, although it occurs in normal children with severe gastroesophageal reflux (GER). Frequent nighttime cough, dyspepsia, and nocturnal chest pain suggest GER.

Recurrent bacterial pneumonia may be due to an abnormality of B-cell function. The most common immune deficiency is **AIDS**, which is caused by the human immunodeficiency virus (HIV). Children with AIDS have abnormalities in both T- and B-cell function. The T-cell function varies directly with the CD4+ count. Although children with AIDS have hypergammaglobulinemia, the circulating gammaglobulins are not functional, and the children have poor antibody responses to bacterial antigens and toxoids. In 1993 the Centers for Disease Control made recurrent pneumonia (two episodes within 1 year) an AIDS-defining illness for people with HIV infection.

Bruton agammaglobulinemia affects males and is associated with a lack of antibody formation. Affected children have recurrent infections in the lung and elsewhere, including deep soft tissue. **Decreased amounts of IgA or IgG subclasses II and IV** are associated with recurrent chest infections. Association of IgG subclass deficiency with "difficult-to-control asthma" somewhat confounds the etiology of the abnormal radiograph. Patients also are at risk for developing recurrent sinus infection.

Finally, abnormalities of the white blood cells may cause recurrent bacterial infections. The most common of these uncommon conditions is **chronic granulomatous disease,** in which the white cells lack the enzymes necessary for intracellular killing of the organism. Less common are deficits in white-cell **phagocytosis** or **chemotaxis.**

The **diagnostic approach** to children with recurrent dense infiltrates starts with a careful history in an attempt to detect asthma, with particular attention to cough, including chronicity, occurrence at night, potential triggers, and persistence after upper respiratory infections. Gastrointestinal symptoms and evaluation of growth measurements over time may suggest CF if abnormalities are found. The family history should address specifically asthma and allergies, CF, early infant deaths, and risk factors for HIV infection. The laboratory evaluation should include pulmonary function tests, sweat tests, and measurement of immunoglobulins. If HIV infection is suspected, testing must be considered.

TABLE 3. Recurrent Diffuse Disease

Asthma
Cystic fibrosis
Gastroesophageal reflux/aspiration syndromes
Idiopathic pulmonary fibrosis
Pulmonary hemosiderosis
Bronchiolitis obliterans
T-cell disorders
Acquired immunodeficiency syndrome (AIDS)
DiGeorge syndrome
Chronic mucocutaneous candidiasis

RECURRENT DIFFUSE DISEASE

Children with recurrent diffuse disease (Table 3) are less likely to have recurrent bacterial disease than viral or noninfectious inflammatory disease. In our experience most patients fit into the second category.

Asthma is the most common etiology of noninfectious diffuse inflammatory disease and the most common underlying etiology in children with recurrent pulmonary infiltrates of any kind. Radiographic changes consistent with pneumonia also can be explained by changes due to asthma. The hallmark of asthma is now recognized as diffuse inflammation of the airways. The radiographic changes may include atelectasis due to mucous plugging and peribronchial thickening from inflammation and edema. Interstitial edema and inflammation cause a pattern of interstitial infiltration (Fig. 2). Furthermore, the clinical manifestations of asthma and atelectasis associated with pneumonia can be similar. Both are likely to be preceded by an upper respiratory infection; in both, fever, cough, tachypnea, and dyspnea are common; physical examination in both may disclose tachypnea, retractions, wheezes, and crackles; and blood counts and blood gas values also may be similar. The inspiratory crackles in asthma arise from closure of the small airways, which is due both to edema, mucus, and inflammation within the airways and to edema and inflammation in the interstitium. Therefore, **aggressive treatment of the asthma usually improves both the symptoms and the radiograph.**

Asthma is often difficult to distinguish from CF. The radiographic patterns and physical examinations are often similar. Normal growth and stool pattern mean only that the child does not have pancreatic insufficiency and do not rule out CF (see chapter 14).

Gastroesophageal reflux (GER) with or without aspiration and with or without a concomitant degree of airway reactivity may cause a similar clinical and radiographic picture. GER may be associated with severe asthma, even in adults. Airway inflammation as a result of **ciliary dyskinesia syndrome** or **IgG subclass deficiency** before bronchiectatic changes appear also may cause a similar radiographic pattern.

Less common forms of noninfectious **interstitial pneumonitis and fibrosis** with chronic or recurrent intestitial patterns include usual interstitial pneumonitis (UIP, e.g., cryptogenic fibrosing alveolitis, Hamman-Rich syndrome), desquamative interstitial pneumonitis (DIP), lymphocytic interstitial pneumonitis (LIP), and sarcoidosis, all of which are usually diagnosed by lung biopsy. These entities frequently worsen when the child has an intercurrent viral illness. LIP is frequently seen in children with AIDS. Although these entities, as well as **bronchiolitis obliterans**, may result from exposure to infections and toxins or may occur in a familial pattern, most of the time no etiology is found.

Pulmonary hemosiderosis must be suspected in infants with a pattern of diffuse lung disease and iron-deficiency anemia. Some children have a pattern of severe intermittent acute lung disease with diffuse infiltrates and severe anemia. In infants with pulmonary hemosiderosis in which milk allergy plays an etiologic role, serum precipitins to milk proteins are detected. Withdrawal of milk products from the diet may

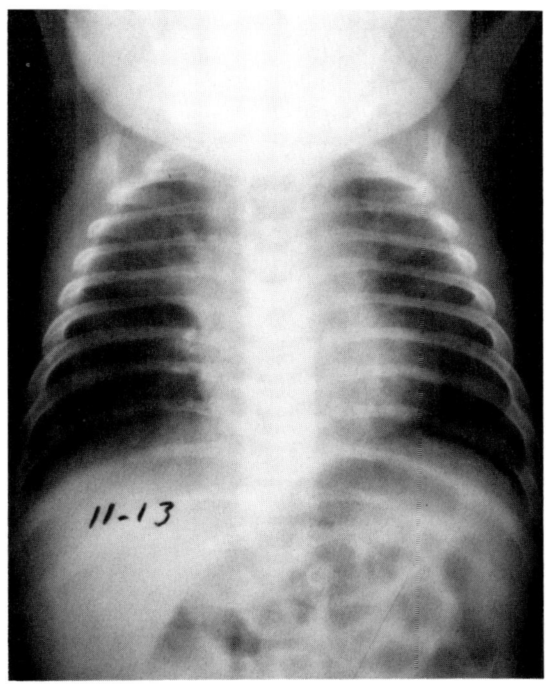

FIGURE 2. Chest radiograph (anteroposterior) shows bilateral, diffuse interstitial infiltration in a child with asthma.

reduce symptoms and normalize the radiograph and lung function in some children. In older children pulmonary hemosiderosis may occur in conjunction with collagen vascular disease. Wegener granulomatosis or Goodpasture syndrome often presents with renal involvement.

T-cell dysfunction, such as occurs in AIDS, DiGeorge syndrome, and chronic mucocutaneous candidiasis, results in recurrent infection with viruses, fungi, and organisms such as *Mycobacterium tuberculosis* and *Pneumocystis carinii.*

The **diagnostic approach** in patients with recurrent diffuse infiltrates starts with the history, evaluating for the possibility of asthma and CF, as discussed above. Recurrent sinusitis or severe otitis media may suggest ciliary dysfunction or IgG subclass deficiency. Nocturnal cough, chest pain, dyspepsia, or symptoms after meals suggest GER. Episodes of cutaneous candidiasis, unusual or prolonged viral infections, and serious varicella infections are clues to T-cell dysfunction. On physical examination, the presence of wheezes strongly suggests asthma but does not exclude CF.

Clubbing of the fingers excludes simple asthma and increases the likelihood of associated bronchiectasis, CF, or interstitial fibrosis. Pulmonary function tests are helpful if the child is old enough and able to cooperate. We have often done a trial of antiasthma therapy and assessed the clinical response. A sweat test is an important part of the evaluation. Other studies may be considered if the initial assessment does not suggest a simple answer or if the asthma proves difficult to control.

Practitioners often fixate on the diagnosis of pneumonia and downplay the asthma. This results in undertreatment of the asthma and furthers a vicious cycle. In evaluating a child with recurrent pneumonia, one first should consider asthma. If the history and physical or laboratory evidence suggest this diagnosis, the "pneumonias" were probably infiltrates due to mucus plugs. In that case, treating the asthma is more helpful to the patient than pondering which antibiotic to use.

SUGGESTED READING

1. Blazer S, Naveh Y, Friedman A: Foreign body in the airway: A review of 200 cases. Am J Dis Child 134:68–71, 1980.
2. Bye MR, Bernstein LJ: Identifying pulmonary sequelae in children with AIDS. J Respir Dis 10:27–39, 1989.
3. Eigen H, Laughlin JJ, Homrighausen J: Recurrent pneumonia in children and its relationship to bronchial hyperreactivity. Pediatrics 70:698–704, 1982.
4. Fan LL, Mullen ALW, Brugman SM, et al: Clinical spectrum of chronic interstitial lung disease in children. J Pediatr 121:867–872, 1992.
5. Landing BH, Dixon LG: Congenital malformations and genetic disorders of the respiratory tract. Am Rev Respir Dis 120:151, 1979.
6. Larsen GL: Asthma in children. N Engl J Med 326:1540–1545, 1992.
7. Orenstein SR, Orenstein DM: Gastroesophageal reflux and respiratory disease in children. J Pediatr 112:847–857, 1988.
8. Rubin BK: The evaluation of the child with recurrent chest infections. Pediatr Infect Dis J 4:88–98, 1985.
9. Turner JAP, Corkey CWB, Lee JYC, et al: Clinical expressions of immotile cilia syndrome. Pediatrics 67:805–810, 1981.
10. Wood RE, Boat TF, Doershuk CF: State of the art: Cystic fibrosis. Am Rev Respir Dis 113:833–878, 1976.

COMMENTARY

by Daniel V. Schidlow, M.D.

The reader is referred to chapter 11 on chronic cough for further information. As one would expect, the approaches to the child with persistent or recurrent abnormalities in the chest radiograph and to the child with chronic cough share many similarities.

In the experience of pediatric pulmonologists, asthma accounts for a significant share of the referrals for chronic respiratory symptoms and radiographic abnormalities of the chest. Cystic fibrosis is always in the differential diagnosis, because it is a relatively common disease with protean manifestations.

One useful observation about the respiratory manifestations of patients with gammaglobulin deficiency and immotile cilia syndrome is the conspicuous severity of the upper respiratory symptoms. Characteristically, discontinuation of antimicrobial therapy in such patients results in almost immediate recrudescence of purulent rhinorrhea and symptoms of sinus and middle-ear disease. Upper respiratory manifestations are frequently more bothersome to the patient than pulmonary manifestations and may require surgical intervention (e.g., tympanostomy, sinus surgery).

Although patients with seasonal or perennial rhinitis or asthma may present in a similar manner, our experience has been that prompt onset of severe upper respiratory symptoms after discontinuation of antibiotics is most characteristic of diseases in which local defenses are impaired.

For the work-up of patients with recurrent pneumonia, we obtain spirometries whenever possible and repeat abnormal tests after administration of bronchodilators. In addition, we frequently obtain sweat tests in such patients. Cultures of pharyngeal secretions or sputum can be useful if distinct pathogens are found. For instance, *Pseudomonas aeruginosa,* particularly the mucoid variety, is essentially pathognomonic of cystic fibrosis. Patients with decreased immunoglobulin levels harbor *Staphylococcus aureus,* nontypable *Hemophilus influenzae,* or even *P. aeruginosa* in their sputum, unlike patients with allergic disease or individuals with normal defense mechanisms. A complete blood cell count showing anemia, leukocytosis, or lymphopenia may steer the physician to the corresponding diagnosis (hemosiderosis, infection, or cellular immune deficiency, respectively).

A considerable portion of the work-up can be done in the physician's office with the aid of community-based resources. Referral to a specialist should be considered for children with atypical or severe symptoms and for those who do not respond to therapy.

18

TUBERCULOSIS

Charles W. Callahan, Jr., D.O. MAJ, MC, USA

Tuberculosis was a major cause of disease and death in children a mere hundred years ago. Since that time, the morbidity and mortality of tuberculosis have declined steadily in the United States. This decline has been especially dramatic over the past four decades with the availability of effective antibiotic therapy. However, the number of new cases of tuberculosis in children has increased over the past several years. This increase in the United States can be attributed to immigration of individuals with tuberculosis from developing countries and to the rising incidence of acquired immunodeficiency syndrome (AIDS).

THE TUBERCULOSIS ORGANISM AND INFECTION

The primary portal of entry for the bacillus *Mycobacterium tuberculosis* into children is the lungs; in more than 95% of cases, the primary lesion in a tuberculosis infection involves the lung parenchyma. **Children are never the primary source of a tuberculosis infection.** They are rarely, if ever, contagious to other children. Children develop the infection from adults with active, bacillus-eliminating lesions. Thus, whenever a child is diagnosed with tuberculosis, every effort should be made to identify the adult source. Transmission is by contact with respiratory droplets, which may dry and remain virulent for months.

The incubation period commonly lasts 1 month, but it may range from 2–10 weeks. Tuberculosis infection of the lung leads to a parenchymal lesion, lymphangitis, and regional lymph node involvement, which are known as the primary complex. Transient bacillemia often occurs with the initial infection. Hypersensitivity to the tuberculous organism develops within 2–10 weeks, thus the delay between primary infection and skin test postivity. **A positive skin test results from infection with tuberculosis, not from "exposure." Therefore, asymptomatic children who have positive skin tests should be considered infected and treated as such.**

As immunity develops, the primary parenchymal lesion is usually encapsulated and gradually disappears. Healed, calcified lesions, along with the affected nodes, are referred to as the Ghon complex. If immunity is delayed or suppressed, the center of the parenchymal lesion or regional lymph node may caseate, liquefy, and empty into the pleura or bronchi. Hematogenous spread to the meninges, bones, joints, or kidneys occurs most commonly during this period of caseation. Hematogenous spread occurs in 3% or less of affected children, usually within 6 months of primary infection. Chronic pulmonary tuberculosis occurs only rarely in childhood. It is seen more frequently in adolescents and represents reactivation of a quiescent, often inadequately treated previous infection.

CLINICAL SIGNS OF INFECTION

Most children do not develop clinical symptoms upon infection with tuberculosis. However, fever, anorexia, weight loss, cough, and sputum production may be present. The clinical presentation of a tuberculosis infection may range from a complete lack of symptoms with positive skin test to overwhelming meningitis. Physical examination may be normal. If lung disease is present, moist crackles may be heard over the affected segment of the lung. In these cases, lymphadenopathy and splenomegaly may be present.

Tuberculosis should be suspected and tested for in symptomatic children with hilar adenopathy as well as in children with pneumonia and infiltrate on chest radiograph (especially when they are unresponsive to antibiotics). However, hilar adenopathy in such children also may be caused by other bacterial pneumonias with adenopathy (*Pneumococcus, Hemophilus*), lymphoma, or histoplasmosis. Pulmonary tuberculosis also should be suspected in children with endobronchial disease and obstructive emphysema or atelectasis; pneumonia with pleural effusion; diffuse (miliary) pneumonia; and calcifications on the chest radiograph. Extrapulmonary tuberculosis is less common in children than in adults. However, it should be suspected in the child with painless cervical adenitis unresponsive to antibiotics; meningitis of insidious onset; and bone or joint disease that is unresponsive to antibiotic therapy (Table 1).

DIAGNOSIS

Smears and Cultures

Mycobacterium tuberculosis can be recovered from sputum smears in 50–80% of patients with primary tuberculosis. Preschool children and children with mild pulmonary disease are frequently unable to produce sputum. In such children, fasting gastric aspirates obtained on 3 successive mornings will recover organisms that have been swallowed in up to 60% of cases.The stomach should be lavaged with 20–60 ml of sterile water. Sterile water is preferred because nontuberculous or atypical *Mycobacterium* can be recovered from tap water in many areas of the United States. Older children and adolescents often are able to produce sputum after aerosol therapy and chest physiotherapy. In addition to rapid diagnosis with stains, such as the Ziehl-Nielsen, sputum or gastric aspirate may be cultured on Lowenstein-Jensen buffered egg-potato medium or the American Trudeau Society egg yolk–potato flour medium. Several additional agar-based media are also available. As with any infection, the diagnosis is based on the recovery of the organism; culture of the organism for confirmation may take as long as 10 weeks and thus may not be helpful in determining the initial treatment.

TABLE 1. When to Suspect Tuberculosis

Asymptomatic hilar adenopathy
Asymptomatic pulmonary calcification
Pneumonia with infiltrate and adenopathy, unresponsive to antibiotics
Endobronchitis with obstructive emphysema
Pneumonia with pleural effusion
Diffuse, nodular pneumonia
Painless, unilateral, cervical adenitis, unresponsive to antibiotics
Meningitis of insidious onset, unresponsive to antibiotics
Bone or joint disease unresponsive to antibiotics

Skin Test

Tuberculosis is diagnosed most often in children through the routine skin testing of individuals at risk. Skin testing for this disease has been available since 1907, when it was introduced by Mantoux and associates. Concentrated broth cultures of the tubercle organism are sterilized with heat to provide the material for multiple puncture devices (called old tuberculin [OT]). The Mantoux technique of intracutaneous injection uses the precipitate from these cultures, purified protein derivative (PPD). The standard test dose of 5 tuberculin units (TU) is based on the immunologic response expected for a given preparation compared with the standard 5-TU PPD-S established in 1939. (This concentration was formerly known as the "intermediate strength" preparation.) Additional unstandardized strengths are available, but they have few indications. Care must be taken in administering either the multiple puncture screening technique (i.e., Monovac, tine) or the intracutaneous Mantoux test. Errors in administration include inadequate pressure or duration with the tine test or accidental subcutaneous administration of the Mantoux injection. A correctly administered Mantoux injection should not result in a blister or bleeding. The needle is advanced, bevel up, until the opening disappears into the

TABLE 2. Reasons for False-negative Skin Tests

Testing during incubation period (2–10 weeks)
Problems with administration technique
Severe systemic tuberculosis infection (miliary or meningitis)
Anergy, immunosuppression, malnutrition, or immunodeficiency
Concurrent infection: measles, varicella, human immunodeficiency virus, Epstein-Barr virus, *Mycoplasma*, mumps, rubella
Recent viral immunization (measles)

TABLE 3. Reasons for False-positive Skin Tests

5–9 mm reaction to 5 TU PPD as result of atypical *Mycobacterium*
Sensitivity to test substance preservative
Incorrect administration technique
Previous immunization with bacille Calmette-Guérin (BCG) vaccine

skin, and the PPD is injected. Tests should be read in 48–72 hours by an experienced individual, not by a parent. Measurement of induration should be by touch, not by sight. Occasionally it may be useful to highlight the edges of the reaction with a ballpoint pen before measurement. **PPD should be used to confirm a positive multiple puncture screening test, except when vesiculation results from the original test.**

Interpretation of Skin Testing

Neither the multiple puncture test nor the Mantoux test has been found to be as sensitive (90–95%) as it is specific. In either case, false-negative and false-positive reactions have occurred (Tables 2 and 3). Atypical *Mycobacterium* (ATM) is sometimes the cause of a false-positive skin test. No commercial skin test is currently available for ATM. A skin reaction to ATM represents immunologic cross-reactivity and is usually smaller than 10 mm. If this reaction occurs in a child suspected of having tuberculosis, he or she should be treated for tuberculosis and retested in 4–6 weeks. A positive test for tuberculosis consists of induration, erythema, or vesiculation of varying degrees. Induration of 15 mm or more is considered positive in any child. Smaller reactions are also possible and may be considered positive in specific settings (e.g., in immune-deficient individuals such as those with human immunodeficiency virus [HIV]). The approach to reactions of different sizes is summarized in Table 4.

Indications for Skin Testing

In addition to their use for the diagnosis of tuberculosis infections in the acute setting, skin tests are used widely to screen persons at risk for infection. Routine yearly skin testing of children with no risk factors who live in low-prevalence areas is not indicated. High-risk groups include black, Hispanic, Asian, American Indian, Polynesian, and native Alaskan children. Children

TABLE 4. Interpretation and Response to a Positive Purified Protein Derivative (PPD) Test

Measurement	Population	Interpretation	Action
≥ 5 mm	Children with: Close contact with known tuberculosis infection Strong suspicion of tuberculosis infection Immunosuppression Human immunodeficiency virus infection Healed tuberculosis on chest radiograph (without treatment)	Positive	1. Treat 2. Evaluate contacts 3. Chest radiograph 4. Repeat PPD in 4–6 weeks
≥ 10 mm	Children with: Age less than four years Chronic disease or malnutrition Frequent exposure to high-risk adults Birth or parents born in high-risk region	Positive	1. Treat 2. Evaluate contacts 3. Chest radiograph 4. Repeat PPD 4–6 weeks
≥ 15 mm	Children ≥ 4 years without risk factors	Positive	1. Treat 2. Evaluate contacts 3. Chest radiograph

TABLE 5. Indications for Tuberculosis Screening

Children in high-risk groups yearly with Mantoux
Children in low-risk groups who reside in high prevalence areas (with Mantoux):
- At 12 months of age
- Before school entry at age 4–6 years
- During adolescence at age 11–16 years

Children in contact with tuberculous adult every 10–12 weeks
Children at the time of exposure to known contact with tuberculosis and 10 weeks later (if initial Mantoux is negative)

who are socioeconomically deprived, who live in areas with a high case rate of tuberculosis, or whose parents immigrated from high-risk areas (Asia, South Pacific, Africa, Middle East, Latin America, or Caribbean) are also at increased risk. Numerous specific guidelines are available to identify children who would benefit most from tuberculosis screening. Children should be screened with the Mantoux and not the multiple puncture test. Current recommendations are found in Table 5.

TREATMENT

Pharmacologic Agents

Treatment should be started in all cases of suspected tuberculosis even before the organism is identified or isolated. It is safer to treat than to wait. Several agents are available for the treatment of tuberculosis in children, including isoniazid, rifampin, ethambutol, streptomycin, and pyrazinamide. Commonly seen toxicities and routine screening procedures for children on therapy are summarized in Tables 6 and 7. Steroid use in pulmonary tuberculosis is controversial. Steroid therapy is generally reserved for children with pleural effusion, endobronchial obstruction, or meningitis.

Children with primary tuberculosis infection (usually pneumonia in the presence of a positive skin test) were traditionally treated with 2 or 3 drugs for up to 1 year or longer. Recently, several short-course and intermittent-dose regimens have been suggested for children, based largely on similar treatment in adults. The regimens generally use 2 or 3 drugs for 4–10 months on daily or weekly dosing schedules. Complete reviews of these regimens can be found in the references. A simple representative regimen is found in Table 8.

Short-course therapy (6 months) should not be used in (1) children who show toxicity to isoniazid or rifampin; (2) children with persistent positive cultures or resistant organisms; (3) children who show no clinical response to therapy; or (4) children who have underlying systemic disease, such as HIV or malignancy. Such children should receive 9–10 months of daily or twice weekly therapy with isoniazid or rifampin.

TABLE 6. Adverse Reactions to Tuberculosis Therapy

Agent	Common Reactions	Serious Reactions	Drug Interactions
Isoniazid	Gastrointestinal upset	Seizures Peripheral neuritis	Phenobarbital Phenytoin Carbamazepine
Rifampin	Orange secretions	Hepatotoxicity	Theophylline Adrenocorticoids Chloramphenicol Oral contraceptives Ketoconazole Fluconazole
Ethambutol		Retrobulbar neuritis Diminished visual acuity Color blindness	
Streptomycin	Pain at injection site	Hearing loss Vestibular dysfunction	
Pyrazinamide		Hepatotoxicity Hyperuricemia	

TABLE 7. Routine Screening of Tuberculosis Therapy

Agent	Screening Parameters	Additional Considerations
Isoniazid	Liver function tests:* Beginning of therapy Midpoint End	Give pyridoxine (10 mg per 100 mg of isoniazid) to children with milk- and meat-deficient diets as well as pregnant or lactating women
Rifampin	Liver function tests*	
Ethambutol	Check visual acuity and visual fields every month on therapy	Avoid use in children too young for visual testing
Streptomycin	Check hearing acuity: Beginning of therapy Midpoint End	Available only as intramuscular injection
Pyrazinamide	Liver function tests*	

* Children with liver disease or clinical hepatotoxicity, on high-dose isoniazid with rifampin, or with disseminated disease.

Children whose symptoms have improved on therapy may be considered noncontagious.

Children known to have had treated tuberculosis should receive prophylaxis with isoniazid for 8 weeks after measles infection or vaccination, during prolonged therapy with corticosteroids, and during surgery with anesthesia. They should also receive prophylaxis for 8 weeks after pertussis infection. A complete summary of dosing regimens for long and short courses of the commonly used agents is found in Table 9.

Additional agents are available for the therapy of tuberculosis in specific clinical situations. Indications for their use, precautions, dosing regimens, and duration of therapy are available in the references provided at the end of this chapter. Practitioners should be aware of the pattern of tuberculosis resistance in their area. Treatment should be adjusted accordingly. The local public health department can usually provide information regarding tuberculosis resistance.

SPECIFIC CLINICAL SITUATIONS

Tuberculosis is not a common disease in children. But the practitioner may be confronted by specific clinical situations in the evaluation and management of tuberculosis infections. Physicians caring for children should be familiar with the approach to a child with a positive or borderline tine or PPD test result, a child with tuberculosis exposure, and the infant born to a mother with tuberculosis infection or skin-test positivity. Tables 10–13 summarize the clinical approach to each of these patients. An approach to a positive multiple puncture test or tine test is presented, although it is likely that these will be replaced entirely by the Mantoux test in the future.

Additional issues often must be considered in the care of newborns whose mothers have tuberculosis or skin-test positivity. Pregnant women with tuberculosis or a positive skin test should be treated aggressively by a practitioner with expertise in the care of tuberculosis. The risk to the fetus from the use of therapeutic agents is minimal. Congenital tuberculosis, although extremely rare, is possible in infants born to women with hematogenous tuberculosis infection. Such infants should be evaluated and begun on isoniazid, rifampin, streptomycin, and pyrazinamide until serial skin tests and chest radiographs prove or disprove the presence of disease. Isoniazid is transferred to breast-milk,

TABLE 8. Suggested Therapy for Pulmonary Tuberculosis in Children

1. Isoniazid (10 mg/kg/day)
   Rifampin (10 mg/kg/day)
   Pyrazinamide (20 mg/kg/day)
2. Treat daily for 8 weeks
3. After 8 weeks:
   Isoniazid (20 mg/kg/day)
   Rifampin (20 mg/kg/day)
   Given twice weekly
4. Treat for a total of 6 months

TABLE 9. Doses in Tuberculosis Therapy

Agent	Daily Short Course (dose per 24 hours)	Weekly Short Course (dose given twice weekly)	Standard Course
Isoniazid*	10–15 mg/kg (max: 300 mg)	20–40 mg/kg (max: 900 mg)	10–20 mg/kg (max: 300 mg)
Rifampin*	10–20 mg/kg (max: 600 mg)	10–20 mg/kg (max: 600 mg)	15–20 mg/kg (max: 600 mg)
Ethambutol	15–25 mg/kg (max: 1500 mg)	50 mg/kg	15–20 mg/kg (max: 2500 mg)
Streptomycin	20–40 mg/kg (max: 1000 mg)	20–40 mg/kg	20–40 mg/kg (max: 1000 mg)
Pyrazinamide	20–40 mg/kg (max: 2 gm)	50–70 mg/kg	20–30 mg/kg (max: 2000 mg)

* When isoniazid and rifampin are used together, no more than 10 mg/kg isoniazid and 15 mg/kg rifampin should be used.
max = maximal dose.

but no adverse effect on infants has been identified. Treatment with this agent is not a contraindication to breast-feeding.

PREVENTION

In many countries, children receive the bacille Calmette-Guérin (BCG) vaccine for protection against tuberculosis. The vaccine is made from an attentuated strain of *Mycobacterium bovis.*

TABLE 10. Child with Exposure to Tuberculosis

1. Obtain PPD and chest radiograph.
2. Begin prophylaxis with isoniazid (10 mg/kg/day).
3. Repeat PPD at 10 weeks:
   If PPD is negative, stop therapy.
   If PPD is positive, treat with isoniazid for 9–10 months total.

PPD = purified protein derivative test.

TABLE 11. Child with Positive Tine Test (Tuberculosis "Converter")

1. Place PPD to confirm positivity.
2. Obtain chest radiograph.
3. Begin prophylaxis with isoniazid (10 mg/kg/day).
4. Search contacts for evidence of disease.
5. Protect against concurrent illness.
6. Repeat PPD at 10 weeks:
   If PPD is negative, stop therapy.
   If PPD is positive, treat with isoniazid for 9–10 months.

PPD = purified protein derivative test.

In the United States, the vaccine has not been widely used, and no consistent efficacy against tuberculosis infection has been demonstrated. The BCG vaccine does not seem to be effective in preventing infection, but rather it appears to prevent severe primary disease and hematogenous spread of disease in children who contract tuberculosis.

Vaccination against tuberculosis should be considered for infants and children who live in households in which compliance is questionable and continued contact with infectious adults is likely. It should also be considered for children in groups at high risk for tuberculosis exposure, such as first-generation immigrants from Asia, Central and South America, American Indians, and Alaskan natives. Children who have been adopted from these areas should be examined for evidence of BCG vaccination: a small 1-cm square scar on either shoulder. Children who have been recently vaccinated may develop mild ulceration at the site or regional lymphadenitis.

The vaccination should not be given to children who are immunocompromised (such as those with HIV) or to children on immunosuppressive therapy (such as prolonged therapy with corticosteroids).

The greatest disadvantage to the use of BCG vaccine is that the resulting skin test reaction is difficult to distinguish from that of a tuberculosis infection. Once a child is immunized, skin-test positivity usually occurs by about 10 weeks but rarely remains beyond 10 years. There is no reason for routine skin tests of children

TABLE 12. Child with Borderline Positive Tine Test

1. Place PPD to confirm positivity.
2. If still borderline, treat children at risk as "converters" (children with human immunodeficiency virus, immunosuppression, close contact with tuberculosis) (see Table 11).
3. Obtain chest radiograph.
4. Repeat PPD at 10 weeks:'
   - If PPD is negative, stop therapy.
   - If PPD is borderline:
     - Treat children at risk with isoniazid for a total of 10 months and
     - Continue observation and serially repeat skin test.
   - If PPD is positive, treat with isoniazid for 9–10 months.

PPD = purified protein derivative test.

who have been vaccinated; however, concern about a mild dermatologic reaction should not prevent testing in the face of possible primary infection. A skin reaction that is larger than 15 mm is not likely to be due to BCG vaccination and probably represents infection. Children who have been vaccinated and who are thought to have had significant tuberculosis exposure should have skin testing and a chest radiograph. If the test is positive in the face of significant risk, the child should be treated as a "converter" for a full course of therapy.

The best means of preventing tuberculosis is by identifying and treating source cases. **All cases of active tuberculosis should be referred to the public health authorities.**

SUMMARY

The primary means of preventing tuberculosis is through the early identification and evaluation of children with exposure to the organism. Prompt initiation of therapy with isoniazid and close monitoring for compliance to the suggested treatment regimens probably have had a significant impact on the incidence of tuberculosis in children in the United States.

Ironically, the same effective public health measures that have made tuberculosis a rare disease in most parts of the United States also may contribute to the physician's low threshold of suspicion. Children who become ill with tuberculosis more often suffer from the lack of efficient recognition and delayed diagnosis than the lack of effective treatment. Physicians who care for children should suspect tuberculosis in the appropriate setting, thoroughly test for it, and be prepared to initiate aggressive treatment.

TABLE 13. Tuberculosis and the Newborn Infant

1. Mother with positive skin test and no disease:
   - Place PPD on newborn at 4–6 weeks and 3–4 months of age.
   - If PPD is positive, treat with isoniazid, 10 mg/kg/day for 9–10 months.
2. Mother with positive skin test and untreated tuberculosis who is felt to be noncontagious:
   - Treat newborn with isoniazid, 10 mg/kg/day. (Discontinue if PPD is negative at 3–4 months of age and if no active disease exists in family members.)
   - Obtain chest radiograph at birth, 4–6 weeks, 3–4 months, and 6 months of age.
   - Place PPD on newborn at birth, 4–6 weeks, 3–4 months, and 6 months of age.
   - Use bacille Calmette-Guérin vaccine (if PPD is negative and continued exposure to tuberculosis is likely).
3. Mother with active or hematogenous tuberculosis who is suspected to be contagious:
   - Separate newborn from mother until she is noncontagious.
   - Treat newborn with isoniazid, and manage as minimal disease when mother is considered noncontagious.
   - Use bacille Calmette-Guérin vaccine (if PPD is negative and continued exposure to tuberculosis is likely).

PPD = purified protein derivative test.

The views expressed by the author should not be construed as official or as reflecting the views of the United States Army or the Department of Defense.

SUGGESTED READING

1. Committee on Infectious Diseases, American Academy of Pediatrics: Screening for tuberculosis in infants and children. Pediatrics 93:131–134, 1994.
2. Diagnostic standards and classification of tuberculosis: Official statement of the American Lung Association. Am Rev Respir Dis 142:725–735, 1990.
3. Inselman LS, Kendig EL: Tuberculosis. In Chernick V (ed): Kendig's Disorders of the Respiratory Tract in Children, 5th ed. Philadelphia, W.B. Saunders, 1990, pp 731–769.
4. Starke JR, Jacobs RF, Jereb J: Resurgence of tuberculosis in children. J Pediatr 120:839–855, 1992.
5. Peter G, Lepow ML, McCracken G, Phillips CF (eds): Report of the Committee on Infectious Disease ("Redbook"), 22nd ed. Elk Grove, IL, American Academy of Pediatrics, 1991, pp 487–508.

19

PLEURAL EFFUSIONS

Caitlin Papastamelos, M.D.

The first step in management of a pleural effusion is to detect its presence. Although symptoms are nonspecific, the physical examination is characteristic. The diagnosis usually can be confirmed by chest radiographs with upright or decubitus views. Once an effusion is diagnosed, the next step is to obtain pleural fluid for laboratory analysis and to determine the cause of the effusion. Treatment entails management of the underlying disease and may also involve drainage of the fluid. Most of this chapter focuses on effusions associated with bacterial pneumonia, which are the most common effusions in children.

Normally, only a few mililiters of fluid are present in the pleural space. Pleural fluid accumulates when excessive fluid leaks from the pleural surfaces or when reabsorption of fluid by the pleural surfaces or lymphatics is ineffective. Ineffective reabsorption occurs when pleural surfaces are inflamed or infected or when lymphatic channels are obstructed by tumor, lymph nodes, or inflammation. Increased hydrostatic or decreased oncotic pressures, such as in congestive heart failure or nephrotic syndrome, also cause accumulation of pleural fluid. Blood and chyle also may fill the pleural space in certain situations, and ascitic fluid or peritoneal dialysate can enter the pleural cavity through small diaphragmatic defects.

DETECTING THE PRESENCE OF A PLEURAL EFFUSION

The symptoms of a pleural effusion are nonspecific. The patient's most prominent symptoms usually are caused by the underlying disease, such as pneumonia, which results in fever, cough, and tachypnea. Large effusions cause dyspnea, dry cough, and orthopnea due to lung compression, but small effusions may be asymptomatic. Symptoms of pleural inflammation include chest pain and ipsilateral shoulder pain, which worsen with deep inspiration or cough.

The physical examination is characterized by decreased breath sounds over the effusion, dullness to percussion, decreased tactile fremitus, and voice egophony (a-to-e changes). Again, small effusions may be difficult to detect.

Every child in whom a pleural effusion is suspected should have a chest radiograph, with bilateral decubitus or upright views. On supine films, effusions cause haziness of an entire hemithorax, with a "pleural stripe" that represents fluid lying between the lung and chest wall (see Fig. 5, chapter 37). Radiographs in the upright position reveal effusions that cause blunting of the costophrenic angles or elevation and lateral displacement of the apex of the dome of the diaphragm (Fig. 1). A distance of more than 2 cm between the gastric bubble and the left lung is another sign of an effusion. On lateral decubitus views, free pleural fluid "layers out," shifting to the dependent aspect of the thoracic cavity (Fig. 2). Loculated fluid and pleural thickening fail to layer out on decubitus views (Fig. 3). Decubitus views also may reveal small effusions that are concealed behind the diaphragmatic shadow on upright views. Similarly, underlying lung and mediastinal abnormalities, such as pneumonia and tumor, may become apparent on decubitus views as fluid shifts away.

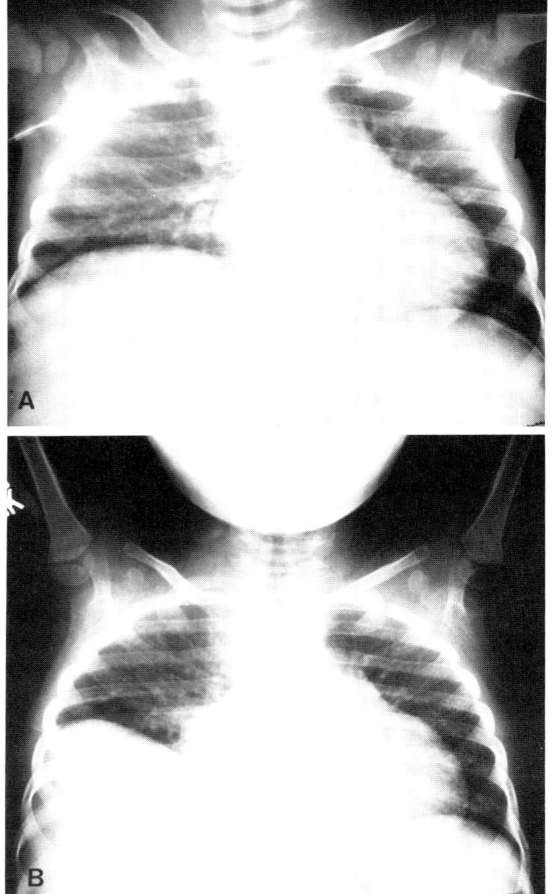

FIGURE 1. *A,* Chest radiograph of a child in upright position shortly after liver transplantation. *B,* A repeat film 1 week later revealed a right pleural effusion, evidenced by upward and lateral displacement of the right hemidiaphragm. The patient at this time had developed ascites due to rejection of the transplanted liver, and the pleural effusion was presumed to be secondary to ascitic fluid traversing the diaphragm.

At times effusions may be difficult to distinguish from various other entities of the chest radiograph, such as pleural thickening, parenchymal consolidation, lung abscess, adenopathy, and tumor. The most frequent problem is distinguishing loculated fluid from thickening of the pleural membrane, because both appear on the radiograph as pleural densities that do not change position on decubitus views. Ultrasound imaging of the chest is the easiest and least expensive means of differentiating loculated fluid from pleural peel and also provides guidance for percutaneous placement of drainage tubes (Fig. 4). Computed tomography (CT) is the diagnostic study of choice when the chest radiograph suggests intraparenchymal or mediastinal abnormalities that require further treatment, such as lung abscess, mediastinal mass, or adenopathy. CT of the chest also should be obtained in any patient with a hemothorax, chylothorax, or lymphocytic effusion of unclear etiology, because adenopathy or masses due to malignancy and tuberculosis are potential causes.

OBTAINING THE PLEURAL FLUID

Diagnostic thoracentesis should be performed in every patient with an effusion. Exceptions to this rule are effusions in patients with diseases known to cause transudative effusions, such as congestive heart failure, nephrotic syndrome, or ascites, or in patients beginning peritoneal dialysis, as long as the patients are afebrile and only minimally symptomatic. In addition, small effusions associated with known, uncomplicated viral or mycoplasmal infection need not be sampled.

Thoracentesis can be safely performed when the thickness of the effusion's layering-out on decubitus views is at least 1 cm. Thoracentesis is used to obtain fluid for diagnostic studies and also may be therapeutic if fluid removal allows lung reexpansion. The procedure is discussed in chapter 38.

When the clinical presentation is consistent with parapneumonic effusion (i.e., acute onset of fever and cough, parenchymal infiltrate), it is advantageous to place a thoracostomy tube before performing thoracentesis. Tube placement is both diagnostic and therapeutic in cases of parapneumonic effusion, and a superfluous thoracentesis can be avoided (see below).

DIAGNOSING THE CAUSE

Once pleural fluid is obtained, its appearance and the results of laboratory studies provide clues to the diagnosis.

Appearance. If the effusion consists of pus, it is nearly always a parapneumonic effusion. Purulent fluid that is also sanguinous is typical of empyema due to Group A *Streptococcus. Staphylococcus aureus* usually produces

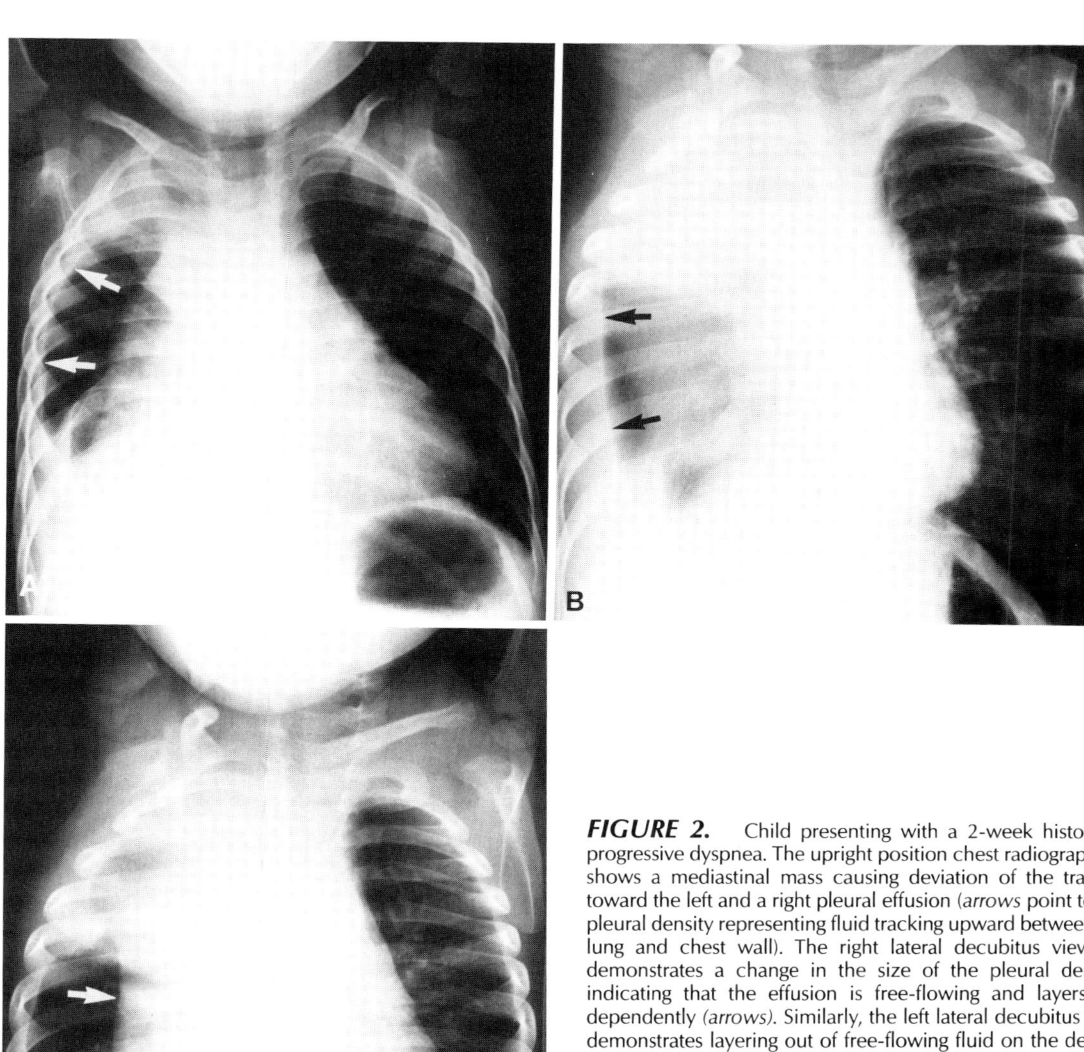

FIGURE 2. Child presenting with a 2-week history of progressive dyspnea. The upright position chest radiograph *(A)* shows a mediastinal mass causing deviation of the trachea toward the left and a right pleural effusion (*arrows* point to the pleural density representing fluid tracking upward between the lung and chest wall). The right lateral decubitus view *(B)* demonstrates a change in the size of the pleural density, indicating that the effusion is free-flowing and layers out dependently *(arrows)*. Similarly, the left lateral decubitus view demonstrates layering out of free-flowing fluid on the dependent or mediastinal surface *(arrows)*. Analysis of pleural fluid revealed blast cells consistent with non-Hodgkin lymphoma.

extremely thick, tan or brown purulent effusions, and anaerobic infections result in effusions with a putrid odor. Milky fluid is consistent with chylothorax, although chylothoraces may appear bloody or even serous, so that the diagnosis must be confirmed by assessment of the triglyceride level in the pleural fluid. Hemothorax is present if bloody fluid has a hematocrit of more than half the blood hematocrit. Bloody effusions that do not qualify as hemothoraces usually are caused by Group A streptococcal empyema, malignancy, tuberculosis, uremia, or traumatic thoracentesis (Table 1).

Laboratory Studies. Laboratory studies, which are nearly always required to confirm the diagnosis, should include the battery of

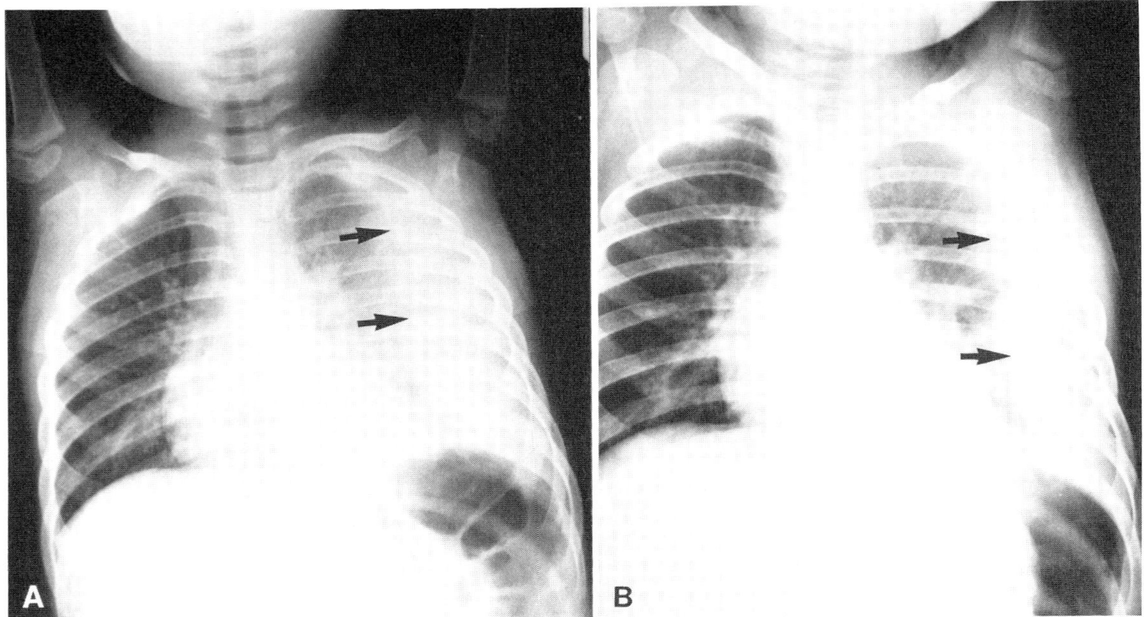

FIGURE 3. Upright *(A)* and right lateral decubitus *(B)* chest radiographs in a patient with persistent fever, tachynea, and chest pain after 7 days of intravenous antibiotics. The left pleural density *(arrow)* does not change in position or location on either view, suggesting loculated fluid or pleural thickening.

tests listed in Table 2. Table 3 lists situations in which additional studies are indicated.

Steps to Making the Diagnosis. In many cases, the appearance of the fluid suggests the diagnosis, which is then confirmed by checking a few of the laboratory results (Table 4). If the diagnosis is not obvious, the laboratory results must be used to categorize the effusion and to narrow the possible diagnoses. **The first categorization to make is whether the effusion is a transudate or an exudate;** this distinction is based on the lactate dehydrogenase and protein levels of the pleural fluid (Table 5). There are only a few causes of transudative effusions in children, all of which are easy to diagnose clinically. If the effusion is an exudate, the number of potential diagnoses is considerably greater, but by far the most common are effusions associated with bacterial pneumonia, followed by those due to malignancy and trauma. Therefore, the most practical first step is to

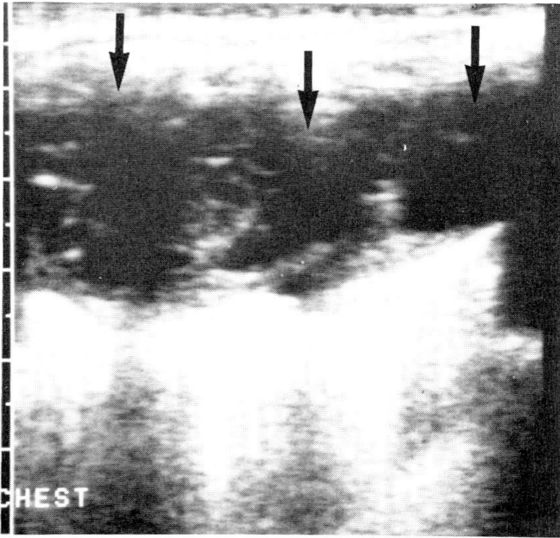

FIGURE 4. Ultrasound of the chest defined several large areas of fluid and debris *(arrows)* consistent with loculated pus. The ultrasound provided guidance for placement of thoracotomy tubes.

TABLE 1. Clues That the Thoracentesis is Traumatic

The fluid clots when blood is introduced during a traumatic tap.
The bloody tinge is not uniform during aspiration of the fluid.
Hemosiderin-laden macrophages are not present unless blood was present in the pleural space for several hours.

TABLE 2. Laboratory Studies to be Obtained in All Cases

Pleural fluid	Protein
	Lactate dehydrogenase
	Bacterial culture and Gram stain
	Glucose
	pH*
	Differential cell count
	Red blood cell count
	Amylase
Serum	Complete blood cell count with differential
	Lactate dehydrogenase
	Total protein
	Glucose

* Use heparinized syringe; pH obtained with blood gas machine.

analyze the cell count of the pleural fluid to determine if the effusion is purulent. Greater than 5,000 leukocytes/μl indicates a purulent effusion and makes the diagnosis of parapneumonic effusion almost certain, because other causes of purulent effusions are rare in children (see below).

If the effusion is not purulent, one should next determine whether the fluid has a lymphocytic predominance. Lymphocytic effusions are due most often to malignancies involving the pleural lymphatics (particularly lymphoma), followed in frequency by uremia and tuberculosis. Another fairly common type of effusion in children is chylothorax, which usually appears milky and has a triglyceride level of at least 50 mg/dl. Hemothorax is confirmed when a bloody effusion has a hematocrit value half that of the blood. Other types of effusions in children are much less common, such as those with a monocytic or eosinophilic predominance and an elevated amylase level. The following sections discuss the causes of different types of effusions, focusing on the most common entities, particularly parapneumonic effusions.

TRANSUDATIVE EFFUSIONS

Transudates form because of disruption of the normal balance of oncotic and hydrostatic pressures governing the accumulation of pleural fluid, as in congestive heart failure or nephrotic syndrome. The formation of a transudate may be just one manifestation of widespread physiologic alterations originating outside the pleural space. Because there is no active inflammatory

TABLE 3. Additional Studies to Be Obtained in Specific Cases

Condition	Additional Studies	Comment
Purulent fluid	Blood culture	
	Nasopharyngeal culture	
Bloody fluid	Effusion hematocrit	If hematocrit >50% of serum value, effusion is a hemothorax
	Pleural fluid for hemosiderin-laden macrophages	Absent if blood in effusion is due to traumatic thoracentesis
	Effusion triglyceride level	Chylous fluid may appear bloody
Lymphocytic effusions	Effusion triglyceride level	Chyle contains a predominance of lymphocytes
	Cytology	Causes of lymphocytic effusions include malignancy, tuberculosis, fungal infection, rheumatoid arthritis, and systemic lupus erythematosus
	Pleural fluid examination and culture for acid-fast bacilli and fungi	
	Tuberculin skin test	
	Consider: pleural and serum antinuclear antibody, rheumatoid factor, and complement	
	Consider fungal titers and skin tests	
Eosinophilic effusions	Effusion bacterial and viral culture	Parapneumonic effusions and viral effusions are occasionally eosinophilic
	Consider examination of fluid for ova and scolices	Paragonomiasis and echinococcus are rare in North America
Effusions with milky appearance	Triglyceride level	

TABLE 4. Most Common Causes of Effusions in Children

Etiology	Transudate vs. Exudate
Parapneumonic effusions	Exudate
Malignancy (especially lymphoma)	Exudate
Nephrotic syndrome	Transudate
Congestive heart failure	Transudate
Uremia	Exudate
Trauma (hemothorax)	Exudate
Chylothorax (neonatal)	Exudate
Tuberculosis	Exudate

process, the protein content of the transudative fluid remains low.

The causes of transudates in children are listed in Table 6. In most cases, the underlying cause is not difficult to determine. Treatment should be directed at the underlying disease. Drainage of transudative effusions is required only when the effusion is large and causes respiratory distress. Reaccumulations of fluid may occur until the underlying disease is controlled.

EXUDATIVE EFFUSIONS

Exudative effusions result from diseases that directly involve the pleural surfaces or lymphatic system (see Table 5).

Purulent Effusions

Purulent effusions contain >5,000 leukocytes/μl with a neutrophilic predominance, although the number of lymphocytes increases after several days. Effusions that have remained undrained for a few weeks may appear purulent, but the cell count is lower than expected because of cell lysis. Parapneumonic effusions are by far the most common cause of purulent effusions in children.

Parapneumonic Effusions

Parapneumonic effusions result when inflammation or infection from bacterial pneumonia spreads to the pleural space. Much less commonly, infections of the retropharyngeal, vertebral, abdominal, and retroperitoneal spaces may spread to the pleurae.

Early in the course of a parapneumonic effusion, the pleurae become inflamed because of adjacent pneumonia, and sympathetic effusion forms as protein, fluid, and leukocytes leak into the pleural space. At this point, the pleural space is free of infection, and Gram stain and culture of the effusion are negative. With time, bacteria invade the pleural space. Leukocytes pour into the effusion, fibrin is deposited, loculations form, and the pleural membranes become covered with a thick layer of inflammatory exudate. The infection and intense inflammation

TABLE 5. Categories of Effusions

Type of Effusion	Appearance	Pleural Fluid Characteristics
Exudates		Fulfills at least one of the following: Pleural fluid : serum lactate dehydrogenase >0.6 Pleural fluid : serum protein >0.5 Pleural fluid lactate dehydrogenase >2/3 upper limit of normal serum value
Purulent	Serous, turbid, or pus	>5,000 leukocytes/μl, predominance of neutrophils
Lymphocytic	Serous, turbid	1,500–5,000 leukocytes/μl with >50% lymphocytes
Chylothorax	Milky	Triglyceride >110 mg/dl confirms <50 mg/dl rules out 50–110 mg/dl questionable
Hemothorax	Bloody	Hematocrit >½ blood hematocrit
Monocytic	Serous	<5,000 leukocytes/μl, monocytic predominance
Eosinophilic	Serous	<5,000 leukocytes/μl, >10% eosinophils
Elevated amylase	Serous-purulent	Pleural fluid amylase >100 mg/dl
Transudates	Serous	Fulfills none of the lactate dehydrogenase and protein criteria of exudates (above)

TABLE 6. Causes of Transudates in Children

Nephrotic syndrome
Congestive heart failure
Ascites
Peritoneal dialysis
Upper airway obstruction
Atelectasis

of the pleural space are reflected by isolation of the organism on Gram stain and culture, an increase in the effusion leukocyte count and lactate dehydrogenase (LDH) level, a decrease in the glucose level to <60 mg/dl, and a decrease in pH to <7.3. The glucose, pH, LDH, and Gram stain may remain normal for many hours after infection of the pleural space has occurred, particularly if the infection is partially treated with oral antibiotics.

Clinical Presentation. Patients with parapneumonic effusion present with the symptoms of the underlying pneumonia: fever, cough, and chest pain. Approximately 70% of parapneumonic effusions occur in children less than 2 years old, who typically present with abrupt onset of fever and progressive respiratory distress. Older children usually have a history of a preceding viral respiratory infection. In general, children with effusions due to anaerobic infections are neurologically impaired; they aspirate chronically and frequently present with a more indolent course.

Causative Organisms. The organisms responsible for parapneumonic effusions are also the most frequent causes of pneumonia and sepsis (Table 7). The prevalence of particular organisms varies with age and underlying medical problems, but no one organism is

TABLE 7. Organisms Causing Parapneumonic Effusions in Children

Organism	Peak Age	Effusion Appearance	Associated Conditions	Course	Duration of Antibiotic Treatment
S. aureus	<1 yr, but prevalent throughout childhood	Thick, tan or brown	Skin infection, postthoracotomy	Severe, complicated by pneumatoceles, bronchopleural fistulas, lung abscess, hydropneumothorax	Minimum of 3 wk intravenously, then 2–3 wk orally
Pneumococcus	6–24 mo, but prevalent throughout childhood			Usually not severe or complicated	Minimum 10 days intravenously, then 1–2 wk orally
H. influenzae	6–24 mo, not after age 7 yr		Meningitis, arthritis, pericarditis	Impressive systemic illness, but empyema usually not complicated	Same as for pneumococcal infection
Group A *Streptococcus*	School age	Serosanguinous or bloody	Pharyngitis, impetigo, after varicella or rubeola infection	Bronchopneumonia on chest radiograph Effusions loculate rapidly Prolonged systemic symptoms: fever, chest pain, myalgia	Minimum of 3 wk intravenously, then 1–2 wk orally
Anaerobes	Usually older than 2 yr	Putrid odor	Neurologic impairment, aspiration, foreign body aspiration, dental work, poor dental hygiene	Complicated course: loculations, bronchopleural fistulas, lung abscesses	Minimum 3–4 wk intravenously, then 1–3 wk orally
Gram-negative enterics	Variable		Hospitalized patients	Underlying diseases and antibiotic resistance predispose to severe course	Minimum 3–4 wk intravenously

responsible for more than 20% of all cases of parapneumonic effusion. The prevalence of organisms causing parapneumonic effusion differs from that of organisms causing uncomplicated bacterial pneumonia. Whereas *S. aureus*, Group A *Streptococcus*, and anaerobes account for a relatively small percentage of childhood pneumonias overall, they account for a considerable portion of empyemas, because of their predilection to result in effusions and other complications. *Pneumococcus*, on the other hand, accounts for the large majority of childhood pneumonias, but only a small proportion of children with pneumococcal pneumonia develop empyema. *S. aureus* is the primary cause of parapneumonic effusions in infants less than 1 year of age. After infancy, empyema due to *Staphylococcus* is less prevalent, but it remains a major entity throughout childhood. *Hemophilus influenzae* causes effusions in infants after 2 months of age, with a peak incidence at 6–12 months. The incidence decreases thereafter; effusions due to *H. influenzae* are unusual after 2 years of age and rare after 7 years. *Pneumococcus* also occurs in infants as young as 2 months old, reaches its peak incidence in infants from 6–12 months of age, and remains a common cause of parapneumonic effusions thereafter, along with *S. aureus* and anaerobes. Empyema due to Group A *Streptococcus* is unusual and occurs most often in school-age children. Anaerobic empyema is usually multibacterial, typically due to anaerobic streptococci, pneumococci, gram-negative anaerobes (e.g., *Bacteroides* sp., especially *B. fragilis*, and *Fusobacterium* sp.), and *Actinomyces* sp. Anaerobic infection usually occurs outside infancy, when dentition allows a higher yield of anaerobes in the mouth and foreign body aspiration is more likely. Anaerobic organisms, gram-negative enteric organisms, and staphylococci are usually responsible for empyema in the hospitalized patient, which most frequently is due to aspiration.

S. aureus should be suspected as the cause of empyema at any age, but especially when the patient is less than 1 year old, the fluid is extremely thick and tan or brown in color, and the course is severe and complicated by loculated fluid, bronchopleural fistula, pneumatocele, lung abscess, or pneumothorax. This organism results in a large amount of tissue necrosis, producing thick pleural fluid that often requires weeks of drainage to resolve the infection.

Group A *Streptococcus* should be suspected when a child older than 2 years develops empyema after impetigo, varicella, rubeola, or pharyngitis, or when empyema fluid is serosanguinous and loculated early in the clinical course. Also typical of empyema due to Group A *Streptococcus* is a prolonged course of prominent systemic symptoms, characterized by up to 2 weeks of fever, myalgia, and chest pain despite adequate treatment.

The typical patient with empyema due to ***H. influenzae*** is an older infant who presents with abrupt onset of high fever, rigors, and ill appearance and may have extrapulmonary sites of infection, such as meningitis. In contrast to the severe systemic illness caused by *H. influenzae*, local pleural and lung involvement is less severe compared with infection by *Staphylococcus* or Group A *Streptococcus*; loculated fluid and pneumatoceles occur less often. Pneumothoraces occur occasionally.

Pneumococcal empyema is usually not associated with systemic illness as severe as that caused by the organism mentioned above. As with *H. influenzae*, effusions are usually not loculated or complicated.

Anaerobic infection should be suspected when the course is indolent, with up to several weeks of progressively worsening respiratory symptoms and fever before presentation. Anaerobes are also likely when the effusion has a putrid odor; complications may include bronchopleural fistulas, lung abscess, and drainage through the chest wall (empyema necessitans) if *Actinomyces* sp. are involved. Effusions are nearly always loculated by the time the patient presents. Factors in the history that support anaerobic infection are neurologic impairment, aspiration (including foreign body aspiration), poor dental hygiene, recent dental procedures, and chronic nasal congestion with possible aspiration of nasopharyngeal contents during sleep. Polymicrobial infection is common and may be associated with a longer course of illness.

Hospital-related parapneumonic effusions are usually associated with aspiration. In addition, the organisms commonly responsible for anaerobic empyema, gram-negative enteric organisms, and *S. aureus* must be considered.

Culture of secretions obtained from an endotracheal tube or bronchoalveolar lavage help to determine the etiology.

The causative organism is isolated in pleural fluid or blood in approximately three-fourths of cases of empyema. The causative organism is not usually isolated when cultures are obtained after even a few doses of an oral antibiotic. Improper handling of specimens for anaerobic culture frequently results in false-negative results; thus the diagnosis of anaerobic empyema is often based on clinical criteria alone. Nasopharyngeal cultures can be misleading, as *Pneumococcus* and *S. aureus* can be commensal organisms. Similarly, isolation of Group A *Streptococcus* on pharyngeal culture is supportive but not diagnostic. Culture of bronchoalveolar lavage fluid adds nothing to results of pleural fluid culture.

Treatment: Antibiotics and Drainage. Choice of an orally administered antibiotic is determined by the organisms likely to be responsible, the age of the patient, and the clinical presentation. Empyema in infants less than 2 months of age is most likely due to *S. aureus,* but coverage for Group B *Streptococcus, Escherichia coli,* and *Listeria* sp. should also be provided. The combination of nafcillin, ampicillin, and gentamicin is an effective initial regimen. From 2 months to 1 year of age cefuroxime plus nafcillin is a good initial choice to provide coverage for *Staphylococcus* as well as beta-lactamase-positive *Pneumococcus* and *H. influenzae.* Children from 1–7 years old may be treated with cefuroxime alone, because staphylococcal infections are less prevalent, and children over 7 years old may be treated with ampicillin alone, because *H. influenzae* is rare. Nafcillin should be added if the presentation is suggestive of *S. aureus* infection (see above) or if gram-positive cocci in clusters are noted on the Gram stain of the effusion.

When the presentation suggests anaerobic infection, clindamycin, ticarcillin-clavulanate, ampicillin-sulbactam, or cefoxitin is a good choice. In situations in which the clinical presentation has characteristics of both anaerobic and aerobic infection—for instance, when a patient with chronic aspiration presents with empyema after a viral respiratory infection or experiences abrupt onset of fever—regimens that provide coverage for both types of infection include ticarcillin-clavulanate and ampicillin-sulbactam.

The presence of a lung abscess suggests infection due to *Staphylococcus* or anaerobic bacteria; thus clindamycin is appropriate. The presence of positive branching filaments on Gram stain is indicative of infection due to *Actinomyces* sp.; clindamycin, ampicillin, or penicillin should be part of the antibiotic regimen, which is given intravenously for at least 4–6 weeks and followed by 6–8 months of oral penicillin. Hospital-associated empyema can be treated with ticarcillin-clavulanate, ampicillin-sulbactam, or cefoxitin. Prior respiratory culture results, a high prevalence of multiresistant gram-negative organisms or methicillin-resistant *Staphylococcus,* or a morbidly ill patient suggests empirical treatment with ceftazidime or piperacillin combined with an aminoglycoside.

In all cases of empyema, if the organism is isolated on Gram stain, culture of blood or pleural fluid, or quantitative culture of bronchoalveolar lavage, the antibiotic regimen should be adjusted to provide the most narrow spectrum of coverage in an effort to prevent overgrowth of yeast and multiresistant organisms. Initial antibiotic choices for treatment of empyema are summarized in Table 8. When choosing antibiotics empirically, it is useful to know the local or institutional prevalence of etiologic agents and their antibiotic resistance, particularly when infection is acquired in the hospital or is due to *Staphylococcus.*

TABLE 8. Initial Choice of Antibiotic Regimens for Treatment of Empyema

Age of Patient	Initial Antibiotic Choice
<2 mo	Nafcillin, ampicillin, and gentamicin
2–12 mo	Nafcillin and cefuroxime
1–7 yr	Cefuroxime*
>7 yr	Ampicillin
Special circumstances:	
Anaerobic empyema	Clindamycin Ticarcillin-clavulanate Ampicillin-sulbactam Cefoxitin
Hospital-acquired empyema	Ticarcillin-clavulanate Ampicillin-sulbactam Cefoxitin Consider piperacillin or ceftazidime plus an aminoglycoside (see text)

* Add nafcillin if *S. aureus* is suspected (see text).

Because empyemas are essentially abscesses of the pleural space, antibiotic treatment alone is not sufficient; drainage of fluid is also required for resolution of infection. The longer the time between onset of infection and drainage by thoracostomy tube, the higher the incidence of loculation, fibrous peel that encases the lung and prevents lung expansion, and spontaneous drainage of pus through bronchopleural fistulas or the chest wall (empyema necessitans). **Because such complications may be avoided by prompt drainage, it is safest to proceed immediately to thoracotomy tube drainage of any purulent effusion.**

Because sympathetic effusions do not absolutely demand drainage, some sources advocate delaying drainage of purulent effusions with normal glucose and pH and negative Gram stain and following these values with repeated thoracenteses. The problem with this approach is that no laboratory criteria are totally reliable determinants of bacterial invasion of the pleural space. There may be a delay of many hours between invasion of the pleural space and the emergence of abnormal pH, glucose, and Gram stain values, particularly if the patient has received antibiotic therapy. By the time an empyema is correctly diagnosed after repeated thoracenteses, many effusions have become loculated and impossible to drain percutaneously. **Therefore, it is safer to drain any purulent effusion with a tube as early as possible.** In addition to preventing possible complications that require open thoracotomy, thoracostomy tubes are generally well tolerated and are preferable to repeated thoracenteses in anxious and uncooperative children.

Duration of antibiotic treatment and tube drainage depends on the clinical response. Children with sympathetic parapneumonic effusions generally experience defervescence and great clinical improvement in the first few days of treatment. Thus 5–7 days of intravenous antibiotics, followed by oral antibiotics to complete a 14-day course, is usually adequate. If the patient becomes afebrile and there is no further drainage, the thoracostomy tube should be removed (usually after 2 or 3 days of therapy). If marked improvement has not occurred in a few days, pleural fluid should be reexamined to determine if the glucose and pH levels have decreased below 60 mg/dl and 7.3, respectively; if so, the effusion is probably an empyema rather than a sympathetic effusion.

Patients with empyema typically have a more prolonged recovery, with response to treatment characterized by gradual improvement of fever, tachypnea, tachycardia, overall well-being, leukocytosis, and effusion drainage. The radiographic appearance should not be used to determine response to treatment, because minimal improvement in pleural opacification for several weeks is typical. If clinical response is adequate, radiographs need to be obtained only before and after tube placement and removal and at discharge from the hospital.

For any empyema, antibiotics should be administered intravenously for a minimum of 10 days—until the patient is afebrile for several days, appears healthy, and does not require supplemental oxygen. Empyema due to *H. influenzae* and *Pneumococcus* typically requires 10–14 days of intravenous antibiotics; in most patients fever and fluid drainage resolve within 5–7 days. In contrast, fever and drainage of pus in empyemas due to anaerobes or *S. aureus* frequently require several weeks for total resolution; 3–4 weeks of intravenous antibiotics and tube drainage are commonly needed. Treatment of empyema due to Group A Streptococcus tyically results in up to 2 weeks of gradually improving fever, tachycardia, and chest pain, even when pus has been adequately drained from the pleural space; intravenous antibiotics are required for at least 2–3 weeks. For all patients with empyema, it is prudent to administer oral anitbiotics for 1–3 weeks after hospital discharge, until the respiratory rate is normal and the patient is free of respiratory symptoms.

Thoracostomy tubes should remain in place as long as there is drainage of fluid. They should be removed if no fluid or only a small amount of serous fluid is drained for 24 hours. A nonfunctioning thoracostomy tube causes unnecessary discomfort, risk of secondary infection, and pleural inflammatory response. **Flushing clogged tubes or reinserting tubes that have partially exited from the pleural space should not be attempted because of the risk of introducing bacteria. If further fluid drainage is required, a new tube should be placed.**

If the patient fails to respond to treatment (no gradual decline in fever, leukocytosis, tachycardia, tachypnea, chest pain, malaise, and anorexia), **treatment must be reassessed. The following possibilities must be considered:**

1. **Antibiotic coverage may be inadequate.** More effective coverage for *S. aureus* or anaerobes should be strongly considered.

2. **The diagnosis may be incorrect.** The patient may have tuberculosis, an intraabdominal abscess, or an additional site of infection, such as pyogenic arthritis. Review of the patient's history and physical examination as well as of the strain for acid-fast bacilli may suggest the diagnosis.

3. **The suction holes of the thoracostomy tube may be outside the pleural space,** a problem easily detected by chest radiograph. The location of the tube in the pleural space is not usually a cause of ineffective drainage as long as the fluid is free-flowing. Because fluid forms a meniscus around the lung and inside the entire surface of the pleural space, fluid may be removed with gentle suction, even when tubes are positioned anteriorly in a supine patient.

4. **The course may be complicated by loculation, lung abscess, or peel formation** with entrapment of the lung that results in persistent atelectasis and retained secretions. Lung abscess usually can be detected by a repeat chest radiograph and confirmed with CT. Loculated fluid should be searched for with ultrasound imaging of the effusion, and thoracostomy tubes can be placed strategically with ultrasound guidance. However, open thoracotomy with lysis of adhesions and removal of pus is indicated if there are many areas of loculation or if the patient does not improve after a 5–7 day-trial of tubes inserted into loculated areas. The presence of pleural peel with lung entrapment may be difficult to detect. On chest radiograph or CT this entity resembles the inflammatory pleural exudate and organizing pneumonia that occur in the course of any empyema. The presence of peel can be only presumed, when the patient fails to experience clinical or radiographic improvement after 2–3 weeks of treatment and no other reasons for treatment failure are found. This complication requires decortication (open thoracotomy and removal of the peel). Patients who undergo open thoracotomy for removal of loculated fluid or pleural peel generally improve rapidly after the procedure and usually can be discharged from the hospital in 5–7 days. **Continued attempts at percutaneous drainage of loculated fluid are usually futile, prolong the patient's illness, and increase the risks associated with protracted illness.**

5. **More time is required for clinical improvement to be obvious.** If a careful search for causes of treatment failure yields nothing, close observation and continued treatment are the best plan.

Prognosis. **Most children with parapneumonic effusions recover with no long-term sequelae.** The overall mortality rate of approximately 5% is usually associated with pulmonary compromise or sepsis as well as underlying conditions (such as chronic aspiration or poor nutritional status). Mortality is higher in infants, with reports ranging from 1–33%. The majority of patients have nearly complete resolution of parenchymal and pleural disease, and only a small amount of pleural thickening remains. On follow-up, lung function evaluation occasionally reveals mild restrictive disease that is rarely symptomatic.

Other Causes of Purulent Effusions

Other causes of purulent effusions in children are very rare, such as pancreatitis, pulmonary infarction or embolism, post cardiac injury syndrome (Dressler syndrome), pulmonary infection with *Nocardia asteroides,* and esophageal perforation.

Patients with pancreatitis present with abdominal symptoms, dry cough, dyspnea and chest pain, and effusions with an amylase level >100 mg/dl.

Lung infarctions and emboli occasionally result in transudative effusions but more often cause bloody effusions with >50,000 leukocytes/μl and an amylase level >100 mg/dl.

Dressler syndrome is characterized by fever, chest pain, dyspnea, rales, pericardial friction rub, and pulmonary infiltrates, 2–86 days after injury to the heart or pericardium, as in chest surgery or closed severe chest trauma.

Pulmonary nocardial infection causes cavitary lung lesions in immunocompromised patients and requires up to 1 year of treatment with sulfonamides. The filamentous, gram-positive organisms can be noted on Gram stain and culture of the pleural fluid.

Esophageal perforation also results in effusions with an amylase level >100 mg/dl. On rare occasions, purulent effusions may be caused by tuberculosis and malignancy. Drainage of such effusions is necessary only in cases of esophageal perforation or with large effusions associated with respiratory compromise.

Lymphocytic Effusions

Lymphocytic effusions appear turbid or serous and typically contain 1,500–5,000 leukocytes/μl with a predominance of lymphocytes. The following conditions may cause lymphocytic effusions in children:

Uremia. Up to one-fifth of patients with acute renal failure develop fever, cough, chest pain, occasionally a pleural friction rub, and pleural effusions. Effusions are less common in chronic renal failure. Effusions due to uremia are usually unilateral, small, and serosanguinous or bloody. Other causes of effusions should be considered because of the patient's predisposition to bleeding, infection, and fluid retention.

Tuberculosis. Tuberculosis is discussed in detail in chapter 18. No specific therapy for effusions is necessary, and resolution usually occurs within 1–2 months after antituberculous drugs have been started. The presence of a pleural effusion does not affect antibiotic choice or duration of therapy. Decortication is rarely necessary.

Malignancy. The childhood malignancies most often associated with pleural effusions are non-Hodgkin's lymphoma, leukemia, neuroblastoma and other neuroectodermal tumors, Wilms' tumor, and a few rare entities (e.g., histiocytosis, rhabdomyosarcoma or Ewing's sarcoma of the chest wall, hepatoma). Patients with malignant effusions typically present with symptoms attributable to the underlying malignancy; occasionally they also have dyspnea on exertion due to the effusion. Effusions are usually unilateral and may have almost any appearance. Tumor cells are often detectable in pleural fluid. The effusions usually resolve with treatment of the tumor, and fluid drainage is not necessary except for relief of respiratory distress. Repeated thoracenteses can lead to protein depletion or secondary empyema. Lack of resolution of effusions is a poor prognostic sign; such patients may require pleurodesis for relief of persistent pain or respiratory compromise.

Chylothorax. Because chyle contains lymphocytes, the triglyceride level of any lymphocytic effusion without a clear etiology should be measured. Chylothoraces are discussed in more detail below.

Autoimmune Disease. Effusions due to autoimmune diseases are extremely rare in children (see chapter 31), but they may be an initial manifestation of such conditions. The rheumatoid factor and antinuclear antibody (ANA) titers of the pleural fluid usually exceed those of the serum and are generally greater than 1:320 and 1:160, respectively. These studies are nonspecific and should be followed by more specific studies, such as LE cells and complement levels of serum and pleural fluid.

Fungal Infection. Effusions due to fungal infection are rare. Infection occurs following inhalation of spores of *Aspergillus nigrans* or *fumigatus, Blastomycosis dermatitidis, Cryptococcus neoformans, Coccidioidomycosis immitis,* and *Histoplasmosis capsulatum*. Patients usually present with subacute or chronic onset of fever, chest pain, cough, and malaise; the chest radiograph shows parenchymal infiltrates. Budding yeasts or hyphae often are noted on silver stain or Gram stain of the pleural fluid, and fungal culture may be positive. Other diagnostic studies include skin tests, fungal serology of serum and pleural fluid, and pleural biopsy. Most cases resolve without treatment. Amphotericin B remains the treatment of choice for immunocompromised patients and severe cases.

Longstanding Parapneumonic Effusion. Parapneumonic effusions are occasionally discovered many weeks after formation, especially if antibiotics have been administered orally or anaerobic infection is present. The presentation can resemble that of malignancy or tuberculosis, because all three produce a subacute course of prolonged fever, malaise, and dyspnea, with predominantly lymphocytic effusions. Clues pointing to a parapneumonic effusion are a history of acute onset of fever and respiratory symptoms, a history consistent with aspiration, and a pneumonic infiltrate. Pleural fluid cytology and acid-fast stain and culture help to rule out other diagnoses.

Chylothorax

Chylous effusions occur when lymphatic channels are obstructed or ligated. Chylous fluid usually appears milky but may appear bloody or even serous in patients who are severely malnourished or who have not had enteral feedings. A pleural fluid triglyceride content >110 mg/dl is indicative of chyle. Levels under 50 mg/dl rule out chyle, and levels between 50 and 110 mg/dl place the diagnosis in question. In such cases, a lymphocyte count in excess of 5,000/μl confirms the diagnosis. After a fat-containing meal, the triglyceride level of a chylous effusion increases. The diagnosis also may be confirmed when an effusion turns blue a few hours after a small amount of methylene blue is placed in the stomach. It is rarely necessary to confirm the diagnosis by identifying chylomicrons in the fluid.

Chylothoraces in children are most often due to severation of the thoracic duct during thoracic surgery or chest trauma (blunt or penetrating). Malignancy, particularly lymphoma, is the second most common cause of chylothorax. Patients without a history of recent thoracic surgery or severe chest trauma should undergo CT of the chest to rule out mediastinal adenopathy or a mass. Diagnostic studies for tuberculosis are also indicated (see Table 3). Occasionally exploratory thoracotomy is required to rule out malignancy or tuberculosis.

Chylothoraces must be drained by tube thoracostomy, regardless of cause. To reduce chyle flow, the patient should receive a trial of enteral feedings with low fat content and medium-chain triglycerides, which are absorbed directly into the bloodstream and do not require uptake as chylomicrons in the lymphatic system. If chyle flow persists, all enteral feeds should be discontinued, and a nasogastric tube should be placed to provide gentle suction of gastric secretions, which stimulates lymph flow.

Chylothoraces due to trauma tend to resolve spontaneously within 2 weeks. If malignancy or tuberculosis is the cause, resolution is less assured. In cases of malignancy, chemotherapy and mediastinal radiation may rapidly decrease chyle leakage. Similarly, antituberculous therapy speeds resolution of tuberculous pleuritis. Optimal nutrition is essential, because chylous drainage may lead to profound losses of protein, fat, water-soluble vitamins, and lymphocytes. Conservative therapy should be considered a failure if chylous drainage has not decreased within 2 weeks of discontinuing enteral feedings or if the chyle flow persists at a daily rate of >100 ml per year of age or 1,500 ml in adolescents. Definitive therapy consists of ligation of the thoracic duct close to the diaphragm, which forces lymph flow through collateral channels.

Hemothorax

Hemothoraces are effusions with a hematocrit value of at least half the blood hematocrit. There are only a few causes, which usually can be determined fairly easily from the clinical presentation. Because some hemothoraces are also chylous (particularly when caused by trauma), the triglyceride level should be obtained for every bloody effusion (see Table 3). **Hemothoraces most often result from trauma, but other causes are malignancy, pulmonary embolus or infarction, Dressler syndrome (post cardiac injury syndrome), and traumatic thoracentesis** (see Table 1). Thoracostomy tube drainage is required, regardless of the cause, to assess blood loss and to allow apposition of the pleural surfaces for tamponade of bleeding sites. Possible complications include secondary empyema, fibrothorax requiring decortication, and massive blood loss (if trauma is the underlying cause).

Monocytic Effusions

Viral and *Mycoplasma pneumoniae* infection occasionally may result in small or moderate serous effusions that contain <5,000 leukocytes/μl with a monocytic predominance and glucose and pH levels similar to those of serum. Influenza, adenovirus, cytomegalovirus, herpes simplex, varicella, and rubeola are the most common viral etiologies. Intranculear inclusions and multinucleated giant cells in the pleural fluid are indicative of infection with the herpes viruses or rubeola. **Viral effusions are usually asymptomatic, are not associated with pulmonary infiltrates, and resolve without therapy.**

Effusions due to *M. pneumoniae* often are associated with an ipsilateral parenchymal infiltrate; they are easily differentiated from parapneumonic effusions by the much lower leukocyte count and monocytic predominance. The diagnosis is confirmed by an 8-fold rise in antibody titers of *M. pneumoniae* over 6 weeks and suggested by a positive cold-agglutinin titer during the illness. Effusions resolve spontaneously, but therapy with erythromycin or doxycycline may speed resolution.

Eosinophilic Effusions

Uremic and parapneumonic effusions occasionally may contain up to 20% eosinophils, representative of acute inflammation. Other causes of eosinophilic effusions in children are rare, such as longstanding hemothorax or pneumothorax, pulmonary infarction, infection due to tuberculosis, viruses, histoplasmosis, echinococcus, paragonomiasis, and certain drugs (especially dantrolene). Treatment depends on the underlying cause.

Effusions with Elevated Amylase Concentrations

Elevated amylase levels (>100 mg/dl) occur in pleural effusions associated with pancreatitis and esophageal rupture.

Pleural Effusions in Neonates

Nearly all pleural effusions in newborn infants are due to infection (parapneumonic effusions) or chylothorax. The organisms that cause parapneumonic effusions are the same that cause neonatal sepsis: Group B *Streptococcus*, gram-negative rods (especially *E. coli*), and rarely *Listeria* sp. *Staphylococcus* is also a consideration, particularly if skin lesions are present. Pneumonia in the neonatal period is discussed in detail in chapter 15. Chylothoraces generally result from traumatic delivery and may be associated with other complications, such as brachial nerve palsy or fractured clavicle; a relative lymphopenia is often present. **Chyle does not appear milky until after the infant receives a feeding that contains fat.** Treatment is the same as for chylothorax in older children, and the expected outcome is favorable.

SUGGESTED READING

1. Banales JL, Pineda PR, Fitzgerald JM, et al: Adenosine deaminase in the diagnosis of tuberculous pleural effusions: A report of 218 patients and a review of the literature. Chest 99:355–357, 1991.
2. Bartlett JG: Bacterial infections of the pleural space. Semin Respir Infect 3:308–321, 1988.
3. Brook I: Microbiology of empyema in children and adolescents. Pediatrics 85:722–726, 1990.
4. Joseph J, Sahn SA: Connective tissue diseases and the pleura. Chest 104:262–270, 1993.
5. Lambert RS, George RB: Fungal diseases of the pleura: Clinical manifestations, diagnosis, and treatment. Semin Respir Infect 3:343–351, 1988.
6. Light RW, Girard WM, Jenkinson SG, George RB: Parapneumonic effusions. Am J Med 69:507–512, 1980.
7. McGloughlin JF, Goldmann DA, Rosenbaum DM, et al: Empyema in children: Clinical course and long-term follow-up. Pediatrics 13:587–593, 1984.
8. Sahn SA: Pleural effusions in the atypical pneumonias. Semin Respir Infect 3:322–334, 1988.
9. Sahn SA: State of the art: The pleura. Am Rev Respir Dis 138:184–234, 1988.
10. Sassoon CS, Light RW: Chylothorax and pseudochylothorax. Clin Chest Med 6:163–170, 1985.

20

RESPIRATORY DISORDERS OF THE NEWBORN INFANT

Eileen E. Tyrala, M.D.

This chapter provides a practical and systematic approach to the care and evaluation of respiratory distress in the newborn infant. The majority of respiratory problems during this period can be related directly to problems during pregnancy, labor, and delivery.

HISTORY: QUESTIONS THAT NEED TO BE ANSWERED

(Table 1)

To evaluate effectively an infant who experiences respiratory distress within the first 24 hours of life, information about the prenatal and perinatal period is of vital importance. If the infant is evaluated in the delivery room, this information should be readily available from the obstetrician and should require only a few moments to gather. If the onset of distress occurs in the nursery, a quick review of the prenatal record and the labor and delivery sheets should answer most of the following questions:

1. **What gestational age was the infant expected to be?**

Of fundamental importance are the accuracy and reliability of the information used to determine the estimated date of confinement (EDC). If the EDC has not been documented by at least two pieces of data (e.g., maternal dates, serial uterine fundal heights, early ultrasound) or if the actual EDC has been in doubt at any time during the pregnancy, an error in calculation of the gestational age may occur. Similarly, inaccurate maternal dates and/or erratic prenatal care may result in underestimation of gestational age and delivery of a post-date infant.

2. **Did the infant show any signs of in utero distress, such as aberrations in heart tones, passage of meconium into the amniotic fluid, or decreased scalp pH?**

Fetal heart tones are an important indicator of the well-being of the fetus and the integrity of the fetal–placental unit. Infants who display loss of beat to beat variability, fetal bradycardia, or late or variable decelerations of fetal heart tones on a persistent basis are at risk for perinatal asphyxia and subsequent respiratory depression at birth. The presence of meconium in the amniotic fluid generally indicates that during the labor process the fetus experienced an hypoxic or otherwise stressful event. This phenomenon, however, may or may not be associated with documented aberrations in fetal heart tones. If the stressful event occurred at or close to the time of delivery, risk for thick meconium in the mouth, nares, and/or trachea and aspiration by the fetus or neonate is significant. Meconium that has been present in the amniotic fluid for a period of hours before delivery is generally thinner and usually is not associated with acute fetal distress; however, it still may cause problems if it is aspirated.

3. **Was oligohydramnios or polyhydramnios present?**

The normal amount of amniotic fluid ranges from 400–600 ml. Either too much or too little amniotic fluid may indicate the presence of a congenital anomaly in the infant. Polyhydramnios is associated with esophageal

TABLE 1. Questions That Need to Be Answered As Part of the Assessment of the Newborn with Respiratory Distress

1. What gestational age was the infant expected to be? How good were the data used to date the pregnancy?
2. Was there evidence of fetal distress?
   Aberrations in fetal heart tone?
   Meconium present in the amniotic fluid?
   Decreased fetal scalp pH?
3. Was polyhydramnios or oligohydramnios present?
4. Was there premature or prolonged rupture of the membranes?
5. Is the maternal cervix colonized with the group B streptococcal bacteria?
6. Did the mother receive medications during labor and delivery that could cause respiratory depression in the neonate?
7. Was the infant delivered vaginally or by cesarean section? If by cesarean section, why?
8. Was there a maternal history of vaginal bleeding?

or high gastrointestinal obstructions, central nervous system anomalies, maternal diabetes, or twin gestation. Oligohydramnios may indicate decreased fetal urine output secondary to genitourinary abnormalities or renal dysplasia. This condition may be associated with lung hypoplasia, which may present with low Apgar scores and early development of a pneumothorax once positive pressure ventilation is applied.

4. **What was the duration of the rupture of the fetal membranes before delivery?**

Rupture of the membranes before onset of labor (premature rupture of the membranes) or rupture of the membranes more than 18–24 hours after the onset of labor (prolonged rupture of the membranes) are risk factors for the development of chorioamnionitis and infection in the fetus or infant. Infants with sepsis in the delivery room may be acidotic and/or depressed at birth. As a result, they may have low Apgar scores and poor transition to extrauterine life. In addition to being septicemic, some infants in this category may already have pneumonia at birth. Either situation may manifest clinically as respiratory distress.

5. **Is the mother known to be colonized with the group B streptococcal bacteria?**

Maternal colonization with group B streptococci in the presence of prolonged rupture of the membranes or prematurity is a serious risk factor for the development of group B streptococcal disease in the newborn infant. This disease may present with respiratory distress in the delivery room or in the early hours of life. It is important to remember, however, that group B streptococcal infections may occur without premature rupture of the membranes.

6. **What medications did the mother receive during labor and delivery?**

Infants born to women who have received narcotic medications for pain control within 1 hour of delivery have some risk, although generally small, for respiratory depression secondary to transplacental passage of drug. Similarly, infants born to mothers who have received large quantities of magnesium sulfate for the control or management of premature labor or eclampsia, as well as infants born to mothers who receive general anesthesia for a cesarean section, also may experience respiratory depression at birth and be at risk for abnormal transition to extrauterine life.

7. **What was the mode of delivery (cesarean section vs. vaginal)?**

The infant born via cesarean section has a much greater risk of experiencing an abnormal transition to extrauterine life compared with vaginally delivered infants. Risk factors include transplacental exposure of the infant to respiratory depressant medications that may delay the onset of breathing and absence of the "vaginal squeeze," which not only forces expulsion of fluid from the trachea but also promotes movement of air into the lung by elastic recoil of the chest. In addition, the potential for aspiration of amniotic fluid and its associated debris is far higher than in a vaginally delivered infant.

Another important question, of course, is why the cesarean section was done. Cesarean section for failure to progress or cephalopelvic disproportion in the mother involves much less risk than cesarean section on an emergent basis for abruptio placentae with decreased fetal heart tones or a similar obstetric emergency. Infants born by cesarean section also have a higher risk for the development of hyaline membrane disease and persistence of fetal circulation if the mother has not experienced labor. The scheduled cesarean done at 38 weeks without determination of fetal lung maturity may lead to delivery of an immature infant with hyaline membrane disease.

8. **Was there a history of vaginal bleeding?** Deliveries complicated by abruptio placentae or placenta previa may result in the delivery of an asphyxiated, hypovolemic infant with implications for the development of severe respiratory distress.

APPROACH TO THE INFANT WITH RESPIRATORY DISTRESS

The priority in any infant in respiratory distress is assessment followed by appropriate therapy as quickly as possible. A quick review of the history should precede evaluation of the infant (Table 2). **Regardless of the cause of the distress, enough oxygen should be delivered to make the infant look pink.** (In the age of pulse oximetry, rarely do we have to guess about an infant's oxygenation status. The ability to judge the presence or absence of cyanosis in an infant, however, is still an important clinical skill.) **In the effort to achieve 90–100% oxygen saturation by pulse oximetry, nothing is gained by holding back. If a full-term infant still is not well saturated with 100% oxygen, the infant has either severe pulmonary disease (meconium aspiration, group B streptococcal sepsis, or persistent pulmonary hypertension) or a congenital anomaly of the heart or lung (cyanotic congenital heart disease or a diaphragmatic hernia).**

Once the infant is pink, evaluation should continue with **quick visual assessment of gestational age. Is the infant premature or full-term? The next step is to assess the degree of the infant's distress.** Is it mild, moderate, or severe? The typical appearance of an infant with respiratory disease to some extent is determined by the infant's gestational age. Normal preterm infants may appear to be in mild distress if judged by standards for full-term infants because of an overly compliant or "frail" chest cage, which causes mild retractions even in the absence of pulmonary disease. Intercostal, subcostal, and suprasternal retractions, however, are characteristic of the infant in respiratory distress. It is primarily the degree of retractions that classifies the infant's distress as mild, moderate, or severe.

TABLE 2. A Practical Approach to the Infant with Respiratory Distress

1. Review the history (quickly).
2. Give the infant enough oxygen to make him or her look pink (O_2 saturations between 90 and 100%).
   If 100% oxygen is required, consider the possibility of persistent pulmonary hypertension or cyanotic congenital heart disease.
3. Assess the gestational age.
4. Assess degree of distress.
   How hard is the infant working?
   How fast is the infant breathing?
5. Assess air exchange and movement of chest.
   Is stridor present? Consider the possibility of airway obstruction.
6. Is a heart murmur present?
   Are the femoral pulses present?
   Is there a hyperdynamic precordium?
7. Is the infant
   Cold?
   Hypoglycemic?
   Mottled?
   In shock?
8. Keep the infant warm.
   Check a Dextrostix.
   Take the blood pressure.
   Draw a blood gas, complete blood count and differential and blood culture.
   Start an intravenous line.
   Order a chest radiograph.
9. Start antibiotics (ampicillin and aminoglycoside).

Abdominal muscles are normal accessory muscles of respiration in both preterm and full-term infants. Increased use of these muscles is readily apparent and indicates distress. Loss of the use of these muscles, which may occur with abdominal pathology, may cause an infant to become apneic or to appear to be in severe distress.

Tachypnea (respiratory rate >60 breaths per minute [bpm]) is usually an important indicator of distress. Infants with aspiration syndromes (particularly meconium) can breathe shallowly at rates exceeding 100 bpm and may appear to be panting. In addition, infants with respiratory distress secondary to cardiac disease typically breathe in a rapid, shallow fashion. Infants with hyaline membrane disease are tachypneic, classically have grunting respirations and retractions, and require significant amounts of oxygen. Infants who are tiring from excessive work of respiration may breathe at rates within or below the normal range (<40 bpm) but also appear to be in great distress.

Nasal flaring is a nonspecific physical finding commonly seen in infants with respiratory distress of any cause and reflects increased work of breathing.

It is important to listen to the infant. **Grunting respirations or expiration against a closed glottis is associated with diseases characterized by decreased lung compliance.** In essence, the infant is attempting to generate his or her own positive end-expiratory pressure to make breathing easier. The syndrome is seen classically in infants with hyaline membrane disease but may occur in any disease associated with decreased lung compliance. Listening to the infant's chest with a stethoscope is a crucial part of assessment. **Decreased air exchange is seen with hyaline membrane disease and other processes associated with poor pulmonary compliance.** Coarse breath sounds may be heard in aspiration syndromes, particularly meconium. Rales, which suggest that fluid is present in the alveoli, may be heard if heart disease or hyaline membrane disease is present. Decreased breath sounds may mean atelectasis, pneumonia, or pneumothorax.

TABLE 3. Causes of Respiratory Distress in the Newborn Infant

Most common
- Transient tachypnea of the newborn infant
- Sepsis/pneumonia—group B streptococcal disease
- Aspiration syndromes
  - Meconium
  - Amniotic fluid
- Miscellaneous
  - Metabolic
    - Hypoglycemia
    - Hypocalcemia
  - Hypothermia
  - Hyperthermia
  - Acidosis

Common
- Hyaline membrane disease (if predisposing factors are present)
- Pulmonary hypertension/persistence of the fetal circulation

Less common
- Nonbacterial pneumonia acquired in utero
  - Syphilis
  - Cytomegalovirus
  - Herpes
- Congenital anomalies
  - Airway
  - Diaphragmatic hernia
- Congenital heart disease
- Pleural effusion
- Birth trauma
- Abdominal problems

On the other hand, because the chest of the neonate readily transmits sounds, normal breath sounds may be heard despite the presence of significant pulmonary disease. **Infants with respiratory distress and abnormal airway sounds such as stridor, hoarseness, or wheezing should be carefully evaluated for airway obstruction.** If stridor is present, the infant may be placed on his or her abdomen to see if this position decreases the noise or distress. A floppy tongue or hypotonic posterior pharyngeal tissue may fall forward with this positioning and relieve the distress.

Does the infant have a heart murmur or a hyperdynamic precordium? If so, the possibility of heart disease should be considered.

It is always advisable to get a chest radiograph of any infant whose respiratory distress does not resolve quickly after birth.

Infants with respiratory distress associated with poor perfusion or poor color may be hypothermic, septic, anemic, or hypoglycemic; they may have decreased cardiac output from hypovolemia, low blood pressure, or congestive heart failure. **It is useful to check temperature and blood pressure, to do a Dextrostix, to determine arterial blood gas values, to obtain a blood culture and complete blood count with differential, to place an intravenous catheter, to administer antibiotics (ampicillin and an aminoglycoside), and, of course, to get a chest radiograph.**

COMMON CAUSES OF RESPIRATORY DISTRESS IN THE NEWBORN INFANT

In diagnosing the cause of respiratory distress in the newborn infant (Table 3), it is important to **remember that common things are common.**

Delayed Transition to Extrauterine Life or Transient Tachypnea

One of the most common causes of respiratory distress in the first 24 hours of life is transient tachypnea of the newborn infant or delayed transition to extrauterine life. The infant has experienced some difficulty in accomplishing one or more of the transitional events necessary to go from intra- to extrauterine life. This condition may occur in both preterm and full-term infants. During passage of the infant's chest through the birth canal, intrathoracic pressures of 60–160 cm of water may be generated. This pressure serves to expel up to 30 ml of tracheal fluid from the mouth and nares as soon as the face is exposed to atmospheric pressure. After delivery of the chest, the chest wall recoils to prelabor proportions and draws in a variable amount of air, sufficient to fill the airways.

It is not difficult to see why infants delivered by cesarean section are always at higher risk for an impaired transition to extrauterine life. Because they totally miss the "vaginal squeeze," they must rely on other factors to expel the fluid. Although total thoracic volume is the same, infants delivered by cesarean section have significantly decreased thoracic gas volumes compared with their vaginally delivered counterparts. Cesarean delivery without labor is a particular hazard; studies have shown that labor-induced increases in fetal catecholamine levels decrease lung fluid secretion and increase lung fluid resorption after birth.

Clinically the infant with delayed transition to extrauterine life shows relatively mild degrees of tachypnea, flaring, grunting, and retractions and may or may not require supplemental oxygen. Such infants generally do not appear to be very ill and recover quickly. If, over a short period of time (2–4 hours), all clinical distress has disappeared, this probably is the diagnosis. **Delayed transition to extrauterine life, however, is a diagnosis of exclusion. If the infant requires supplemental oxygen from the beginning and the clinical symptoms are prominent, it is necessary to consider other diagnoses, such as group B streptococcal sepsis and pneumonia.** The chest roentgenogram in infants with transient tachypnea generally shows the presence of fluid in the fissures and exaggerated perihilar marking that probably represent engorgement of lymphatics (Fig. 1). As suggested by its name, the problem is usually short-lived (i.e., <24 hours in duration), but on occasion it may last for 48–72 hours. Transient tachypnea, although not limited to infants born by cesarean section, is more common in this group.

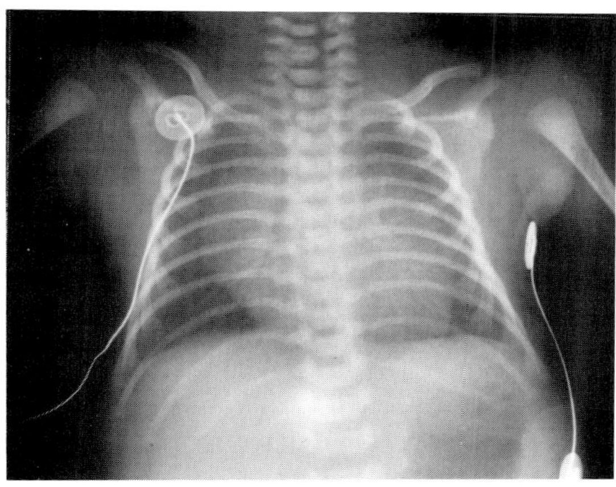

FIGURE 1. Transient tachypnea of the newborn infant.

Sepsis/Pneumonia

Group B Beta-Hemolytic Streptococcal Disease

Group B streptococcal disease, the most common cause of early-onset pneumonia and sepsis in the neonatal period, should be part of the differential diagnosis in every infant with respiratory distress. Although prolonged rupture of membranes in association with maternal group B streptococcal colonization statistically increases the risk, disease also may occur with membranes ruptured at the time of a normal vaginal delivery. The affected infant may present with respiratory distress and shock (usually from severe ascending disease acquired in utero) in the delivery room or, more commonly, with respiratory distress alone in the first 12–24 hours of life. The first chest radiograph may show only unilateral or bilateral streaky densities or focal pneumonia, or it already may show signs of a severe disease process, radiographically indistinguishable from hyaline membrane disease. (The inability to distinguish hyaline membrane disease from severe bacterial pneumonias, particularly group B streptococcal infection, has made it common practice to treat all infants with respiratory distress with antibiotics for at least 72 hours). Group B streptococcal disease is known to occur in approximately 1% of infants whose mothers are colonized. If the maternal colonization rate is 20%, the incidence of infants with disease is 2/1,000 live births. Some populations, however, have colonization rates as high as 40%; thus the incidence is doubled. Current strategies for prevention of disease in the newborn infant include selective chemoprophylaxis for mothers with known group B streptococcal colonization who present with premature labor, prolonged rupture of the membranes, or intrapartum fever. Because the disease carries a mortality rate of 20–50%, it must be viewed as a major risk to the susceptible newborn infant. Because the mortality rate is even higher in the preterm infant, selective chemoprophylaxis for the woman in preterm labor who is known to be colonized with group B streptococci has become the standard of care. Infants with this disease can become overwhelmingly ill very quickly. Many of them later require positive pressure ventilation and maximal levels of supportive care.

Other Causes of Bacterial Infection

Any bacteria in the maternal genital tract may cause a perinatally acquired infection that presents with pneumonia and respiratory distress in the newborn infant. Prolonged rupture of the membranes (>18–24 hours), maternal fever, and chorioamnionitis are associated with a significantly increased risk for the development of neonatal sepsis and pneumonia secondary either to ascending infection or to aspiration of contaminated debris at delivery.

The organisms most commonly associated with this mode of transmission include Group B *Streptococcus, E. coli, Klebsiella* sp., *Listeria* sp., *H. influenzae, Enterobacter* sp., *S. aureus, S. agalactiae, Proteus* sp., and *Chlamydia* sp. Their clinical presentations are indistinguishable and follow the pattern described above for group B streptococci. An antibiotic regimen that includes both ampicillin and an aminoglycoside (in addition to other supportive measures) is the standard approach to treatment.

Meconium and Other Aspiration Syndromes

With a history of meconium staining of the amniotic fluid, meconium aspiration should be considered as a cause of respiratory distress. Its presence is usually confirmed by the classic appearance of the chest radiograph, the presence of rapid, shallow respirations, and the clinical course.

Depending on the nature of the obstetric population, passage of meconium into the amniotic fluid occurs in 8–20% of all deliveries, but it is associated almost exclusively with full-term infants. Risk factors for in utero passage of meconium include a dysmature or postmature fetus, cord complications, or any situation associated with compromise of placental circulation, such as preexisting maternal preeclampsia, toxemia, or essential hypertension. The timing of the stressful or hypoxic event that precipitated the passage of meconium may be impossible to determine, because such events are usually not recorded on monitoring strips. The thickness of the meconium may be a clue: the more recent the event, the thicker the meconium. In addition, yellow or greenish staining of the infant's nails and/or the umbilical cord implies exposure to meconium over a period of hours. In general, the more distant the stressful event from the time of delivery, the less likely a major postnatal aspiration event, although the possibility of in utero aspiration can never be excluded.

The combination of the passage of thick meconium with aberrations in fetal heart tone shortly before delivery is cause for concern because of the increased likelihood that a depressed infant will be born with thick meconium in the mouth and nares. Under these circumstances **suctioning of the nares, mouth, and airway is of vital importance before initiation of positive pressure or the first breath to prevent the aspiration of meconium into the airway.** For the prevention of meconium aspiration, the oropharynx should be thoroughly suctioned at the perineum, preferably before delivery of the shoulders and chest and before the first breath. If the meconium is thick, if the infant has experienced fetal distress or is depressed at birth, or if the oropharynx has not been suctioned adequately at the perineum, direct tracheal suctioning should be done.

The typical clinical picture of meconium aspiration involves a full-term infant who experiences progressive respiratory distress over the early hours of life. The respiratory pattern of the infant is frequently characterized by very rapid, shallow breaths. (In particularly severe cases, it is not uncommon for the respiratory rate to exceed the heart rate.) **Retractions, flaring,**

and the need for an oxygen-enriched environment are also typical. Meconium aspiration usually can be distinguished from other aspiration syndromes not only by the clinical history but also by the chest radiograph. Classically, the radiograph shows overaeration with flattening of the diaphragm and diffuse, irregular pulmonary densities (Fig 2). Over the years, **I have been impressed with how difficult it is to predict the clinical course of meconium aspiration on the basis of the early chest radiograph alone.** The classic radiographic picture of "cannon balls" in the lung may clear dramatically in a relatively short period of time with or without significant improvement in the clinical picture. In addition, regardless of the radiograph, if chest physiotherapy, postural drainage, and pulmonary suctioning and toilet are not successful in mobilizing debris from the airway, complications associated with air trapping, such as pneumothorax, may worsen the clinical picture significantly.

Once the meconium has migrated to the distal parts of the lung, little can be done to enhance its ultimate removal by phagocytosis. **Although meconium is sterile, the use of antibiotics is recommended, because meconium causes a chemical pneumonitis and may predispose to the development of a superimposed bacterial infection.** In addition, infection of the fetus may have been the factor that precipitated the in utero passage of meconium. Corticosteroid therapy has not been shown to be effective in the management of this disease.

Oxygen should be administered liberally with the goal of maintaining arterial oxygen tension in the range of 80–90 torr. Infants are at significant risk for the development of persistence of the fetal circulation because of preexisting fetal distress or perinatal asphyxia; thus it is important to maintain an environment that favors maximal dilation of the pulmonary vascular bed (i.e., high oxygen tensions and normal acid/base status). Assisted ventilation should be undertaken when evidence of respiratory failure is clearly present, on the basis either of inability to maintain adequate oxygen tensions despite administration of high concentrations of oxygen or of increasing tensions of CO_2. Unacceptable levels of clinical distress in the infant and the need to ensure adequate pulmonary toilet are also factors that must be considered in the decision to provide ventilator support.

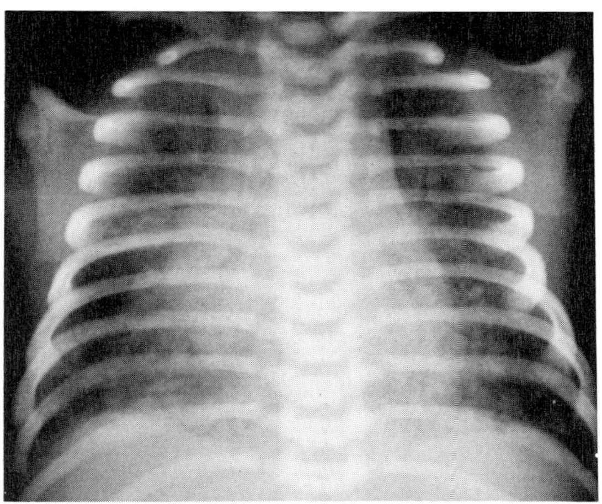

FIGURE 2. Meconium aspiration syndrome. Note the diffuse densities present throughout all lung fields.

The newborn infant is potentially at risk to aspirate not only meconium, but any fluid or debris that may be encountered during passage through the birth canal. Aspiration of amniotic fluid is a particular risk for the infant born by cesarean section with intact membranes. As soon as the first breath is taken, any substance (e.g., blood, hair, nails, desquamated skin) that has not been adequately suctioned from the nose and mouth may enter the airway and produce an aspiration syndrome. In general, unless large quantities have been aspirated, aspiration of blood or amniotic fluid does not cause severe clinical disease, because each is reabsorbed relatively quickly and does not produce chemical pneumonitis. If the amniotic fluid is purulent, however, the infant is at risk of aspirating bacteria directly into the lung with implications for development of neonatal pneumonia. Aspiration of large quantities of blood may result in the inactivation of surfactant in the lung and cause a clinical picture that resembles hyaline membrane disease. It may be difficult to establish a definitive diagnosis of pneumonia by chest radiograph obtained during the first 24 hours of life. Frequently follow-up studies are required for accurate diagnostic classification and for guidance relative to duration of antibiotic therapy.

The degree of distress and severity of illness in infants with aspiration syndrome vary considerably from mild distress with a low-grade oxygen requirement to severe distress requiring positive pressure ventilation and maximal supportive care.

Metabolic and Other Causes of Respiratory Distress

Other conditions that at first may seem unrelated are also important causes of respiratory distress in the newborn infant. Hypothermia and hypoglycemia, two of the most common events in newborn infants, may present with either apnea or respiratory distress. Thus it is important to ensure that the infant is kept appropriately warm at all times and given dextrose intravenously to avoid hypoglycemia.

Hyperthermia may cause tachypnea as the infant attempts to rid himself or herself of excess heat. Because hyperthermia usually results from a malfunctioning warmer bed, equipment should be checked immediately if it occurs. Anemia or polycythemia may result in an increased effort of breathing because of either heart failure, as with severe anemia, or pulmonary hypertension, which may be seen with hyperviscosity syndromes. Any cause of metabolic acidosis from sepsis to inborn errors of metabolism also may present with respiratory distress. With appropriate bedside and laboratory monitoring, it should not be difficult to determine whether any of these conditions is present.

Hyaline Membrane Disease

Hyaline membrane disease or respiratory distress syndrome is a disease process related to impaired or delayed synthesis of surfactant. **The incidence of hyaline membrane disease varies inversely with advancing gestational age, although other risk factors, such as maternal diabetes, perinatal asphyxia, male sex, and family history, are also involved. Exogenous substances, such as hemoglobin, red blood cell membranes, albumin, plasma proteins, phospholipases, and meconium, have been shown to inhibit surfactant function and may account for hyaline membrane disease in infants who otherwise are not considered to be at risk.**

Surfactant deficiency produces an increase in surface tension forces at the alveolar level, which leads to secondary atelectasis and inequality of ventilation/perfusion ratios. The classic results are hypoxemia and retention of CO_2, with development of acidosis, pulmonary vasoconstriction, pulmonary hypoperfusion, and capillary endothelial leak as well as deposition of fibrin and cellular debris (e.g., hyaline membranes) in the alveolar space. Respiratory support is offered with an oxygen-enriched environment, end-expiratory pressure, and/or positive pressure ventilation, as needed. The goal is to sustain the infant until the surfactant production system matures, while doing as little damage as possible to the lung with oxygen and barotrauma. **The classic picture of hyaline membrane disease involves a preterm infant who presents with grunting, retractions, and cyanosis either at birth or within the early hours of life. The chest radiograph shows hypoaeration, air bronchograms, and ground-glass appearance to the lung fields** (Fig. 3).

The introduction of exogenous surfactant for treatment of hyaline membrane disease has decreased dramatically the severity of the disease process. The most immediate benefit is improvement in survival rates for infants at greatest risk. Decreased requirements for oxygen and positive airway pressure and a decreased incidence of air leak syndromes also have been demonstrated in treated infants. To date, however, these improvements have not translated into a decreased incidence of chronic lung disease or bronchopulmonary dysplasia for most infants. Several studies have provided data to support the prophylactic administration of surfactant in the infant of $\leq$26 weeks' gestation in the delivery room, before a definitive clinical diagnosis of hyaline membrane disease is made. In infants of $>$26 weeks' gestation, most studies support the use of surfactant after the diagnosis has been made (i.e., rescue treatment) because of the high percentages of infants who will need no treatment at all.

Surfactant should be administered only by personnel experienced in offering respiratory support to preterm infants. In particular, the need for reduction in respiratory support after surfactant has been administered may be rapid and dramatic. If the reduced need is not recognized immediately and treated accordingly, severe air leak syndromes may result. Figure 3 shows chest radiographs of an infant with classic hyaline membrane disease before and after the instillation of exogenous surfactant into the trachea. Clinical results can be equally as dramatic.

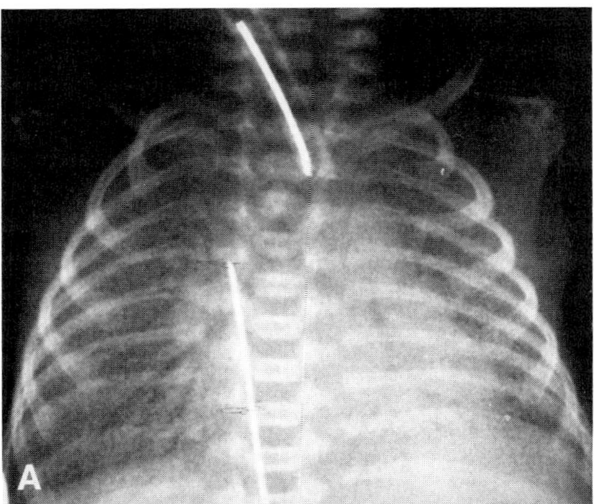

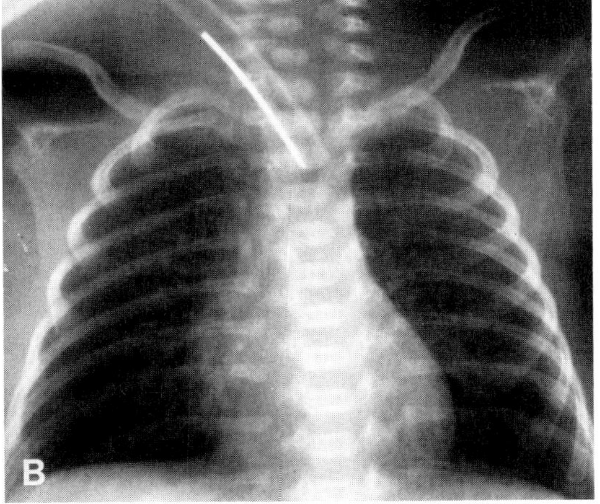

FIGURE 3. *A,* Hyaline membrane disease. Note the presence of air bronchograms and the diffuse ground-glass appearance of the lung fields. *B,* After surfactant treatment. Note the dramatic improvement in aeration and appearance of lung fields.

Air Leak Syndromes

Air leak syndromes associated with respiratory distress include pneumothorax, pneumopericardium, pneumoperitoneum, and pulmonary interstitial emphysema. (Although technically a type of air leak, pneumomediastinum is not included, because, by itself, it rarely causes respiratory distress.) Air leaks that occur in the delivery room or in the first 24 hours of life are generally associated with application of positive pressure to the airway of an infant with one of the following conditions: hypoplastic lungs, meconium-filled airway, misplaced endotracheal tube, diaphragmatic hernia, or requirement of a high mean airway pressure to achieve adequate oxygenation. The application of positive pressure to an airway in any situation may result in the development of a pulmonary air leak, most commonly a pneumothorax (Fig. 4).

The diagnosis should be suspected when, despite the use of all appropriate measures to improve oxygenation, poor color and decreased arterial oxygen saturations persist. Decreased breath sounds on the affected side, a shift in location of the heart tones, or increased transillumination of light through the chest on the affected side also may be present. Radiographic confirmation of a pneumothorax is not always necessary if one or more of the above features are present in the appropriate high-risk settings or if the clinical situation is so extreme that the need to rule out this possibility is urgent. Tension pneumothoraces and those that involve a continuing need for positive airway pressure almost always require placement of a thoracostomy tube and application of appropriate suction and drainage. Before placement of the chest tube and in less acute situations, tapping of the chest with a butterfly needle attached to a three-way stopcock and syringe evacuates the air and may be used as either a temporizing measure or as definitive treatment, according to the clinical situation.

Some infants develop spontaneous pneumothoraces (usually *not* under tension) during the normal birth process with no obvious predisposing conditions. Such infants generally present with tachypnea and usually require only

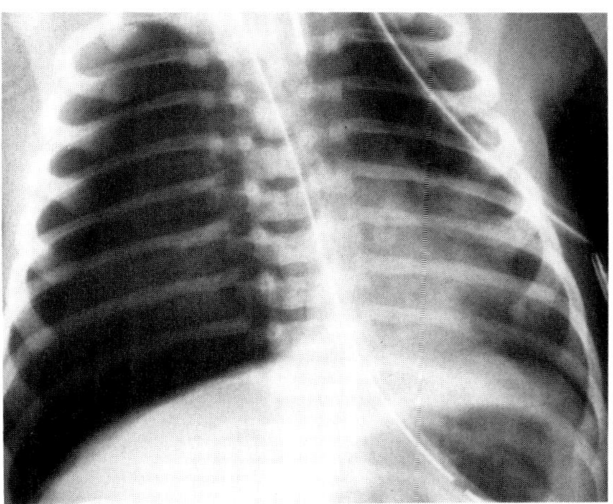

FIGURE 4. Pneumothorax complicating meconium aspiration syndrome, and initiation of positive-pressure ventilation.

a small amount of oxygen (i.e., <30%). Most such air leaks resolve on their own within 24 hours. Placing the full-term infant in a 100% oxygen-enriched environment (nitrogen washout technique) may be useful to accelerate the process. Infants with spontaneous pneumothoraces should have a renal ultrasound examination, however, to rule out renal dysplasia with secondary lung hypoplasia.

Pneumoperitoneum is a relatively rare condition that occurs when air dissects from the mediastinum into the peritoneal cavity. It is generally seen when a significant degree of underlying pulmonary disease already exists and the infant or child is receiving positive pressure. If large quantities of gas are present in the abdomen, respiratory compromise may result from impeded diaphragmatic excursion. On rare occasions, evacuation of the peritoneal air to relieve the tension on the diaphragm may be required.

Pneumopericardium, the most severe and life-threatening of all the air leak syndromes (and fortunately a very rare event), results from air tracking along pleural reflections around the great vessels and into the pericardial sac. It generally presents with signs and symptoms of cardiac tamponade (i.e., decreased cardiac output, reduced stroke volume, and decreased venous return) in conjunction with either a pneumomediastinum or a pneumothorax. Immediate relief of the cardiac tamponade by tapping of the pericardium or by placement of a pericardial tube is indicated.

Pulmonary Hypertension/ Persistence of the Fetal Circulation

The ultimate example of poor transition to extrauterine life, fortunately, is not a common cause of respiratory distress, However, an obstetrics service that delivers 2,000 infants per year will see at least 1 or 2 cases of persistent pulmonary hypertension (PPH) per year. Early identification and appropriate management of affected infants are crucial for a good outcome. **Clinically these full-term infants with respiratory distress are cyanotic in 100% oxygen.** For various reasons, they have not been able to establish successfully normal pulmonary blood flow during the all-important transition to extrauterine life.

In this context it is appropriate to review the physiology of the lung as the first few breaths of life occur. At the time of the first breath, an immediate and profound decline in pulmonary vascular resistance must occur to allow the normal and necessary increase in pulmonary blood flow. Work by Rudolph in the newborn calf has elegantly showed the sensitivity of the pulmonary vascular resistance in the first 24 hours of life to changes in pO_2 and pH. In the condition called pulmonary hypertension or persistence of the fetal circulation, in utero levels of pulmonary vascular resistance persist after birth, resulting in right-to-left shunting through fetal channels (e.g., the foramen ovale and ductus arteriosus); hence the name. **The classic picture of PPH involves a full-term or postterm infant who experiences fetal distress during labor with passage of meconium into the amniotic fluid.** The chronically stressed, growth-retarded fetus is at particular risk for these events, because chronic oxygen deprivation in utero has been shown to stimulate the development of abnormal pulmonary vascular constriction and hypertrophy of the smooth muscle surrounding the arteriolar bed.

Clinically the disease is characterized by severe respiratory distress and profound cyanosis, despite the administration of high concentrations of oxygen, within the first 24 hours of life. On physical examination an excessively loud second heart sound (indicative of increased pulmonary vascular resistance) and a systolic heart murmur (the flow through a patent ductus arteriosus) are frequently appreciated. M-mode echocardiographic studies demonstrate a prolongation of right ventricular systolic time intervals. The classic chest radiograph shows overly lucent lungs with diminished pulmonary vascularity and no evidence of pulmonary disease (Fig. 5). More often than not, however, parenchymal lung disease is also present in the form of meconium aspiration or pneumonia. Beta-hemolytic streptococcal sepsis and pneumonia also have been associated with this syndrome. **Other factors associated with PPH include polycythemia; chronic in utero exposure to prostaglandin inhibitors, such as salicylates and indomethacin; diaphragmatic hernia; and elective repeat cesarean deliveries.** The complex management of this important but fortunately relatively uncommon entity is beyond the scope

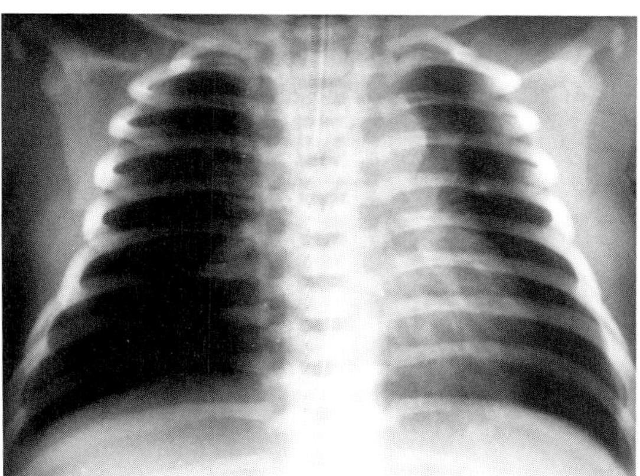

FIGURE 5. Persistence of the fetal circulation. Note the increased lucency of the lung fields.

of this chapter; the interested reader is referred to the standard texts of neonatal medicine. Such infants clearly need to be transferred to a level-3 neonatal intensive care unit as quickly as possible.

Nonbacterial Pneumonia Acquired In Utero

Nonbacterial pneumonia acquired in utero may occur in any infant of any gestational age. It primarily includes infections that can be acquired by transplacental passage of microorganisms from the mother to the fetus.

Currently, in the United States, the most common transplacentally acquired infection is syphilis. Fortunately, respiratory distress and pneumonia are relatively uncommon presentations for congenital syphilis. If present, however, it is generally associated with a severe disease process, in association with other physical signs such as hepatosplenomegaly, jaundice, and petechiae. A check of the maternal serology can eliminate or support the diagnosis fairly quickly.

Cytomegalic inclusion disease in the newborn infant (associated with primary maternal infection during pregnancy) may present with a respiratory component, because the lung is a primary target organ in approximately 35% of cases. Involvement of other organ systems usually dominates the clinical picture (e.g., hepatosplenomegaly, jaundice, petechiae). The diagnosis may be confirmed by isolation of the virus from the urine of the infant.

Congenital rubella, toxoplasmosis, and disseminated herpes simplex infection present with primary lung involvement in slightly less than 20% of cases. Of the three, herpes is the most common cause of respiratory distress. Infection is generally acquired by exposure of the fetus to virus during passage through an infected birth canal. Herpes must be considered as a possible cause of pneumonia and respiratory distress in any neonate, even if cutaneous vesicles are not present. Infants with herpes pneumonia, however, are always very ill.

The infant born to a mother with active varicella infection at the time of delivery is at risk for acquisition of transplacental varicella with possible pulmonary involvement. Such infants should be given varicella immunoglobulin immediately after birth to prevent perinatal infection.

Congenital Anomalies and Early-Onset Respiratory Distress

The list of congenital anomalies that may contribute to the early onset of respiratory distress in the newborn infant is long and varied. Although a full discussion of each is beyond the scope of this chapter, a list is presented in Table 4, according to anatomic location.

Choanal atresia, or obstruction of the nasal passage by osseous or membranous tissue, may occur unilaterally or bilaterally. **Bilateral choanal atresia classically involves the infant whose respiratory distress is relieved with crying and in whom suction catheters cannot be passed down the nares.** In approximately 50% of cases, it is associated with other anomalies that are part of the CHARGE, Apert, or Treacher-Collins syndromes.

The most common anatomic locations of congenital anomalies that may produce respiratory distress in the neonate are the larynx, mouth, and jaw. The degree of respiratory distress, however, is related to the degree and site of obstruction. Such problems should be considered when stridor, hoarseness, or other upper airway findings dominate the clinical picture. **Laryngomalacia, or a floppy epiglottis, is statistically the most common airway abnormality in the neonate and may present with inspiratory stridor, with or without respiratory distress.** Vocal cord paralysis is next in frequency, usually

TABLE 4. Congenital Abnormalities as Causes of Respiratory Distress in the Newborn Infant

Nose
- Choanal atresia/stenosis
  - CHARGE syndrome
  - Apert syndrome
  - Treacher-Collins syndrome

Mouth and jaw
- Pierre-Robin syndrome
- Hypoplastic mandible
- Enlarged tongue—Beckwith-Wiedemann syndrome
- Cysts: thyroglossal, gingival

Larynx
- Laryngomalacia
- Vocal cord paralysis
- Laryngeal web
- Congenital subglottic stenosis

Trachea and bronchi
- Tracheomalacia
- Tracheal stenosis
- Tracheal cyst
- Bronchostenosis
- Bronchial atresia
- Bronchomalacia
- Lobar emphysema
- Bronchogenic cyst

Lung
- Cystic adenomatoid malformation

Extrinsic compression syndrome
- Goiter
- Vascular rings
- Aberrant vessels
- Hemangiomata
- Cystic hygroma
- Teratoma
- Esophageal atresia

Mediastinal masses
- Neuroblastoma
  - Ganglioneuroma
  - Neurofibroma

Others
- Diaphragmatic hernia
- Diaphragmatic paralysis due to cervical nerve root injury
- Eventration of the diaphragm
- Thoracic cage and skeletal abnormalities
  - Asphyxiating thoracic dystrophy
  - Thanatophoric dwarfism
  - Achondroplasia
- Neuromuscular disease
  - Neonatal myasthenia gravis
  - Werdnig-Hoffmann disease
  - Dystrophia myotonica

without a readily definable etiology. Disorders related to the size and/or tone of the tongue, mandible, and hypopharynx, such as Pierre-Robin or Beckwith-Wiedemann syndromes, also may present with respiratory distress.

Abnormalities of the trachea and bronchus are fortunately rare; most are not readily amenable to surgical treatment or correction.

Entities that produce external compression on the airway and that can be diagnosed by physical examination include goiters, cystic hygromas, and teratomas. Careful inspection and palpation of the neck of any infant with respiratory distress should be a routine part of the physical examination. Other causes of extrinsic compression, however, are not so obvious. Esophageal atresia, generally associated wih tracheoesophageal fistula, may cause airway obstruction secondary to overdistention of a blind esophageal pouch with compression on the airway. Vascular rings, aberrant vessels, and other mass-related lesions also fall into this category.

With increased use of prenatal ultrasound, initial diagnosis of diaphragmatic hernia in the delivery room should occur less frequently. However, even under the best circumstances, this condition occasionally presents without advance notice. **The classic physical findings in the infant with a diaphragmatic hernia are respiratory distress and a scaphoid abdomen.** Ordinarily, in the early minutes after birth, physical expansion of the stomach and upper intestinal tract occurs rapidly as gas is swallowed and migration of air throughout the intestinal tract begins. In the infant with a diaphragmatic hernia, air in the gastrointestinal tract functions as a space-occupying lesion in the chest (Fig. 6). Respiratory function, which already may be marginal because of the presence of hypoplastic lungs on one or both sides of the chest, deteriorates even further. Bag-and-mask ventilation should be avoided to minimize the quantity of gas pushed into the gastrointestinal tract. Rapid placement of an orogastric tube to vent gas from the gastrointestinal tract is also important. If the diagnosis is made prenatally, such steps should be taken immediately in the delivery room to avoid further compromise to the infant.

Eventration of the diaphragm does not generally present in as vivid a fashion as diaphragmatic hernia, but it may cause respiratory distress in the newborn infant.

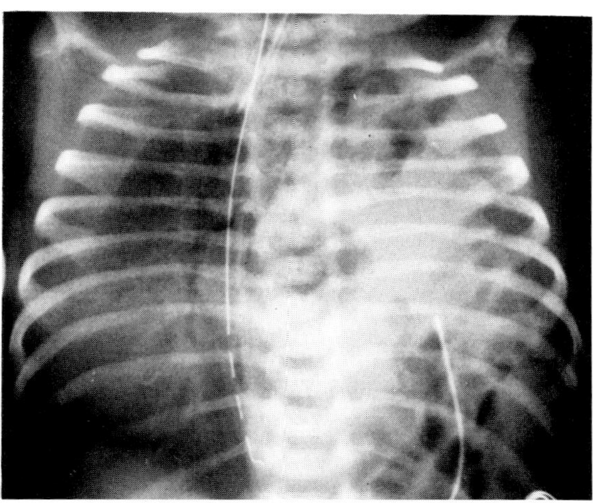

FIGURE 6. Diaphragmatic hernia. Note the air-filled loops of bowel in chest.

Thoracic cage and skeletal anomalies are not common but should be mentioned for the sake of completeness. They are usually evident on physical examination or strongly suspected after radiographic review of the bones and chest.

Neuromuscular disorders such as neonatal myasthenia gravis, Werdnig-Hoffmann disease, or dystrophia myotonica are very uncommon but should be considered when persistent hypotonia or muscle weakness is evident by physical examination. A prenatal history of decreased fetal movement is usually present.

Congenital Heart Disease

Congenital heart disease is generally the most significant of all congenital anomalies that can result in respiratory distress in the early neonatal period. **The most common clinical presentation of infants with congenital heart disease includes poor color, tachypnea, and respiratory distress. The presence of a heart murmur, a hyperdynamic precordium, an abnormal chest radiograph, and enlarged liver make the diagnosis more likely. Full-term infants with a normal birth history who present with profound cyanosis in the early days of life and who do not improve with administration of 100% oxygen should be considered to have cyanotic congenital heart disease until proved otherwise.** In such situations, however, it is best to start an infusion of prostaglandin E (0.1 μg/kg/min). If a ductal-dependent lesion is present, this therapy should reopen the closing ductus and may be life-saving. **In addition, the infant who seemed normal for the first few days of life but who then presents with poor color and poor peripheral perfusion may have coarctation of the aorta or hypoplastic left heart syndrome. A heart murmur may or may not be present.** The rapid initiation of prostaglandin therapy under such circumstances can be life-saving. Heart lesions with decreased pulmonary blood flow, which may present in the first 24 hours of life with profound cyanosis, include pulmonary atresia, pulmonary stenosis, tricuspid atresia, and the severest forms of tetralogy of Fallot. Chest radiographs classically show decreased pulmonary blood flow. Infants with the severest forms of truncus arteriosus may present with cyanosis, depending on the degree of pulmonary blood flow. Infants with transposition of the great vessels have adequate pulmonary blood flow but inadequate mixing of oxygenated blood at the atrial level. Such infants present with profound cyanosis. They may have a normal-size heart on chest radiograph, absence of an audible heart murmur, and normal or increased pulmonary blood flow. **In general, given the level of the cyanosis, an important distinguishing clinical feature in infants with cyanotic congenital heart disease is that the degree of respiratory distress is less than would be expected if the cause were primarily pulmonary in origin.**

Birth Trauma as a Cause of Respiratory Distress

Birth trauma to the third, fourth, and fifth cervical nerve roots with resultant phrenic nerve paralysis and diaphragmatic palsy may result in respiratory distress. It is usually seen in conjunction with an Erb's palsy. **Classic cervical nerve root injuries are seen after a difficult breech extraction, in which lateral hyperextension of the neck results in overstretching or avulsion of the affected cervical nerve roots. It may occur, however, with any traumatic delivery.** Large, asphyxiated infants are particularly vulnerable to excessive separation of bony segments and overstretching and injury of soft tissues.

Infants with this problem present with irregular and labored respirations and require supplemental oxygen. The chest radiograph shows an elevated diaphragm on the affected side (Fig. 7). The diagnosis may be confirmed by fluoroscopy or ultrasound. The clinical significance of this lesion varies considerably. In some cases, a transient need for oxygen and care not to position the infant on the affected side are the only treatment required. Spontaneous recovery usually occurs over 2–3 months. Other infants are not as fortunate and may require assisted ventilation and surgical plication of the diaphragm.

Primary trauma to the spinal cord resulting from difficult deliveries, with secondary thoracic nerve root injury, is fortunately rare; consequences for the newborn infant are often serious. Neurologic manifestations vary from profound respiratory depression with shock to paraplegia. Breech position and significant dystocia are predisposing factors.

Abdominal Disorders

Because the diaphragm and the abdominal musculature are primary muscles of respiration of the newborn infant, any situation that hampers the ability to use these muscles for respiration may cause respiratory distress. Ascites from fetal hydrops or urinary tract obstruction may cause significant abdominal distention and produce pressure on the diaphragm with secondary respiratory compromise. In extreme situations, paracentesis may be required to relieve the pressure. Peritonitis, as with necrotizing enterocolitis, also decreases use of the abdominal muscles of respiration and thus causes respiratory distress or failure.

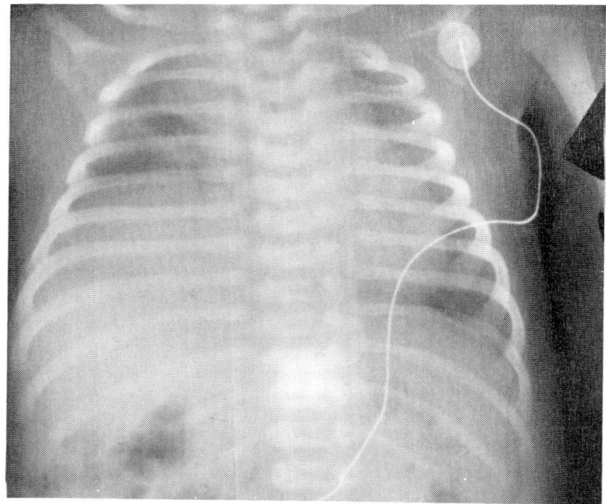

FIGURE 7. Elevated right hemidiaphragm in infant with paralyzed diaphragm secondary to phrenic nerve injury.

Pleural Effusions

Pleural effusions, although not a common occurrence, may cause significant respiratory distress in the immediate neonatal period. In the pre-Rhogam era, Rh isoimmunization with secondary anemia, hypoproteinemia, and hydrops of the fetus was easily the most common cause of pleural effusions. At present, nonimmune hydrops secondary to fetal cardiac arrhythmias, severe anemia, Turner syndrome, chromosomal anomalies, intrauterine infections, and urinary abnormalities, among others, are the most common causes. Congenital chylothorax, secondary to congenital abnormalities of the thoracic duct and lymphatic system, should also be considered in the differential diagnosis. Hemothorax may also ocur; thoracentesis is both diagnostic and therapeutic.

SUGGESTED READING

1. Boyer KM, Gotoff SP: Prevention of early-onset neonatal group B streptococcal disease with selective intrapartum chemoprophylaxis. N Engl J Med 314:1655–1669, 1986.
2. Brown MJ, Oliver RE, Ramsden CA, et al: Effects of adrenaline and of spontaneous labour on the secretion and absorption of lung fluid in the foetal lamb. J Physiol 344:137–152, 1983.
3. Fox WW, Duara S: Persistent pulmonary hypertension in the neonate: Diagnosis and management. J Pediatr 103:505–514, 1983.
4. Gray BM, Egan ML, Pritchard DG: The group B streptococci: From natural history to the specificity of antibodies. Semin Perinatol 14:10, 1990.
5. Linder N, Aranda JV, Tsur M, et al: Need for endotracheal intubation and suction in meconium-stained neonates. J Pediatr 112:613–615, 1988.
6. Moya FR (ed): Prevention and treatment of respiratory distress syndrome. Semin Perinatol 17, 1993.
7. Nelson NM: Respiration and circulation after birth. In Smith CA, Nelson NM (eds): The Physiology of the Newborn Infant. Springfield, IL, Charles C Thomas, 1976, pp 117–262.
8. Walsh-Sukys MC: Persistent hypertension of the newborn: The black box revisited. Clin Perinatol 20:127, 1993.
9. Wiswell TE, Tuggle JM, Turner BS: Meconium aspiration syndrome: Have we made a difference? Pediatrics 85:715–721, 1990.

21

BRONCHOPULMONARY DYSPLASIA

Henry L. Dorkin, M.D.

The success rate of the neonatologist in saving children of profoundly low birth weight and gestational age is a singular achievement. Currently, many infants with birth weights below 1 kg and gestational age below 30 weeks are able to go home. Nevertheless, despite the increasing use of artificial surfactant and increased survival of such infants, the number of children with significant respiratory disease secondary to prematurity—i.e., bronchopulmonary dysplasia (BPD)—has remained too large.

The general pediatrician can expect to be called on for primary care of children with severe respiratory compromise. The initial contact for health care maintenance and intercurrent illness is often the pediatrician in the community. Therefore, it is useful to have an understanding of the guidelines for hospital discharge, home care, and maintenance as well as a list of parameters that ensure appropriate growth and detect decompensation.

CASE PRESENTATION

A 23-year-old woman gave birth by spontaneous vaginal delivery to a 27-week-old infant weighing 800 gm. Apgar scores were 4^1 and 5^5. The infant was given oxygen by hood in the delivery suite. Artificial surfactant was administered, but the infant became progressively tachypneic with nasal flaring, retractions, cyanosis, and mottling. Respiratory rate was 75 breaths per minute with poor air entry bilaterally and paradoxical abdominal wall movement. Within hours the infant was reintubated and ventilated with elevated airway pressure and an FiO_2 of 60%. Over the next 7 weeks the infant's course was complicated by group B streptococcal sepsis, grade II intraventricular hemorrhage with seizures, hyperbilirubinemia treated with phototherapy, continuous nasogastric feeding, necrotizing enterocolitis, patent ductus arteriosus that required surgical closing, anemia corrected twice by packed-cell transfusion, grade I retinopathy of prematurity (ROP), and mild nephrocalcinosis secondary to diuretic therapy.

At 10 weeks of age, the infant was weaned from the ventilator but continued to require nasogastric feedings. A gastrostomy tube was placed electively because of concerns that further presence of the nasogastric tube would delay acceptance of oral feeding. On an aggressive nutritional schedule, a growth rate of 25 gm/day was maintained. Additional therapy included oxygen at 1 L/min by nasal cannula; spironolactone, 2.5 mg/kg/day; chlorothiazide, 25 mg/kg/day; albuterol, 150 μg/kg/dose in 1 ampule of sodium cromoglycate 4 times/day by nebulizer; iron, 2 mEq/kg/day; and multivitamins, 1 cc/day by mouth.

The social setting was a young family with two other children aged 2 and 4 years. Almost no extended family support was available, and visits by the family were difficult because of distance and child care expenses.

DISCHARGE PLANNING

In planning for discharge (see chapter 43 for details about home ventilation), it is helpful to hold an interdisciplinary team meeting with all individuals involved in the patient's care, including the primary physician, home health care agency representatives and consultants, and a third-party payer's case manager. The early establishment of a solid communication between the hospital-based team and the community physician is a high priority, especially because in most cases it is not possible for the primary care physician to attend such meetings. The ability of the family to care for the infant, the existence of basic necessities such as a telephone in the home, and determination of insurance coverage and needs for home services should be addressed at this time.

In the case described above, the age of the siblings and the fact that the mother appeared overwhelmed made nursing support a crucial element in ensuring successful transfer of care. This fact may not have been readily apparent to third-party payers, who assume that parents can provide appropriate care with only periodic nursing support. The combined efforts of the case manager, social worker, discharge planner, and other professionals are usually sufficient to meet basic requirements.

Subsequently, members of the team need to meet with family members to discuss the plans and to ascertain the family's readiness to assume care. It is often important for the primary caretakers of the family (most often the mother and father) to spend a few days living in the hospital with the infant and performing all of the duties that they will be required to fulfill at home, under supervision of nursing personnel. This process, which can take place in the hospital or in extended care facilities designed for such purposes, allows detection of strengths and weaknesses and concentrated teaching in needed areas. In most cases it also improves parental confidence and increases the rate of successful discharge.

The father, who worked all day, was overconfident that the infant could be cared for at home by the mother without much support and failed to appreciate how much effort was involved. More than one spouse has rethought the discharge plan and come to appreciate the work involved after spending 2–3 days in complete charge of the infant's care.

Early selection of a home care company is important. The company's capabilities must be assessed and availability of suitable equipment identified. Last-minute changes of major equipment, such as ventilators, feeding pumps, and oxygen systems, or of minor accessories may generate significant parental anxiety and make support much more difficult. The infant should have home equipment similar to that used at least in the last few weeks of hospitalization.

Home nursing and number of nursing hours can be a particularly difficult point of contention with reimbursement companies. Nursing plans must be realistic and include consideration of the time of the year when the infant is discharged (infants tend to be much more unstable during the winter and respiratory syncytial virus season), the possibility of missed shifts, and related problems. Plans should also attempt to describe projected reductions in care as the infant improves.

A problem-oriented note describing a complete physical examination, growth curve, and recent laboratory tests should accompany the infant at the time of discharge, which should be viewed as a transfer to a step-down unit at home. No one would transfer an infant without proper records, and home discharge under such circumstances is no exception. Immunizations should be given early enough to ensure that the most problematic side effects occur under supervision before the infant goes home. Subsequent immunizations, when the infant is more stable, are provided by the physician in the community.

MONITORING THE PATIENT IN THE HOME

Once the infant has arrived home, an attempt should be made to duplicate the growth rate and to continue or surpass the growth curve achieved in the hospital. As care becomes routine, the infant should be examined at home or in the office by the primary care physician. Any discrepancies between the pediatrician's examination and hospital records should prompt contact with the hospital-based team. A schedule of primary care visits should be intertwined with visits to the hospital-based team. In time, as support is weaned and the child becomes more stable, the visits to the hospital team should decrease until the child is discharged from follow-up.

Various signs and symptoms should be followed to detect destabilization (Table 1). Many can be observed by parents and ancillary personnel in the home, whereas others require the expertise of the pediatrician.

One of the earliest signs of respiratory destabilization is a rise in the resting respiratory rate, which is best assessed while the child is sleeping. Many variables affect the resting respiratory rate, and every attempt should be made to guarantee a consistent time of assessment. To ensure that day-to-day comparisons are valid, one should try to control for the following factors that affect respiratory rate: (1) recent feeding history (recent feedings of large volume may increase respiratory rate significantly); (2) recent alterations in oxygen dose (a recent decrease in the FiO_2 may be the real reason for perceived tachypnea); and (3) a rough estimate of sleep phase (respiratory rates may vary as a function of rapid eye movement [REM] vs. non-REM sleep). If, after taking these factors into consideration, there is a consistent increase in ventilation rate, one should reassess the child for presumptive respiratory destabilization.

More obvious evidence of decompensation includes increased nasal flaring, copious respiratory tract secretions (often from a tracheostomy site), use of accessory respiratory muscles, wheezing, cyanosis or increased oxygen requirement, paradoxical abdominal or chest wall motion, and increased sub-, inter-, or supracostal retraction. Other signs include decreased urine output and diaphoresis.

In the face of respiratory decompensation, one first should look for an overt cause and correct it if possible. If the decompensation appears to be chronic and subtle, one first should confirm that medications and ventilator/oxygen settings are optimal.

Commonly used diuretics are furosemide, chlorothiazide, and spironolactone. The action of these medications ranges from the obvious effects of diuresis and decreased interstitial lung edema to less obvious effects on pulmonary mechanics. The dosage as well as the advantages and disadvantges of each has been previously reviewed.[1]

One should review the fluid intake to see if a recent increase is temporally associated with the deterioration. Sometimes it may take several days or a week for the changes to occur, and one should have a low threshold for reassessing fluid status rather than rely on bolus doses of diuretics above maintenance levels. It is much better to avoid overuse of diuretics than to address their effect on sodium and chloride homeostasis. Judicious addition of potassium chloride to replace chloride losses in the presence of low or low-normal potassium is acceptable with appropriate monitoring.

TABLE 1. Signs and Symptoms of Respiratory Destabilization in Children with Bronchopulmonary Dysplasia

Primary signs and symptoms
- Increased resting respiratory rate
- Nasal flaring
- Retractions
- Paradoxical chest-abdominal motions
- Use of accessory muscles
- Increasing adventitious sounds
  - Crackles
  - Wheezes
  - Rhonchi
- Cyanosis

Others
- Irritability
- Poor feeding
- Fatigue
- Decreased playfulness and activity
- Diaphoresis
- Decreased growth rate

Oxygen and ventilator support may be increased to manage a short-term event and then reduced when the acute episode is over. One should auscultate the chest before making such changes to assess the alteration in ventilation before and after the adjustment. An increase of a few breaths per minute or a few centimeters of water peak pressure per breath can make a significant difference. A chronic increase in support suggests that either weaning was too rapid or the child's baseline respiratory function has shifted.

A decrement in the rate of growth suggests that either basal caloric requirements have changed or that the child is not taking in as many calories/kg/day as previously recorded during the phase of healthy growth. Assuming that intake is adequate, an etiology for increased calorie utilization should be sought, such as interstitial lung edema from subtle fluid overload, increased hyperinflation, intercurrent febrile respiratory illness, or even a simple

TABLE 2. Growth Failure in Bronchopulmonary Dysplasia

Causes	
Insufficient calorie intake	
Increased metabolic expenditure	
Infection	
Increased work of breathing	
Increased activity	
Management	
Increase volume of formula (beware of fluid overload and abdominal distention)	
Increase concentration of formula (1 cal/cc or higher)	
Increase respiratory support	
Diuretic	Start or increase dose or frequency
Bronchodilators	Start or increase dose or frequency
Oxygen	
Mechanical ventilation	

increase in activity as the child begins to move around (Table 2).

The usual response to increased caloric needs is to increase the volume of formula and nutritional support. However, if standard concentration formulas are used, a significant load of fluid volume is also added and may tax the child's respiratory effort in two ways:

1. Feeding with a bolus of large volume may cause distention in an abdomen already compressed by pulmonary hyperinflation. Such distention may be acutely uncomfortable and lead to emesis and possible aspiration. Continuous feedings may mitigate the problem but represent a retrograde step if the child has already moved from continuous feedings to intermittent bolus nutrition.

2. Excessive fluid may be drawn into the interstitium and further increase the work of breathing, thus negating the effect of added calories. A more aggressive diuretic therapy to solve the problem may result in chloride losses and metabolic alkalosis.

If, however, the formula is concentrated and attention is given to the glucose and protein limits of kidney function and dietary requirement, additional fluid is markedly diminished and the cycle is broken. Often this approach is sufficient to restore weight gain. Occasionally, however, maximal adjustment in a marginal patient leads to reinstitution of ventilation, which resolves the dilemma. This step is never taken in an offhand manner and is perceived by the family as a major setback. Nevertheless, such patients often have a residual tracheostomy, and the event is more emotionally than medically traumatic.

Poor feeding, fatigue, and decreased playfulness also may be manifestations of respiratory decompensation. Any child may be irritable or feed poorly for many reasons, such as teething, otitis, viral enteritis, or transient viral infection of the upper respiratory tract. All of these factors either have obvious sources or are of short duration. When symptoms persist, respiratory decompensation should be suspected.

WEANING SUPPORT AT HOME

Once it has been established that the child is growing well in the home environment, possibly demonstrating stability in the face of a viral infection, the family members develop confidence in their ability to care for the child. They begin to take excursions with the child and to suggest how nice it would be if certain cumbersome aspects of the treatment and equipment could be discontinued. After reviewing all of the reasons for the various components, one may try to decrease support. However, **it is important to attempt only one modification of the care routine at a time**, and sufficient time should pass to assess the effect of such a maneuver before deciding on further weaning. It is all too easy to wean several modalities in rapid succession, only to find that the child has ceased growth and that the causative modification is obscure.

Clearly the most difficult item in the child's therapeutic regimen is the ventilator. With all else constant, we decrease the ventilation at a rate of 0.5–1 breath/minute/week. Evidence of decompensation, either subtle (respiratory rate, weight gain) or overt (flaring, use of accessory muscles, retractions), is monitored. When the rate is low enough, one may consider short blocks of 1 or 2 hours off the ventilator, again looking for the same warning signs. Eventually the child may be weaned from the ventilator during awake hours, with replacement of ventilatory support during rest, sleep, or intercurrent respiratory tract infection.

Oximetry is often used to monitor respiratory function during weaning of support, but signs of inadequate minute ventilation may be missed with the use of oximetry alone. End-tidal carbon dioxide measurements are effective, yet sometimes cumbersome, and one must have a device with an adequate response time to determine if the recorded value is truly end-tidal. Determination of the serum bicarbonate value also may be useful as an integrated measure of CO_2 excretion. Subjective measures of activity, fatigue, and irritability should not be ignored.

After the ventilator has been removed, one then turns attention to weaning the oxygen dose. This step assumes that the initial oxygen requirement is less than 50%; a higher dose raises concerns of long-term oxygen toxicity. The hemoglobin oxygen saturation should be kept on the "flat" portion of the oxyhemoglobin desaturation curve (approximately 91–94%). Below this range, there is little reserve for increases in oxygen consumption associated with activity, feeding, and diminished respiratory excursion during phases of sleep. Above this range, there is little need to use excessive oxygen stores, and if the child chronically retains CO_2, one may suppress the respiratory drive.

Oxygen is administered as either a fixed percentage (blender, tracheostomy mask, ventilator) or as a fixed liter flow through a nasal cannula. For weaning from the former, decrements of 3–5% may be used until the percentage is below 30–35%. At this point smaller increments (2%) are appropriate, because they allow confirmation of continued growth. With the nasal cannula, the concentration of inspired oxygen can be measured with a complex formula that takes into account liter flow rate, respiratory rate, inspiratory flow rate, inspiratory/expiratory ratio, and degree of mouth-breathing. This result, based on several variables, provides only an estimated range and is used predominantly to prevent the FiO_2 of the nasal cannula from exceeding a safe range. One may reduce the flow rate by increments of 0.25 L/sec until the rate is below 0.5 L/sec, at which point increments of 0.1 L/sec are more appropriate.

Oximetry is an effective monitor for determination that the given oxygen dose is appropriate, excessive, or inadequate. **One should not rely on "spot checks"; instead one should measure the child's oxygen saturation in various situations: sleep, feeding, active play, and crying.** In this manner, one is not falsely conficent that the child's oxygen dose may be lowered.

There are three instances when the dose of oxygen needs to be raised:

1. Children experience intercurrent illnesses and may need more oxygen during the compromised period. When the illness is resolved, unless it is so severe that the child has a new baseline oxygen requirement, the child should be returned to the previously tolerated dose of oxygen and the weaning procedures resumed.

2. A child who seems to wean well may suddenly stop growing, suggesting that oxygen has been reduced below the threshold necessary for growth.

3. A child who grows actually increases tidal volume and minute ventilation; in a few instances this process may lead to an increased oxygen requirement secondary to growth rather than to lung deterioration. Differentiation between the two is important because of the varying levels of parental anxiety.

In the case study described above, the child thriving on 1.0 L/sec of nasal oxygen did well until the dose was dropped to 0.25 L/min. At that point, growth seemed to reach a plateau, and daily activity seemed to diminish. Return of the oxygen to 0.5 L/sec reversed the trend, and 1 month later the child tolerated the reduction without difficulty. The family understood that this was not a setback but simply a limitation of the child's ability to oxygenate at a given time.

After the child has been removed from ventilatory or oxygen support without decline in growth, other agents may be reduced. The data regarding bronchodilators in BPD suggest that efficacy varies from patient to patient. One can either measure pre- and posttherapy lung function in the laboratory or attempt a clinical trial without bronchodilator therapy. If the results suggest little maintenance effect, the agent may be discontinued. However, a beta agonist should be reconsidered during an acute respiratory illness associated with wheezing, because it may be more effective at that time. Studies of antiinflammatory agents demonstrate their potential efficacy as preventive measures to reduce severity of BPD, but data are as yet scarce about their long-term benefit in the absence of overt bronchospasm. Diuretics are among the last agents removed, and in many instances the patient simply is allowed to outgrow the dose.

PROBLEMS WITH OTHER ORGAN SYSTEMS

Various medical complications of prematurity and BPD are well known to primary care physicians but often require involvement of consultants, usually those who helped to care for the child as an inpatient in the neonatal unit. Contact with consultants is as important as contact with the BPD clinic team; thus the arrangement is often a three-way collaboration. Complications include but are not limited to the following:

- Developmental delay with or without anoxic encephalopathy
- Apnea
- Impairment of hearing, sight, or speech
- Seizures
- Hydrocephalus
- Gastroesophageal reflux
- Short bowel secondary to resection for necrotizing enterocolitis
- Cholestasis
- Disseminated viral systemic infection
- Congenital heart disease with or without congestive heart failure
- Pulmonary hypertension
- Cor pulmonale
- Tracheobronchial abnormalities, both congenital and acquired

SUPPORT TEAM

The model for outpatient care of the patient with chronic BPD is based on the team approach for care of the multiply handicapped child (birth defects service) and the patient with cystic fibrosis (cystic fibrosis center). Although a single physician may be able to perform many tasks of other team members, it is clearly much more efficient and cost-effective to use ancillary medical personnel for specific functions. Like the inpatient team, the support team includes physicians with expertise in chronic lung disease and BPD, developmentalists, pulmonary nurse specialists, social workers, nutritionists, physical/respiratory therapists, psychologists, and occupational therapists (feeding experts). By meeting on a regular basis to discuss the patient from all perspectives, the team continually updates and modifies the treatment plan and communicates with the child's personal physician in the community. The frequency of visits is logarithmic in nature: they are more frequent shortly after discharge from the hospital but decrease until eventually the patient is discharged from the follow-up program.

SURGICAL REPAIRS

Surgical correction of various BPD complications is a function of the extent of surgery (herniorrhaphy vs. intracardiac repair), stability of the child, and potential for postoperative complication. The gastrostomy site may be closed at any time the child is feeding well and no longer requires supplemental nutrition to grow. Conversely, closure of a tracheostomy requires preoperative proof that the child can maintain ventilation and oxygenation while breathing in a relatively normal fashion, has good growth potential without the device, can move secretions adequately (good cough) without access to the lower respiratory tract, and has little potential for developing severe respiratory illness that may require intubation in the near future. For example, a child with a good potential for closure may fare better with surgery in the spring at the end of the winter respiratory illness and RSV season than at the beginning of the fall.

CONCLUSION

As newer therapies evolve to treat the infant with prematurity and respiratory distress syndrome, the incidence of BPD decreases in the larger infants but increases in the youngest infants who are rescued. Until chronic lung disease is preventable in the survivors of the nursery, we need to plan for the care of such patients and their families as they battle the consequences of a war that is partially won. Many patients will need to deal with residual effects of their illness well into adulthood, but with a careful, collaborative approach among the primary care physician, pulmonary specialist, BPD team, and family, the best possible outcome—a meaningful and productive life—can be achieved.

SUGGESTED READING

1. Davis JM, Sinkin RA, Aranda JV: Drug therapy for bronchopulmonary dysplasia. Pediatr Pulmonol 8:117–125, 1990.
2. Hageman JR (ed): Update on neonatology. Pediatr Clin North Am 40:1105–1115, 1993.
3. Merritt TA, Northway WH, Boynton BR: Bronchopulmonary dysplasia. In Contemporary Issues in Fetal and Neonatal Medicine. Boston, Blackwell Scientific Publications, 1988.
4. Northway WH Jr: An introduction to bronchopulmonary dysplasia. Clin Perinatol 19:489–495, 1992.
5. Singer L, Martin RJ, Hawkins SW, et al: Oxygen desaturation complicates feeding in infants with bronchopulmonary dysplasia after discharge. Pediatrics 90:380–384, 1992.

COMMENTARY

by Howard B. Panitch, M.D.

Bronchopulmonary dysplasia (BPD) affects infants at varying stages of lung development, from preterm to term. In addition, it has been described in association with various diseases, such as pneumonia or meconium aspiration syndrome. Differences in treatment, such as early intubation for carbon dioxide retention or use of paralyzing agents in intubated infants, have also been implicated in the pathogenesis. Thus, it is not surprising that presentation is so heterogeneous, ranging from mild tachypnea to chronic respiratory insufficiency and mechanical ventilator dependency. All patients with BPD, however, improve over time. Whereas the infant with BPD may suffer acute respiratory exacerbations (e.g., from viral illnesses), episodes should be infrequent and not affect long-term progress. If the infant with BPD does not follow a course of gradual improvement, complications must be suspected, including reactive airways disease, gastroesophageal reflux, congenital or acquired heart disease, congestive heart failure, pulmonary interstitial edema, and episodic or chronic hypoxemia.

The nursery graduate must be viewed differently from the ill preterm infant in regard to therapies. The pulmonologist's view of oxygen therapy is quite different from that of the neonatologist. Whereas dangers of oxygen toxicity in the underdeveloped infant, such as retinopathy of prematurity and lung injury, are driving forces to wean sick preterm infants from supplemental oxygen in the intensive care nursery, long-term sequelae of hypoxemia, including pulmonary hypertension, cor pulmonale, and growth failure, are reasons to treat infants with oxygen for prolonged courses after discharge. Our experience has proved that most parents can learn complex medical regimens and administer multiple medications when given adequate training. Thus, discontinuation of diuretics, bronchodilators, or even mechanical ventilation should not be a prerequisite for discharge from the nursery. Weaning of therapies should be a natural consequence of the infant's improved health status and maturational process instead of an abstract goal to be reached. Withdrawal of treatment is based on the infant's ability to tolerate less support. The order in which treatment is withdrawn varies from center to center. For example, Dr. Dorkin chooses to withdraw oxygen support before discontinuing diuretic therapy. In our center, the opposite order is preferred. In either case, close monitoring of the child's condition after withdrawal of any therapy is important. As the author states, excessively aggressive withdrawal of support can result in both acute (respiratory distress) and chronic (growth failure) problems and should be avoided.

Although the short-term outcome for infants with BPD is generally good, the effects of early lung injury on aging are unknown. Normally, the lung loses elasticity with age, and some degree of emphysema occurs after the fourth decade of life. This process may be accelerated in children with BPD, who sustain loss of elastic tissue during infancy and undergo abnormal postnatal lung development. As demonstrated in a 25-year follow-up of the first patients described with BPD, adults are smaller in stature and weight than other adults born prematurely without BPD. In addition, a majority of these young adults have signs of fixed or reversible airway obstruction. Children with BPD may represent the next generation of patients with chronic obstructive pulmonary disease (COPD). Rather than coming to medical attention in their 50s or 60s, they may present during young adulthood with respiratory insufficiency.

22

APNEA

Laurie Varlotta, M.D., and Julian Allen, M.D.

DEFINITIONS

Apnea is the cessation of respiratory air flow. The three types of apnea are central, obstructive, and mixed. Central apnea is defined as an absence of chest or abdominal wall movement with no air flow through the nose or mouth (no respiratory effort). Obstructive apnea is the presence of increased chest or abdominal wall movement without air flow through the nose or mouth (Fig. 1). Mixed apnea is central apnea followed by obstructive apnea or vice versa.

Pathologic apnea is a prolonged respiratory pause of 20 seconds or greater or cessation of respiration of any duration associated with cyanosis, marked pallor or hypotonia, or bradycardia.

Periodic breathing is a pattern with 3 or more respiratory pauses of greater than 3 seconds' duration and less than 20 seconds of respiration between pauses (Fig. 2). Periodic breathing may be a normal event at any age. The maximal percentage of time spent in periodic breathing varies with age (Table 1).

In infants apnea may be classified as apnea of prematurity, apparent life-threatening events, and apnea of infancy. In 1987 the National Institutes of Health (NIH) Consensus Panel defined the types of apnea as follows:

> **Apnea of prematurity** (AOP) is characterized by abnormal periodic breathing which may be associated with apnea (obstructive, central, or mixed) and hypoxemia in preterm infants.
>
> **Apparent life-threatening event** (ALTE) is an episode that is frightening to the observer, characterized by apnea (central or obstructive), color change (usually cyanosis or pallor but occasionally erythema or plethora), marked change in muscle tone (limpness), choking, or gagging. In some cases, the observer fears that the infant has died. Previously used terminology such as "aborted crib death" or "near-miss SIDS" should be abandoned because although it is felt that ALTE may be a risk factor for SIDS, this has not been proven.
>
> **Apnea of infancy** (AOI) is an unexplained episode of cessation of breathing for 20 seconds or longer, or a shorter respiratory pause associated with bradycardia, cyanosis, pallor, and/or marked hypotonia. The terminology "apnea of infancy" generally refers to episodes of apnea in infants who are greater than 37 weeks' gestational age at onset of pathologic apnea. Therefore, premature infants are not placed in this group (see AOP). AOI should be reserved for those infants for whom the etiology of the ALTE is not found.

In older children, the most common apnea syndromes during sleep are obstructive sleep apnea and hypoventilation syndrome. Obstructive sleep apnea is the presence of chest or abdominal wall movement without airflow through the mouth or nose because of upper airway obstruction during sleep. Hypoventilation is a decrease in minute ventilation that results in carbon dioxide retention; it is usually defined by an increase in arterial carbon dioxide >45 mmHg.

APNEA IN INFANCY

Apnea of Prematurity

Apnea is a common problem in preterm infants. The incidence of apnea of prematurity

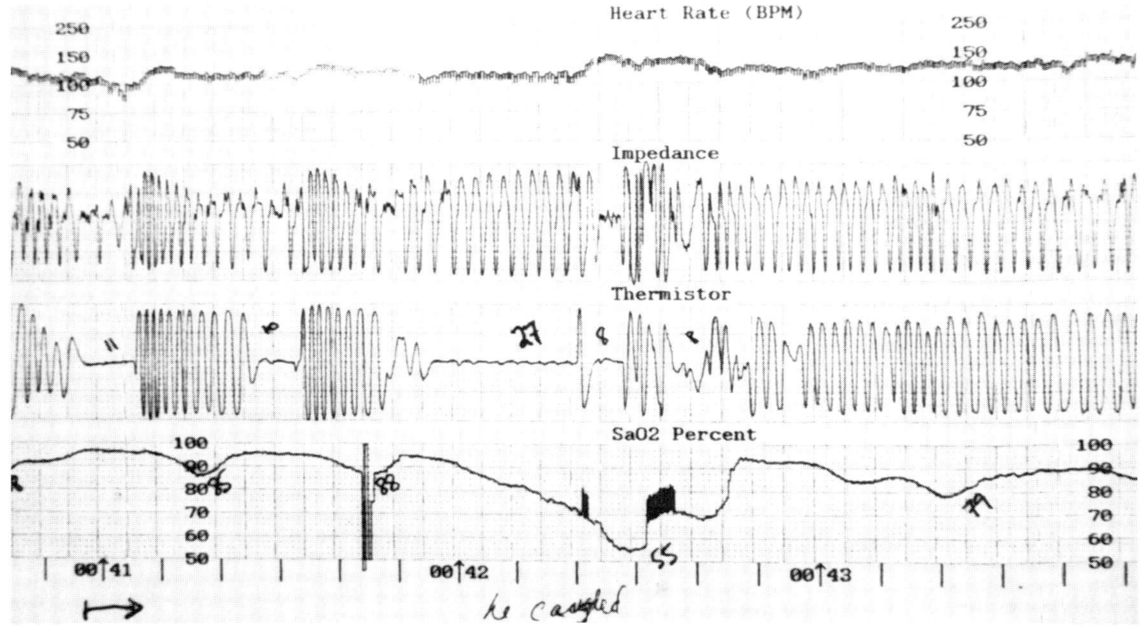

FIGURE 1. Polysomnogram with the following channels: Heart rate (EKG), chest wall impedance, nasal thermistor, and oxygen saturation (SaO_2). Multiple episodes of obstructive sleep apnea (chest wall movement without airflow through the thermistor) with significant desaturation are recorded. The longest episode is 27 seconds with an increase in heart rate and oxyhemoglobin desaturation to 55%.

(AOP) increases with decreasing gestational age from 80% in infants born under 30 weeks' gestation to 7% at 34–35 weeks' gestation. AOP usually appears within the first week of life and resolves by 37 weeks after conception, although it may persist for 50–55 weeks after conception.

The main cause of AOP is immaturity of the respiratory control center. Contributing causes include intraventricular hemorrhage,

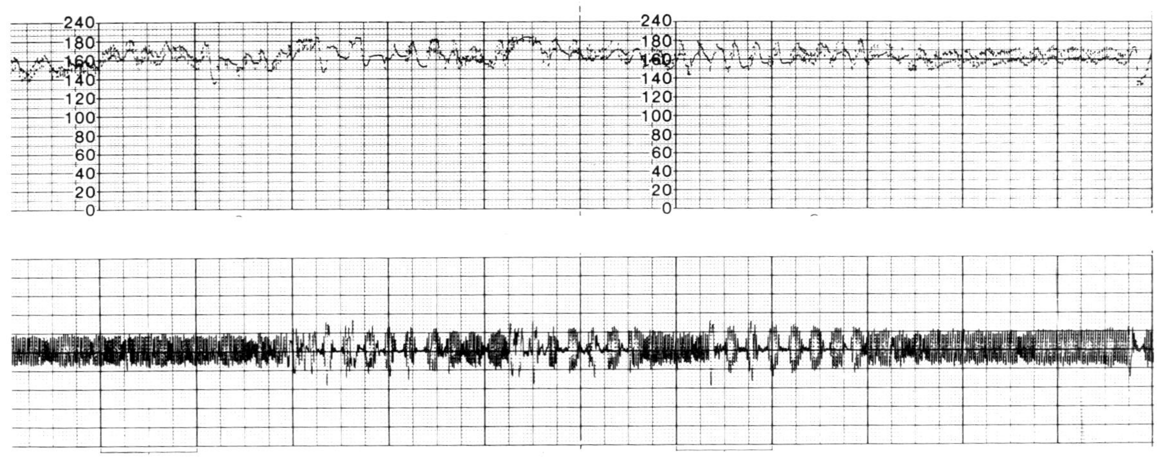

FIGURE 2. Pneumogram demonstrating periodic breathing. The two channels are heart rate *(top panel)* and chest wall impedance *(bottom panel)*.

hydrocephalus, seizures, and gastroesophageal reflux.

Bradycardia occurs in most infants with AOP during or after the apnea or periodic breathing. Bradycardia is defined as a 30% or greater decrease in the heart rate from baseline. This abrupt slowing of the heart rate is due to a vagal reflex. The longer the apnea, the more likely bradycardia will occur. Because oxygen desaturation is common during these events, it is important to diagnose as well as to treat the apnea or periodic breathing.

Apparent Life-threatening Event and Apnea of Infancy

Various etiologies may cause an apparent life-threatening event (ALTE) (Table 2). In about two-thirds of cases, a specific medical or surgical condition can be determined. The other one-third are idiopathic and are termed apnea of infancy (AOI).

Relationship between Sudden Infant Death Syndrome and Apnea

According to the NIH definition, sudden infant death syndrome (SIDS) is "the sudden death of any infant or young child, which is unexplained by history and in which a thorough postmortem examination fails to demonstrate an adequate explanation of the cause of death." The infant is older than 1 month of age and younger than 1 year.

The incidence of SIDS is 1.3/1,000 live births in the general population but higher for African-Americans (5.1/1,000) and native Americans (2.3/1,000). SIDS accounts for 7,000 deaths/year. Risk factors include the following maternal characteristics: young age, smoking, illicit drug use, inadequate prenatal care, low weight gain, perinatal stress, illness 2 weeks before delivery, and low socioeconomic status. Other risk factors include prematurity, ALTE, SIDS in a sibling or twin, age between 2 and 4 months, and male gender. SIDS occurs more commonly in winter months. Some evidence suggests that sleeping in a prone position is a risk factor for SIDS; the American Academy of Pediatrics, therefore, recently recommended that all healthy infants be positioned on their side or back for sleep.

TABLE 1. Periodic Breathing—Normal Values

Age (weeks)	Term Infants (%)	Preterm Infants (%)
0–4	0–3.5	0–5
4–8	0–2.5	0–3.5
8–20	0–1.5	0–2.5
>20	0–1.0	0–1.5

Although prematurity is a risk factor, AOP is not an independent risk factor for SIDS. There is no difference in the incidence of SIDS between infants with a history of AOP and preterm infants without AOP matched for birth weight and ethnicity. However, the incidence of SIDS has been shown to increase with decreasing birth weight.

Although an ALTE is a risk factor for SIDS, only 4% of infants presenting with ALTEs subsequently die of SIDS. Although this rate represents a 30-fold increase over the general population, clearly the vast majority of infants with ALTEs do not die of SIDS. It has been suggested that infants presenting with apnea during sleep and requiring resuscitation may have a higher mortality (10%) than infants who present with apnea while awake (<1%), even if vigorous stimulation is required.

Evaluation of the Infant with Apnea

In the diagnosis of apnea the infant's history and physical examination are of paramount importance. The history should include natal and perinatal events, characteristics of the apneic episode, and various other questions listed in Table 3. Questions about the event should be open-ended and not lead the parent.

TABLE 2. Common Causes of an Apparent Life-Threatening Event (from Most to Least Common)

Gastroesophageal reflux (GER)
Neurologic: seizure disorder
Meningitis
Respiratory factors: respiratory syncytial virus (RSV), pertussis, pneumonia, congenital central hypoventilation syndrome (CCHS)
Airway abnormality or obstruction
Vasovagal syndrome
Cardiac factors: Wolff-Parkinson-White syndrome/arrhythmia
Metabolic/endocrinologic factors
Münchausen syndrome by proxy

TABLE 3. Evaluation: History of the Infant with Apnea

Clinical Situation	Relevant to
Apneic episode	
Awake	GER
Asleep	AOI, CCHS
Position: supine, prone, seated	GER
Last feeding	GER
Noise: obstruction, struggling to breathe, choking	Obstruction, GER, neurologic, respiratory infection, airway abnormality
Color: Cyanosis	Hypoxemia, seizure disorder, airway abnormality/ obstruction
Plethoric	Obstruction, GER
Pallor	Infectious, cardiac, AOI
Tone: Stiff	GER, seizure disorder, obstruction, vasovagal
Limp	GER, infectious, CCHS
Eyes: dazed, upward deviation	Seizure disorder, GER, infectious
Fluid at mouth or nose: Formula	GER
Mucus	Respiratory infection, seizure
Length of episode and intervention: shaking, CPR	Severity of episode
Aftermath: Sluggish	Seizure, vasovagal syndrome, infectious, metabolic, endocrinologic
Normal	GER, obstruction
Excessive sweating	CCHS, vasovagal, metabolic, cardiac
Abnormal body movement	Neurologic, vasovagal, obstruction, torticollis (GER)
Cough ± paroxysms	Pertussis
Wheezing or bronchiolitis	Respiratory syncytial virus (RSV)
Other history	
Prenatal and perinatal history, including drug history of infant and mother	Drug use, neurologic, SIDS, meningitis, sepsis
Gestational age/Apgar scores	Prematurity, neurologic, GER
Family history, including history of apnea, SIDS	Increased risk for SIDS
Feeding history: Difficulty feeding	Airway abnormality/obstruction, infectious, GER
Regurgitation*	GER
Overfeeding	GER
Trauma	Neurologic, CNS hemorrhage, shaken baby syndrome
Irritability	Meningitis, infectious, GER

*Many infants with apnea due to reflux do not have significant regurgitation. GER = gastroesophageal reflux; AOI = apnea of infancy; CCHS = congenital central hypoventilation syndrome; SIDS = sudden infant death syndrome; CNS = central nevous system.

Subsequent laboratory studies depend on the history and physical examination. Infants with apnea are usually hospitalized during the evaluation.

Various laboratory tests are performed in infants with apnea (Table 4). Although all tests may be useful in determining an etiology, none can be used to predict SIDS. The evaluation depends on the history; not all tests need to be performed in all patients.

The pneumogram (see Fig. 2), a recording of heart and respiratory rate, is often used in the evaluation of an infant with apnea. This study can determine if periodic breathing or apnea occurs, but it cannot determine the type of apnea (central or obstructive) or, more importantly, the severity (i.e., if the event is associated with hypoxemia or hypercarbia). We use pneumograms for follow-up and monitoring rather than diagnosis or determination of physiologic consequences.

A polysomnogram (see Fig. 1) is a recording of 3 or more variables, which include chest wall impedance and heart rate as well as any of the

TABLE 4. Evaluation of the Infant with Apnea

Laboratory Tests	Possible Diagnosis
Complete blood count (CBC) with differential	Infection, metabolic
Electrolytes, calcium, glucose, serum bicarbonate	Metabolic, infection, confirmation of event
Chest radiograph	Respiratory abnormality, infection, cardiac
Electrocardiogram (EKG)	Cardiac arrhythmia
Urinalysis and culture	Infection, metabolic
Electroencephalogram (EEG)	Seizure disorder
Polysomnogram ± pH probe	Cardiorespiratory abnormality (obstructive apnea or CCHS), hypoxemia, GER
Barium swallow*	Airway abnormality, GER
Milk scintiscan	GER
Additional laboratory tests (depending on the history)	
Sepsis work-up (blood, CSF, urine culture)	Infection
Capillary or arterial blood gas	CCHS, metabolic, endocrinologic
(RSV) culture/fluorescent antibody	RSV infection or bronchiolitis
Pertussis culture/fluorescent antibody	Pertussis
Laryngoscopy/bronchoscopy	Airway abnormality
Cardiology evaluation	Cardiac abnormality
Neurology evaluation	Neurologic disorder

*A barium swallow is obtained to rule out any anatomic abnormalities that would cause either pathologic reflux or apnea; it is not used to diagnose reflux. CCHS = congenital central hypoventilation syndrome; GER = gastroesophageal reflux; CSF = cerebrospinal fluid; RSV = respiratory syncytial virus.

following: nasal thermistor to detect air flow; capnograph to measure CO_2 for detection of hypercarbia; esophageal pH probe to measure acidity and gastroesophageal reflux; and pulse oximetry to detect hypoxemic episodes, with or without concomitant electroencephalography (EEG). During either pneumogram or polysomnogram studies, sedatives (e.g., chloral hydrate and narcotics) cannot be given for at least 24 hours. Studies should not be done in the immediate postoperative period (24–48 hours) if general anesthesia is used. Both sedatives and general anesthesia can change the results of the study.

Management of the Infant with Apnea

The therapy for apnea of prematurity is the administration of methylxanthines: theophylline or caffeine, both of which are central respiratory stimulants that effectively decrease the frequency of periodic breathing and apnea. The loading dose of theophylline is 5 mg/kg followed 12 hours later with a maintenance dose in preterm infants of 1–2 mg/kg/day divided every 12 hours and in term infants of 2–4 mg/kg/day divided every 12 hours. Blood levels should be maintained at 8–12 μg/dl. The loading dose of caffeine citrate is 20 μg/kg followed 24 hours later with a maintenance dose of 5 mg/kg/day. The therapeutic range is 8–20 μg/dl. Levels of theophylline or caffeine should be obtained every 2 weeks after a steady state is achieved, because the metabolism of the methylxanthines changes significantly with growth. Caffeine is preferable to theophylline, because it is a more potent stimulator of the central nervous system and respiratory system, has a greater therapeutic range, and is given only once a day.

We continue therapy for 3 months or until the infant reaches 40 weeks of gestational age. If the infant has had no apneic events during this period, the medication is withheld. A 4-channel polysomnogram is performed 4 days (if treated with theophylline) or 7 days (if treated with caffeine) after medication is discontinued. If the study is normal, the medication is discontinued. If the study is abnormal, the medication is resumed for another month.

Preterm infants who have refractory disease with obstructive or mixed episodes of apnea may benefit from continuous positive airway pressure (CPAP). This technique is used to overcome the negative pressure in the hypopharynx during inspiration. A pressure of 4–6 cm H_2O via nasal prongs is used. Some preterm infants with refractory apnea of prematurity require mechanical ventilation.

Doxapram, an analeptic respiratory stimulant used in refractory apnea, acts mainly through stimulation of the carotid chemoreceptors, although larger doses also stimulate the respiratory center. An initial loading dose of 2.5–3 mg/kg is given intravenously over 15–30 minutes and followed by 1.0 mg/kg/hr continuous infusion. The continuous infusion may be increased by 0.5 mg/kg/hr to a maximum of 2.5 mg/kg/hr. Blood pressure should be measured frequently because of hypertension noted with infusions >1.5 mg/kg/hr or at plasma levels >5 mg/L. When the apneic episodes are under control, the infusion rate may be decreased. The serum concentration should be 1.5–5 μg/ml. Doxapram has a wide margin of safety, but its use is limited to hospitalized patients.

In older infants treatment depends on the underlying cause—e.g., anticonvulsant therapy, antibiotics, oxygen, antireflux medication. Therapy for infants with GER consists of small, frequent, thickened feedings as well as prone positioning with the head elevated during sleep. Thickened feedings are controversial. **Situations that increase intraabdominal pressure, such as placing the infant in a seated and supine position (e.g., infant car seat), should be avoided.**

Pharmacologic management includes metoclopramide, 0.1 mg/kg/dose 4 times/day (30 minutes before meals and at bedtime) and cimetidine, 10 mg/kg/dose 4 times/day, or ranitidine, 1–2 mg/kg/dose twice daily. If the infant continues to have apneic events, a reflux scintiscan/milk scan is performed. If GER continues to be present, bethanecol, 0.1–0.2 mg/kg/dose every 6–8 hr, can be used in place of metoclopramide. Fundoplication is indicated in rare instances if medical management has failed and the patient continues to have apneic events.

Infants with acute episodes of apnea due to an infectious cause (RSV/sepsis) may require mechanical ventilation as well as other medical therapy (antibiotics). **Infants with apnea due to an infectious cause must be hospitalized.**

Home Monitoring

No universally accepted criteria determine when to prescribe a monitor. However, the NIH consensus panel recommends cardiorespiratory monitoring for certain groups of infants at high risk for sudden death. This group includes infants with one or more severe apneic episodes that require resuscitation, vigorous stimulation, or cardiac massage; preterm infants who continue to have pathologic apnea; siblings of two or more SIDS victims; and infants with certain diseases or conditions (e.g., CCHS, uncontrolled seizure disorder). Even though the NIH recommendation suggests monitoring of an infant after 2 siblings have died, most siblings of SIDS victims are monitored, usually because of family anxiety. **Routine monitoring of preterm infants without AOP is not indicated.**

Home monitoring is best carried out as part of a comprehensive, multidisciplinary program in conjunction with the primary physician. Having a technology-dependent infant at home is a stressful experience, and a team approach gives the family the needed support. Before an infant is discharged, parents and caregivers must be trained in the use of the monitor and cardiorespiratory resuscitation.

Two types of monitors are available: a standard cardiorespiratory monitor, which sounds an alarm when an apneic or bradycardic event has occurred, and the Smart Monitor (Healthdyne Technologies, Inc., Marietta, GA), a cardiorespiratory monitor with memory. The Smart Monitor records apnea or bradycardia as well as provides a record of compliance. We prefer the Smart Monitor. Events and compliance reports ("downloads") are obtained from the Smart Monitor monthly and whenever an event occurs. The tracings include chest wall impedance and heart rate a few seconds before, during, and a few seconds after the episode. In our program infants remain on the monitor for 3 months and are then reevaluated. If no events have been witnessed or recorded by the Smart Monitor for 3 months, a 4-channel polysomnogram is obtained at home. If the infant is receiving theophylline or caffeine, medications are withheld as discussed above. If the study is normal, the monitor (along with medication, if applicable) is discontinued. If the polysomnogram shows any abnormality, the monitor is continued for another 3 months. Three event-free months are recommended before discontinuation of the monitor; it is recommended that the infant experience a stressful event (i.e., upper respiratory infection or immunization) before discontinuation.

In siblings of children who succumbed to SIDS the length of monitoring is controversial. The monitor should be continued at least until the age of death of the sibling, although some authors have proposed continued monitoring until 1 year of age.

APNEA IN CHILDREN AND ADOLESCENTS

The most frequent cause of apnea in children and adolescents is obstructive sleep apnea (OSA).

Obstructive Sleep Apnea

Factors that may cause OSA include decrease in tone of the pharynx and hypopharynx and anatomic obstruction. The most common cause is hypertrophy of tonsils and adenoids.

Craniofacial malformations are also associated with upper airway obstruction, including mandibular hypoplasia and glossoptosis (Pierre-Robin, Treacher-Collins, and Crouzon syndromes). Disorders associated with macroglossia, nasal septal defects, choanal stenosis, nasal hematomas, polyps, and even allergic rhinitis may also cause obstruction and OSA.

Obesity is a common contributing factor in upper airway obstruction. The exact mechanism is unclear, but pharyngeal narrowing and external compression of the pharyngeal walls by an obese neck may be involved.

With inspiration the upper airway muscles should contract to maintain a patent airway during sleep. Several drugs, such as chloral hydrate, narcotics, opiates, and anesthesia, decrease the tone of the upper airway muscles. Neuromuscular disorders, myopathies, and brainstem lesions also may cause a decrease in muscle tone, with collapse of the upper airway during inspiration. The result is obstruction, especially during sleep.

The patient with OSA may become progressively asphyxiated until arousal from sleep by hypoxemia and hypercarbia. With arousal, patency of the upper airway is restored, along with air flow. The patient returns to sleep and the sequence is repeated up to hundreds of times a night. This repetitive sequence gives rise to most of the common signs and symptoms listed in Table 5. Complications of OSA include failure to thrive, systemic hypertension, cor pulmonale with heart failure, and neurobehavioral disturbances.

Evaluation

The history and physical examination are crucial to the evaluation of OSA. Diagnosis may be delayed for years, with development of serious complications.

Evaluation includes a lateral neck film to assess the patency of the upper airway, a complete blood count to detect polycythemia, and electrolyte measurement; elevated bicarbonate is an indication of chronic hypercarbia. Laryngoscopy and bronchoscopy help to determine the patency of the airway. If long-term hypoxemia is indicated, an EKG and echocardiogram are performed to rule out cor pulmonale. If OSA is suspected, polysomnography is indicated.

Treatment

The treatment of OSA depends on the cause of the obstruction. Adenoidectomy and tonsillectomy should be performed to relieve obstruction caused by enlarged adenoids or tonsils.

TABLE 5. Signs and Symptoms Associated with Obstructive Sleep Apnea

Nighttime	Daytime
Most common	
Loud snoring	Excessive sleepiness
Difficulty breathing	Increase in naps or length of nap
Pauses in breathing and arousals	Behavior or personality changes*
Others	Inability to concentrate
Restless sleep	Learning difficulty
Sweating	Morning headache
Enuresis	Frequent upper respiratory tract infections
Nightmares	
Night terrors	Mouth breathing

*Personality changes may range from aggressiveness or irritability and hyperactivity to depression and social withdrawal.

Repeat polysomnography should be performed in patients with severe obstructive apnea (hypoxia or hypercarbia) or if symptoms persist.

Nasal CPAP in younger children and inspiratory pressure with lower expiratory pressures supplied by face- or nose-mask system (BiPAP) are among the preferred methods of stenting the airway with positive pressure during sleep. This approach is indicated when a sleep study demonstrates airway obstruction or hypoventilation and the underlying cause of obstruction is not correctable. In the adolescent, we usually institute BiPAP with inspiratory pressure of 10–15 cm H_2O and expiratory pressure of 5 cm H_2O. Measurements of chest wall motion may be used as a guide in adjusting pressure settings. When the ribcage/abdominal asynchrony or paradox secondary to upper airway obstruction is abolished, adequate ventilator settings have been achieved. A subsequent sleep study is performed with CPAP or BiPAP before discharge from the hospital. The length of treatment varies with each patient, depending on the underlying cause of hypoventilation. Periodic reevaluation is warranted.

Many patients with severe OSA and craniofacial malformations require surgical intervention with tracheostomy or correction, although other less invasive forms of treatment are used when appropriate. In obese patients weight loss is recommended; however, this recommendation is usually unsuccessful.

Alveolar Hypoventilation

The major categories of alveolar hypoventilation seen in infants, children, and adolescents include impairment of ventilatory control, obesity, and neuromuscular disorders, all of which may be congenital or acquired. Congenital central hypoventilation syndrome (CCHS; Ondine curse) and obesity hypoventilation syndrome are discussed below.

Congenital Central Hypoventilation Syndrome

CCHS is a rare disorder with a broad spectrum of manifestations. It was originally described as a failure of automatic or metabolic control of breathing due to an insensitivity of the central chemoreceptor responses to carbon dioxide. Most affected children present in the newborn period with central apnea, failure to maintain adequate ventilation during sleep, or an ALTE.

In general, diagnosis of CCHS depends on documentation of central apnea or hypoventilation during sleep. Absent or blunted responsiveness to carbon dioxide is necessary to diagnose CCHS. Muscle dysfunction and lung disease must be ruled out.

The treatment of CCHS is limited. There is no cure, and the syndrome is lifelong. Support can be maintained with positive-pressure ventilation from portable ventilators. Positive-pressure ventilation requires a tracheostomy to maintain a stable airway.

Phrenic nerve pacing may be an alternative to positive-pressure ventilation in patients with CCHS. It is used when continuous pacing is not required or for daytime support in ambulatory patients requiring full-time ventilatory support. Patients who require full-time support are then supported during sleep with positive-pressure ventilation via tracheostomy.

Children with CCHS may have prolonged survival with a good quality of life as a result of the technology for home ventilation.

Obesity Hypoventilation Syndrome

Obesity hypoventilation syndrome (pickwickian syndrome) is a form of OSA due to obesity and abnormal control of breathing. It is characterized by obesity, somnolence as well as hypoventilation with carbon dioxide retention, cyanosis, pulmonary hypertension, and erythrocytosis. It is seen in patients with longstanding obesity, OSA, and Prader-Willi syndrome.

Symptoms are similar to those of OSA (see Table 5). Complications include right ventricular hypertrophy and pulmonary hypertension with heart failure as well as neurobehavioral disturbances.

Arterial blood gases should be measured in all patients suspected of having obesity hypoventilation syndrome. Noninvasive methods, such as pulse oximetry or end-tidal CO_2 monitoring, are not sufficient but may be helpful in subsequent management. Evaluation also should include exclusion of hypothyroidism and pulmonary function tests to determine if restrictive lung disease due to obesity is involved. Polysomnography should be used to determine the severity of the disease as well as in subsequent management of the patient.

Progesterone stimulates the ventilatory drive by increasing the sensitivity of the respiratory center to CO_2 and increasing minute ventilation. Medroxyprogesterone, 1.5–2.0 mg/kg/day (ideal body weight) orally or intramuscularly, is the agent of choice. A repeat polysomnogram is performed 1 week after therapy is initiated. Supplemental oxygen should be used during sleep to maintain an oxygen saturation >95%.

If pharmacologic treatment is unsuccessful in correcting the hypoxemia and hypercarbia, CPAP or BiPAP is used. Positive pressure ventilation with tracheostomy may be used if CPAP or BiPAP is not tolerated or unsuccessful. Behavioral modification and weight reduction should be attempted, but such attempts rarely succeed. Even with weight loss, hypoventilation may not be corrected immediately because of the change in the response to CO_2; it may correct over a period of months to years.

SUGGESTED READING

1. Beckerman RC, Brouillette RT, Hunt CE: Respiratory Control Disorders in Infants and Children. Baltimore, Williams & Wilkins, 1992.
2. Bradley TD, Phillipson EA: Pathogenesis and pathophysiology of the obstructive sleep apnea syndrome. Med Clin North Am 69:1169, 1985.
3. Kriter KE, Blanchard J: Therapy review: Management of apnea in infants. Clin Pharm 8:577, 1989.
4. Little GA, Ballard RA, Brooks JG, et al: Infantile Apnea and Home Monitoring: Report of the NIH Consensus Development Conference. NIH publ. no. 87-2905. Bethesda, MD, National Institutes of Health, 1987.
5. Mark JD, Brooks JG: Sleep-associated airway problems in children. Pediatr Clin North Am 31:907, 1984.
6. McElroy E, Steinschneider A, Weinstein S: Emotional and health impact of home monitoring on mothers: A controlled prospective study. Pediatrics 78:780, 1986.
7. Sheldon SH, Spire JP, Levy HB: Pediatric Sleep Medicine. Philadelphia, W.B. Saunders, 1992.
8. Spitzer AR, Fox WW: Infant apnea: An approach to management. Clin Pediatr 23:374, 1984.

23

PNEUMOTHORAX

Rohinton K. Balsara, M.D., F.A.C.S., F.A.C.C.P., and Gulnar R. Balsara, M.D.

In human embryology, the paired pleural cavities become separated from the pericardial cavity by the development of the pleural pericardial membranes. The paired pleural cavities are closed spaces. Each pleural space extends from the cervical area superiorly to the diaphragm inferiorly; anteriorly it extends to the retrosternal area in the midline and posteriorly to the level of the spine. Medially the visceral and parietal pleura fuse over the hilar structures. The normally expanded lung projects into the entire pleural cavity and converts it into a virtual space, but in diseased states the pleural cavity may contain increased amounts of air, fluid, or tumors, which cause compression of the lung parenchyma. Intrapleural pressure within the intact thorax is negative (subatmospheric) at all times and becomes more negative during inspiration. Pneumothorax may result in a mild change in pleural pressure with minimal lung collapse or in a large air accumulation with total lung collapse, shift of the mediastinum, and severe respiratory distress.

ETIOLOGY

Pneumothorax may be caused by trauma or associated with chronic inflammatory disease, such as cystic fibrosis and asthma; it also may occur spontaneously.

Traumatic pneumothorax may be due to penetrating injuries, such as stab wounds and gun shots, or nonpenetrating injuries, such as fractured ribs and tracheobronchial lacerations. The term *closed pneumothorax* is occasionally used to describe the second category, whereas *open pneumothorax* describes the first. In the present age of high-speed travel and high- and low-velocity injuries, pneumothorax should be considered as a possible complication of chest injuries. Another cause of traumatic pneumothorax is continuous positive-pressure ventilation in the care of the critically ill patient. In some instances of serious chest injury, esophageal perforation may cause pneumomediastinum and subsequent pneumothorax.

Spontaneous pneumothorax usually results from rupture of subpleural blebs located at the apex of the upper lobe or in the superior segment of the lower lobe. However, many patients develop spontaneous pneumothorax with no apparent cause of air leaks from the lung parenchyma. Although trauma has been incriminated as a precipitating factor in some cases, spontaneous pneumothorax usually occurs when the patient is at rest. It is seen more frequently in males than females, and the incidence is highest between the ages of 15 and 30 years, usually in tall, asthenic individuals.

Catamenial pneumothorax is a rare entity in which spontaneous pneumothorax occurs concurrently and repeatedly with the menses. The right side is involved more frequently than the left. Endometriosis involving the diaphragm has been occasionally demonstrated during thoracotomy. In an estimated 5% of women who sustain spontaneous pneumothorax during their child-bearing years, a relationship to menses is reported.

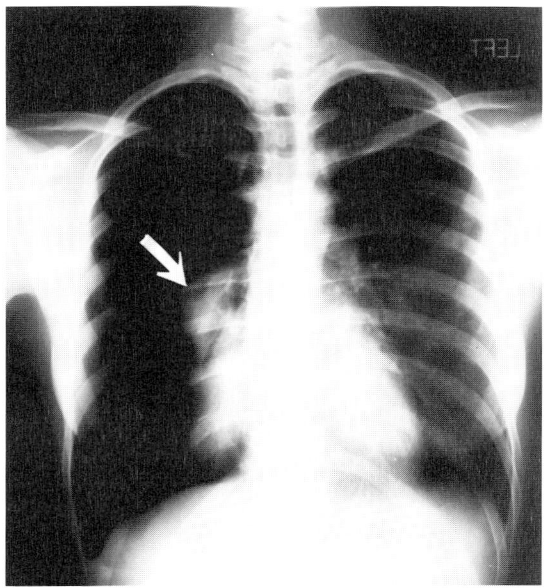

FIGURE 1. Anteroposterior chest roentgenogram shows tension pneumothorax on the right. Arrow shows completely collapsed right lung.

Pneumothorax may occur in association with pulmonary neoplasm. Metastatic osteogenic sarcomas have a high propensity to cause pneumothorax, because they are frequently located in the subpleural areas and may lead to necrosis and rupture of the lung parenchyma.

Pneumothorax occasionally results from rupture of inflammatory or congenital blebs in

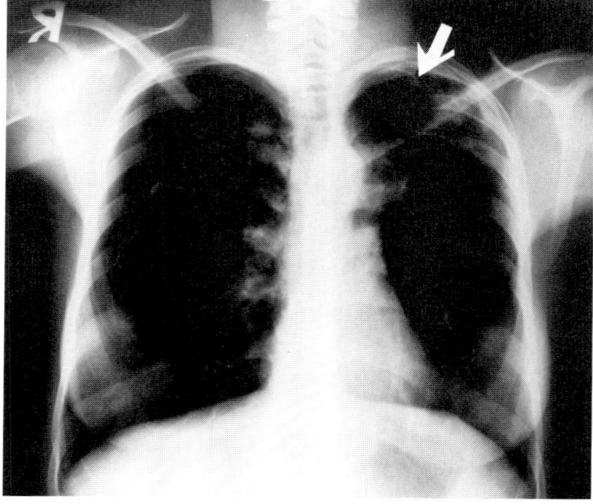

FIGURE 2. Anteroposterior chest roentgenogram shows pneumothorax with partial collapse of the right lung. Arrow shows stapling of blebs at apex of left lung.

conditions such as pneumatocele, lung cysts, bronchopulmonary dysplasia, and asthma.

In the newborn infant, interstitial emphysema is often the consequence of overstretching and rupture of the patent alveoli, while a major portion of the lung remains atelectatic. This situation often results when overzealous pressure ventilation during resuscitative efforts leads to dissection of air along the bronchi and perivascular spaces, which then ruptures into the free pleural space and causes pneumothorax.

In cases of tension pneumothorax (Fig. 1), the severe shift of the heart and mediastinal structures to the opposite side may lead to cardiovascular collapse and, if unrecognized and untreated, even to rapid death. On rare occasions, pneumothorax may be bilateral. In patients with pleural adhesions due either to previous infections, such as cystic fibrosis, or to surgery, the pneumothorax tends to be localized (Fig. 2). A tear of the adhesions or small vessel in the bleb wall occasionally may result in hemothorax. Rarely is the bleeding severe enough to require blood transfusion or emergency exploratory thoracotomy.

CLINICAL PRESENTATION

Clinical signs and symptoms accompanying spontaneous pneumothorax depend in large part on the magnitude of the pulmonary collapse. Although the onset may be insidious and the condition disclosed during an incidental physical examination or chest roentgenogram, more often the event is signaled by sudden, severe chest pain and dyspnea. Usually there is no relationship to activity, and pneumothorax may occur without warning during quiet time. Pneumothorax occurs much less commonly during bouts of coughing or vigorous activity. In patients with a propensity for pneumothorax or a history of previous pneumothoraces, high-altitude flying or deep-water diving may precipitate rupture of a subpleural bleb and cause pneumothorax.

The pain associated with pneumothorax is sharp, knifelike, and aggravated by normal respiratory movement. The pain is located most often in the lower lateral chest wall, but it may radiate to the anterior abdominal wall, simulating an acute abdominal crisis.

In cases of penetrating chest injuries, a hissing sound due to the egress of air from the open chest indicates obvious violation of the pleural space. Other clinical findings include a shift of the trachea to the side opposite to the lesion, hyperresonance on percussion, and absent or decreased breath sounds on the side of the pneumothorax. Chest radiographs (preferably posteroanterior in an upright position) may be diagnostic. In the differential diagnosis of pneumothorax in infants, one should always include a rapidly expanding congenital cystic lesion, such as congenital lobar emphysema.

NEONATAL PNEUMOTHORAX

Pneumothorax, especially in a small premature infant, can be diagnosed at bedside with the transillumination technique. If the chest cavity transilluminates when a lighted flashlight is applied against the patient's chest wall in a darkened room, the patient has pneumothorax. This test may not be useful in full-term neonates, who have fair amounts of soft tissue over the chest wall.

TREATMENT

The treatment of pneumothorax depends on its cause, the extent of the collapse, and the number of episodes of collapse in an individual patient.

A small, asymptomatic pneumothorax needs only observation and no intervention. If the pneumothorax encompasses 25% or more of the lung volume, as grossly determined by examining the radiograph (a lung margin >2 cm from the chest wall), needle aspiration may suffice. However, if the patient has apical blebs or a complicating underlying condition, or if one suspects a high risk for a persistent air leak, a tube thoracostomy should be performed.

Thoracentesis is the drainage of air or fluid from the thoracic cavity through a needle or catheter inserted through the chest wall. If performed early and effectively, it may eliminate the need for chest tube insertion and surgical therapy. The most common error in thoracentesis is to insert the needle too low. The operator has to remember that the dome of the diaphragm normally rises to the sixth interspace during expiration and may remain elevated during inspiration if the patient has atelectasis, diaphragmatic paralysis, or subphrenic pathology. Penetration of the diaphragm by the thoracentesis needle occurs more commonly than realized, and this fact should be suspected if dry tap or bloody tap (traumatic) occurs. Use of low tap in the sitting position is frequently based on two erroneous beliefs: (1) the needle has to be inserted below the level of percussed dullness or below the fluid level visible on chest radiographs to avoid injury to the lung, and (2) the needle has to be directed downward in the pleural cavity to evacuate the most dependent drainage. Both of these premises have proved to be invalid.

The authors prefer the decubitus position for thoracentesis, especially in children, because of five distinct advantages: (1) a sedated child does not tolerate an upright position well; (2) the patient can be better restrained, if necessary, with the arms raised above the head; (3) the chest can be entered with the needle in the midaxillary line as high as possible (usually the fourth interspace) without obstruction by the scapula; (4) the needle can be directed either inferiorly (caudad) or posteriorly (toward the spine) to maximize fluid drainage; and (5) both pneumothorax and effusion can be aspirated safely, effectively, and, in most cases, completely by this route.

Materials for Thoracentesis

Thoracentesis and chest-tube insertion trays can be prepared by the central sterilization services of the hospital, or disposable, commercially available packs may be used. Each pack usually contains:

1. Applicators (sponges or pads) soaked in iodophor for antiseptic cleaning of the skin
2. Sterile gloves
3. Sterile towels
4. Xylocaine 1% without epinephrine (1 vial)
5. Disposable needles, ½-in 25-gauge and 1½-in 21-gauge
6. Plastic needle
7. Three-way stopcock and 12-in extension tubing
8. Test tubes, 3, for specimens
9. Fluid collection chamber

Procedure

After adequate sedation, the patient is placed in a supine position with the head of the bed elevated to an angle of 30°. The sterile tray is unwrapped on a sidetable, and the equipment is checked with sterile technique. Then a wide area of the skin is prepared with antiseptic solution and draped with sterile towels. The optimal interspace to be entered is selected by digital palpation, and the skin and soft tissues of the rib cage are anesthetized with 1% xylocaine. Next, the plastic needle with stylus is introduced into the chest, always aimed at the rib below, and gently advanced superiorly over the top of the lower rib. This approach avoids injury to intercostal vessels located in the undersurface of the upper rib. One must always aspirate for blood as the needle is advanced, because discovery of blood in the syringe suggests injury of an intercostal vessel or puncture of the liver and spleen.

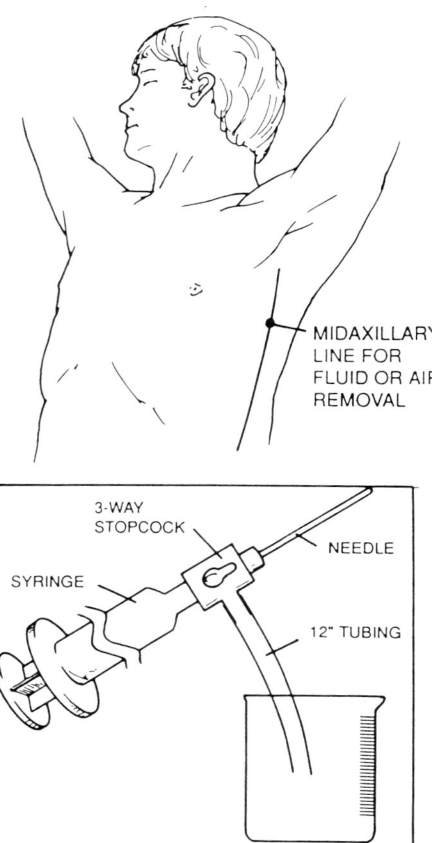

FIGURE 3. Technique of thoracentesis.

The needle must be withdrawn, and if the operator is in doubt, the chest must be entered in the next higher interspace. Once free flow of fluid is obtained, the stylus is removed, the needle is connected to a 3-way stopcock, and extension tubing with a syringe attachment is connected to complete the procedure (Fig. 3). The depth of the needle in the chest cavity should be carefully controlled with one hand while the other hand performs the aspiration. At the conclusion of the procedure the needle is removed. Clinical and radiographic evidence of residual fluid and/or pneumothorax must be obtained.

Chest Tubes

A chest tube is like a drain. Its purpose is to evacuate air, blood, or fluid from the pleural cavity. Chest tubes have been known from the days of Hippocrates, but only in the last few decades has their use been better defined. Early chest tubes were made of red rubber, because it was believed that a stiff, irritating tube would help to seal the air leaks and to stimulate pleural adhesions. Currently the ideal chest tube is nontoxic, nonthrombogenic, and pliable. Pliability helps to avoid laceration of tissue during insertion, to prevent pressure necrosis of the tissue while in place, and to maintain enough rigidity to avoid obstruction by external kinking. The tube should have multiple eyelets spirally arranged in the distal third to facilitate drainage, and it should be radiopaque for identification of eyelets and position of the tube on chest radiographs.

Technique for Insertion of Chest Tubes

The patient must be prepared with injection of a local anesthetic, as for thoracentesis. Before insertion of the chest tube, it is always safe first to aspirate and obtain free flow of liquid with a needle. Once this is accomplished, a skin incision about 5–10 mm long is made, depending on the size of the chest tube. A curved "mosquito" hemostat is inserted, and the soft tissues are spread gently, with care to stay just above the lower rib, and the pleura is punctured. The hemostat and the desired trocar chest catheter are inserted through the previously created tract. Once the chest is entered, the trocar is retracted about 1 cm and the chest tube is advanced in any desired position within the pleural cavity. The trocar is removed, and the tube is clamped to prevent air from entering or fluid from spilling out.

The tube is secured to the chest wall first with a suture and then with tapes. The proximal end of the tube is connected to a drainage collection chamber, and the clamp is released. Hourly measurements of quantity and quality of fluid are recorded. The chest tube connections should be well secured and taped to avoid inadvertent disconnection and resultant pneumothorax.

If two tubes are inserted (possibly connected to the same suction source), it is preferable to use a Y connector rather than a T connector to avoid accidental kinking, which results in impaired drainage. Milking of chest tubes implies gentle, alternate compression and release of the latex tubing between the Pleur-Evac and the chest tubing. This procedure causes a momentary short burst of suction within the tube and helps to dislodge or propel clots and fibrinoid exudate forward. Stripping, on the other hand, implies much vigorous compression and release of the tube. **Stripping should be avoided, because it may generate unnecessarily high negative intrapleural pressures that can traumatize the lung parenchyma. Clamping of chest tubes for transportation should be discouraged, especially in patients with suspected persistent air leak, because clamping causes the air to accumulate in the pleural cavity and results in tension pneumothorax.**

If at any time a fluid specimen is needed for laboratory tests, the fluid should be aspirated under sterile conditions by puncturing the self-seal diaphragm present in the collection chamber of the Pleur-Evac. Specimens should *not* be obtained by (1) breaking the system and disconnecting the connectors or (2) puncturing the chest or latex tubing, because the tubes are not self-sealing.

Removal of Chest Tube

Before removal of any chest tube, one must make sure that there is no air leak. The chest tube may be temporarily clamped and the patient observed for respiratory distress, which may indicate reaccumulation of pneumothorax. A chest radiograph also may be obtained to confirm presence or absence of pneumothorax. Once the decision is made to remove the tube, the operator cuts the suture used to anchor the tube to the chest wall and asks the patient to perform a Valsalva maneuver while removing the tube rapidly and smoothly. The chest-tube site is occluded with Vaseline gauze, which is held in place with a wide tape tightly applied by an assistant to create an air-tight seal.

Three-bottle Chest Drainage System

In the three-bottle chest drainage system, the various bottles are interconnected, but each serves a separate function (Fig. 4A). The first bottle is the volumetrically graduated collection bottle, which is nearest the patient and collects the drainage from the chest through a short glass tube at the top.

The second bottle is the water-seal bottle, which is the most important component of the system. It acts as a one-way valve, allowing air and fluid to leave the pleural cavity but not to reenter, and thus maintains negative pressure. Water can be drawn up the tube only to a height equal to the negative intrathoracic pressure, which rarely exceeds -20 cm H_2O. The apparatus, therefore, must be kept far enough below the patient to prevent suction of water into the chest (100 cm is sufficient under any circumstance). The end of the tube must be covered with water at all times, or the water seal will be broken. The usually recommended depth is 2 cm below the surface of the water in the bottle, but if the end of the tube remains far below the surface, the resistance offered to the expulsion of air and fluid from the chest equals the underwater length of the tube; for example, if the tube is 20 cm below the surface, 20 cm H_2O positive pressure is required to drive the air out of the pleural space, and the lung simply would not be capable of expanding.

Caution: If the collection bottle (bottle 1) were to be eliminated from the system, then fluid entering the water-seal chamber (bottle 2) would steadily increase the water level; this, in turn, would increase the resistance to expulsion of air from the pleural cavity, thus making the system ineffectual after a time.

The third bottle is the suction regulator, a sealed container with an atmospheric vent that

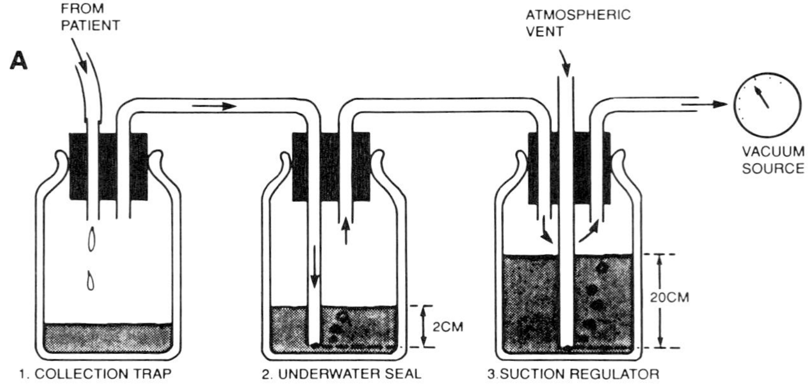

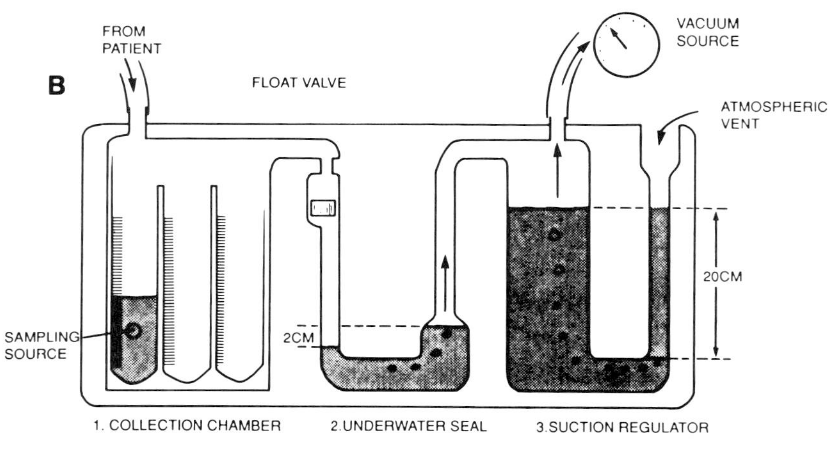

FIGURE 4. *A,* Three-bottle chest drainage system. *B,* Pleur-Evac system.

is used to measure and control suction applied from an external source. The maximal force of suction is determined by the underwater depth of the vent tube in bottle 3. For example, to obtain a suction of -20 cm H_2O, the tip of the vent tube should be set 20 cm below the surface of the fluid in bottle 3. By applying vacuum to the short arm of bottle 3 (Fig. 4A), the water column in the vent tube is pulled down, and further increase in vacuum allows the atmospheric air to enter the bottle and to bubble at a constant rate. **Further increase in vacuum increases the rate of bubbling in bottle 3 but in no way increases the negative pressure.** Excessive wall suction not only causes loud bubbling, which may disturb the patient, but also hastens evaporation of water from bottle 3, thus decreasing the suction applied.

As one can imagine, this system has several drawbacks: (1) the system needs resterilization after each use; (2) it is cumbersome and bulky, thus preventing freedom of ambulation for the patient; (3) the unit has multiple connections that may easily become undone; and (4) breakage and spillovers are quite common.

Pleur-Evac

Pleur-Evac, a currently available system, has reduced the three-bottle set-up to a single, disposable, light-weight, and compact unit (Fig. 4B). The chest drainage enters directly into the collecting chamber, which is analogous to bottle 1. This chamber is marked in graduated increments for determining the rate and volume of drainage. The underwater seal chamber is analogous to bottle 2. The seal is formed by an asymmetric U tube. The narrow arm of the U is equivalent to the underwater tubing, whereas the wide arm represents the water reservoir in bottle 2. When the water level is 2 cm above the seal in the U tube, the same effect is achieved as with the submerged tubing in bottle 2 of the three-bottle system.

The suction regulation chamber (analogous to bottle 3) also has an asymmetric U-shaped configuration. The narrow arm acts as the atmospheric vent and the wide arm as the reservoir. Application of external suction raises the fluid in the reservoir and pulls the fluid down the vent. If sufficient negative pressure is applied, then atmospheric air comes down the air vent and bubbles through the reservoir. It is recommended that the reservoir be filled to the 15–20 cm water level for general Pleur-Evac usage. Again, as in the three-bottle system, increasing the negative wall vacuum does not increase the negative intrapleural pressures. In fact, a large negative pressure may have the adverse effect of collapsing the system; the system may even explode under atmospheric pressure.

On-the-spot management of tension pneumothorax can be accomplished simply by inserting a sterile needle into the pleural cavity and allowing the tension to be relieved. Once this is accomplished, intermittent occlusion of the needle hub with a finger allows the lung to expand while arrangements are made to insert the chest tube. Sometimes a finger cot (with a tiny hole at its tip) may be attached to the hub of the needle. This acts as a one-way valve that allows the air from the pleural cavity to escape but prevents entrance of atmospheric air.

Heimlich Valve

The Heimlich valve is a commercially available disposable unit with a one-way valve mechanism connected to a chest tube. This unit is useful in patients in whom the chest tubes must be kept in place for prolonged periods. It also may be useful while transporting a patient with multiple trauma to the hospital. The Heimlich valve eliminates the need for a Pleur-Evac.

TABLE 1. Troubleshooting

Problem	Cause	Solution
No chest drainage	Patient unstable	
	Tube kinked or filled with clots	Free tube of kinks
	Rapid reaccumulation of fluid	Reposition Pleur-Evac at least 3 ft below patient level
		Milk or strip tube of clots
	Patient stable	
	Absence of fluid in chest (clinically and radiographically)	No action Discontinue chest tube
Patient accidentally pulls out tube	Not restrained	No distress—apply occlusive dressing Distress or air leak—reinsert new chest tube
Collection chamber full	Continued fluid drainage	Replace with new unit (fill new unit with water first to reduce change over time)
New or unexpected air bubbling	Tube connection loose or cracked	Retighten or replace connection
	New pleural leak	Keep lung expanded and avoid development of new pneumothorax
	Air sucked in from tube tract	Apply new occlusive dressing Seal tube tract with additional suture
No bubbling in water seal chamber	Not enough water in chamber	Add additional water
No bubbling in suction control chamber	Suction not turned on	Connect and turn suction on
Unit tips over and spills	Not properly placed or anchored	Refill unit Replace with new unit

TROUBLESHOOTING

All chest drainage systems have three components: the chest tube, the drainage system, and the Pleur-Evac. Whenever a problem arises, one should check systematically each part of the system, starting with the patient (Table 1).

NONRESOLVING PNEUMOTHORAX

Patients with a persistent air leak and patients suspected to be at risk for recurrent pneumothoraces (e.g., recurrent spontaneous pneumothorax, pneumothorax associated with cystic fibrosis) may need further intervention. Chemical pleurodesis with various agents used to be recommended. The increasing lack of availability of sclerosing agents, the variable results, the excruciating pain resulting from chemical pleuritis, and possible impairment of diaphragm motion have made this procedure less desirable. A transaxillary, muscle-sparing minithoracotomy with stapling or excision of blebs and pleurodesis by pleural abrasion or pleurectomy is preferable. Video-assisted thoracoscopic surgery is currently gaining acceptance among surgical specialists for the management of pneumothorax.

SUGGESTED READING

1. Almind M, Large P, Viskum K: Spontaneous pneumothorax: Comparison of simple drainage, talc pleurodesis, and tetracycline pleurodesis. Thorax 144:627–630, 1989.
2. DeLauriers J, Beaulieu M, Despres JP, et al: Transaxillary pleurectomy for treatment of spontaneus pneumothroax. Ann Thorac Surg 30:569–574, 1980.
3. Durtschi MB: Use of thoracoscopy in clinical practice. Am J Surg 165:592–594, 1993.
4. Erickson RS: Mastering the ins and outs of chest drainage. Part I. Nursing May:37–44, 1989.
5. Erickson RS: Mastering the ins and outs of chest drainage. Part II. Nursing June:47–50, 1989.
6. Fagalu O, Braun R: Spontaneous pneumothorax as first manifestation of bronchial carcinoma and mesothelioma. Contemp Surg 31:39–42, 1987.
7. Kuhn LR, Bednarak FJ, Wyman ML, et al: Diagnosis of pneumothorax or pneumomediastinum in the neonate by transillumination. Pediatrics 56:355–360, 1975.
8. Miller KS, Sahn SA: Chest tubes: Indications, technique, management and complications. Chest 91:258–264, 1987.
9. Olson PS, Anderson HO: Long term results after tetracycline pleurodesis in spontaneous pneumothorax. Ann Thorac Surg 53:1015–1017, 1992.
10. Plans WJ: Delayed pneumothorax after subclavian vein catheterization. J Parenter Ent Nutr 14:414–415, 1990.
11. Rodgers BM: Pediatric thoracoscopy: Where have we come and what have we learned? Ann Thorac Surg 56:704–707, 1993.
12. Shearin RPN, Hepper NG, Payne WS: Recurrent spontaneous pneumothorax concurrent with menses. Mayo Clin Proc 49:98–101, 1974.
13. Wakebayaski A: Expanded application of diagnostic and therapeutic thoracoscopy. J Thorac Cardiovasc Surg 102:721–723, 1991.

24

CHEST TRAUMA

John Loiselle, M.D.

Injuries are the leading cause of death in children over 1 year of age. Chest injuries occur in up to 30% of children hospitalized for trauma and are second only to head injuries for associated mortality among injured children under 15 years of age. The overall mortality rate in all children with moderate or severe chest trauma ranges from 4–14% and is even higher in children under 5 years of age. The majority of deaths occur within 1 hour of presentation.

Despite these disturbing statistics, the overwhelming majority of chest trauma in the pediatric patient is minor and rarely results in significant injury. The vast majority of thoracic injuries that a general practitioner is likely to encounter in an ambulatory care setting consists of inconsequential contusions and abrasions. Futhermore, the few pediatric patients with serious chest injuries almost always can be managed without surgical intervention or with a simple thoracostomy.

It is, however, important for the practitioner to recognize children likely to have more significant chest injuries and to be prepared to initiate temporizing measures in the rare instances of severe chest injuries. Careful attention to the mechanism of injury, a thorough physical assessment, and knowledge of unique pediatric anatomic features are necessary for accurate diagnosis and management of such patients.

UNIQUE FEATURES OF THE PEDIATRIC CHEST

Specific features of pediatric chest anatomy in conjunction with the common mechanisms of injury in pediatric chest trauma result in a different response to injury and a different pattern of injuries from what is observed in adults. The chest wall of a child is more compliant because of the less mineralized and more cartilaginous rib cage. The smaller anteroposterior diameter, paucity of soft tissue, and underdeveloped musculature allow a greater transfer of energy to the internal organs. The mediastinum is fairly mobile, placing the child at greater risk of cardiovascular compromise when it is compressed.

ETIOLOGY

Children sustain chest injuries in different ways from adults. Over 80% of serious chest injuries in children are the result of blunt trauma, and subsequent chest trauma is frequently only part of a multisystem injury. **The head and extremities are the two most commonly injured areas associated with chest trauma in children.** As in the adult population, chest injuries in children are predominantly the result of motor vehicle accidents (Fig. 1). Unlike adults, **the majority of children sustain injuries as pedestrians rather than motor vehicle occupants.** Steering wheel impact contributes to a large number of adult chest injuries, whereas children are more likely to become injured by wandering into the street.

Mechanisms of injury vary even within the pediatric population. **Of all significant chest injuries, 5–10% are due to child abuse, with the vast majority occurring in children under 3 years of age.** Pedestrian-motor vehicle accidents

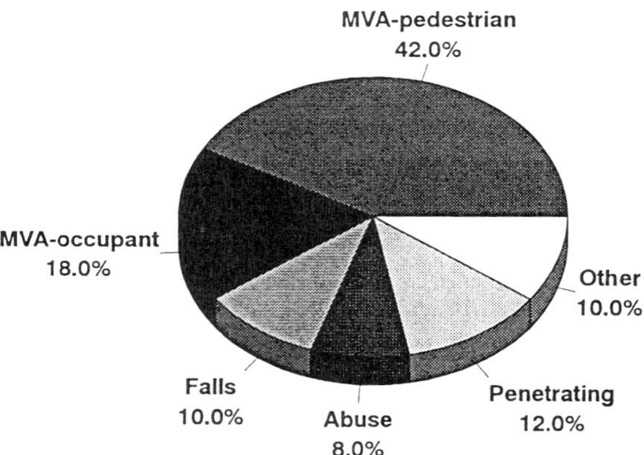

FIGURE 1. Chest trauma in children—mechanisms of injury. MVA = motor vehicle accident.

predominate in the 5–10-year-old age group. This is also the age at which sports injuries appear. The adolescent years see an increase in passenger-related motor vehicle accidents, falls, bicycling accidents, and penetrating trauma.

GENERAL APPROACH

History

The amount of kinetic energy expended on the internal organs is the major determinant of the severity of intrathoracic injury. A careful determination of the energy involved is therefore an important factor in the assessment of a child with chest trauma. Kinetic energy is proportional to the mass of an object and the square of its velocity. A baseball is capable of inflicting a different severity of injury, depending on whether it is thrown by a 5-year-old child or an adult. Similarly, an automobile traveling at 25 miles per hour causes greater damage than a football traveling at the same speed. A detailed description of the mechanism of injury and a subsequent estimate of the applied force are important factors in the anticipation of potential injuries.

A recent history of chest trauma may not be related to the patient's complaint of chest pain. The physician should consider additional etiologies if the degree of chest pain is incompatible with the mechanism of injury or if additional symptoms, such as fever, are present.

Physical Examination

Physical findings in children with intrathoracic injuries may be obvious, subtle, or virtually nonexistent. Evaluation always begins with the primary survey of airway, breathing, and circulation (the ABCs), followed first by necessary resuscitative measures and then by the secondary survey. The early physical assessment of thoracic trauma includes inspection, auscultation, and percussion.

The patient should be undressed for adequate inspection. The back should be visualized to avoid overlooking any injuries. Inspection begins with the measurement of the resting respiratory rate. A posttraumatic respiratory rate that is out of proportion to the child's age and degree of anxiety provokes concern and suggests intrathoracic injury. **Malformations of the bony chest wall and contusions or abrasions should be noted, but their absence does not rule out intrathoracic injury.** An increased work of breathing is further indicated by the use of accessory muscles of inspiration or the presence of nasal flaring. Evidence of splinting helps to focus the examination, especially in the young child. Very severe injuries are suggested by tracheal deviation, neck-vein engorgement, and asymmetric expansion of the chest. Cyanosis is generally an ominous sign that occurs late in respiratory failure.

Auscultation at the midaxillary lines accentuates any differences in breath sounds. Abnormalities include asymmetry of breath sounds or presence of rales. Muffled heart sounds or a pericardial friction rub suggests significant cardiac injury. Palpation may elicit localized tenderness or instability of the chest wall. Both the neck and the chest wall are palpated for evidence of subcutaneous emphysema. Percussion is useful in differentiating intrathoracic accumulation of fluid versus air.

The child with a low-impact mechanism of injury, normal vital signs, no point tenderness, no signs or symptoms of respiratory compromise, and only a small contusion or abrasion has suffered only mild chest trauma and can be adequately assessed with a thorough history and physical examination. A child with a moderate- or high-impact injury, signs and symptoms of intrathoracic injury, or abnormal vital signs requires additional evaluation (Table 1).

TABLE 1. Mechanisms and Clinical Presentations of Chest Trauma

	Minor	Moderate	Severe
Mechanism of injury	Wrestling Short fall (stairs) Occupant in minor MVA Low-speed projectile (baseball, stone)	Moderate-speed projectile (baseball, stone) Fall >8–10 ft	Pedestrian–MVA Penetrating high-speed projectile (bullet) Fall >20 ft Multisystem trauma with head and abdominal injuries
Vital signs	Normal	Elevated respiratory rate Normal heart rate Normal blood pressure	Elevated respiratory rate Abnormal heart rate Abnormal blood pressure
Physical examination	Minimal tenderness Normal lung sounds	Localized tenderness Splinting Decreased breath sounds	Abnormal mental status Absent breath sounds Unstable rib cage Cyanosis Tracheal deviation Chest wall asymmetry Distended neck veins
Potential injuries	Abrasions Contusion	Rib fracture Pulmonary contusion Myocardial contusion Costochondral separation Pneumothorax	Tension pneumothorax Cardiac tamponade Esophageal rupture Flail chest Massive hemothorax Tracheobronchial tree injury

MVA = motor vehicle accident.

A high-quality upright chest radiograph is necessary in the evaluation of a child in whom moderate or severe chest trauma is suspected on the basis of the historical or physical evidence. An electrocardiogram should be obtained when cardiac injury is suspected on the basis of the mechanism of injury, substernal pain, or findings on examination such as a pericardial friction rub, tachycardia, muffled heart sounds, or irregularities of heart rate.

CHEST INJURIES

Pulmonary Contusions

Pulmonary contusions are the most commonly reported intrathoracic injuries resulting from chest trauma in the child. They are present in more than 50% of all pediatric patients with thoracic injuries. They occur most frequently as the result of automobile-pedestrian accidents, although they have been reported secondary to abuse and falls from significant heights. Pulmonary contusions are injuries to the lung parenchyma that involve local hemorrhage and edema (Fig. 2). External chest wall findings are frequently absent. Symptoms are often subtle and may be delayed. Patients may present with tachypnea, splinting, or localized lung findings on examination. More severe cases may present with hemoptysis or hypoxia secondary to ventilation-perfusion mismatch.

The majority of pulmonary contusions are visible as densities on a radiograph, although in some cases the onset of findings may be delayed up to 48 hours. A repeat film and a period of observation are necessary if the initial radiograph is negative but suspicion of injury is high or respiratory symptoms are present.

Treatment for pulmonary contusions includes supplemental oxygen, elevation of the head of the bed so that gravity may help to improve lung expansion, and limitation of fluids. No evidence suggests that the administration of prophylactic antibiotics prevents subsequent infection. In severe or extensive contusions endotracheal intubation and positive-pressure ventilation may be necessary.

Rib Fractures

Rib fractures, the second most frequent injury resulting from pediatric chest trauma,

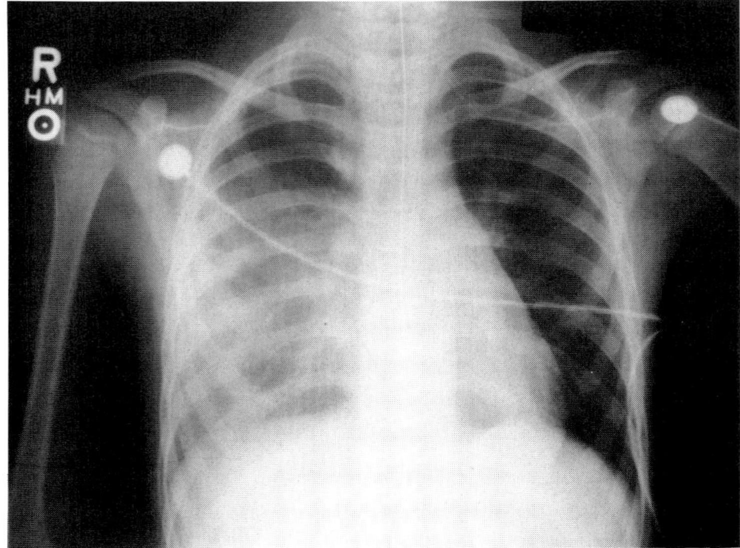

FIGURE 2. Large right-sided pulmonary contusion in a 7-year-old boy struck by a car. Note the absence of rib fractures.

are present in 30–50% of thoracic injuries. They are produced by a direct blow or crushing impact. Because of the resiliency of the ribs at younger ages, however, fractures are significantly less common in children than in adults, in whom they occur in approximately 75% of all thoracic injuries.

The presence of rib fractures in children is a marker of the severity of injury. An increasing number of rib fractures is associated with an increasing likelihood of additional thoracic injuries and a corresponding rise in mortality. However, significant intrathoracic injury *can* occur in children without rib fractures.

The diagnosis is based on clinical findings, including localized tenderness, palpable deformity, and instability of the rib cage. Patients commonly splint the affected side and experience pain with deep inspiration, cough, or changes in position. If a rib fracture is suspected, a chest radiograph should be obtained to rule out additional intrathoracic injuries rather than to document the fracture. Complications that may accompany rib fractures include pneumothorax, hemothorax, or pulmonary contusion. **Fractures of the lower ribs may be associated with lacerations of the liver or spleen. A thorough abdominal examination in such patients is essential.** In addition, rib fractures are associated with ventilatory compromise from excessive splinting and predispose to atelectasis and pulmonary infection. Fortunately, rib fractures are generally well tolerated in the healthy child.

Rib fractures in children require 3–6 weeks to heal. The goal of treatment is relief of pain to improve ventilation. Oral analgesics such as codeine or ibuprofen are adequate in the majority of cases. Intercostal nerve blocks are useful in extremely painful cases. External splinting devices may improve comfort but are not recommended because they further restrict ventilation. Deep-breathing exercises are encouraged, although vigorous exercise and sports participation are discouraged. Pillows held against the injured area minimize pain during breathing exercise. Hospitalization is indicated for children with multiple rib fractures, significantly inhibited ventilatory effort, or underlying pulmonary or cardiac injury.

Rib fractures in an otherwise healthy child under 3 years of age, without a history of severe chest trauma, are pathognomonic of child abuse (Fig. 3). Flail chest, in which multiple rib fractures result in loss of continuity of sections of the rib cage, occurs in less than 1% of children with chest injuries. The paradoxical chest wall motion has a significant impact on ventilation by preventing adequate expansion of the lungs. Flail chest in children is associated with underlying parenchymal injury, which poses a greater threat to respiratory function.

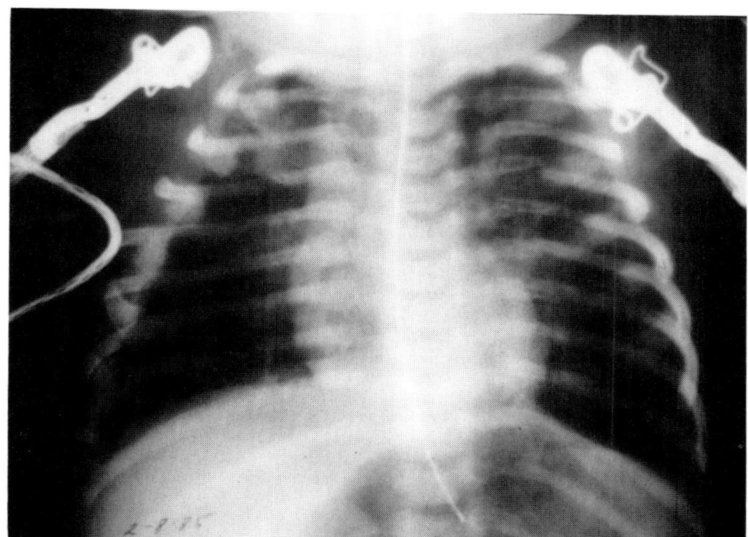

FIGURE 3. Six-month-old child with multiple posterior rib fractures from abuse.

Sternal fractures are also rare in children, because the sternum is comprised mainly of compliant cartilage. Sternal fractures result most commonly from direct impact of a hard object, such as a steering wheel. The injury produces local tenderness with palpation or motion. Swelling is frequently present, and crepitus may be elicited. The fracture is best demonstrated on a lateral chest radiograph, and its presence is an indication for evaluation of possible cardiac injury, including an electrocardiogram. Treatment includes analgesics and hospitalization for potential delayed manifestations of pulmonary or cardiac injuries.

Costochondral separation occasionally results from a particularly forceful tackle. Tenderness is localized to the area where the anterior rib meets the costocartilage. Patients frequently report a clicking or snapping sensation with motion. The diagnosis must be made clinically, because the cartilaginous structures are not visible on radiographs. Treatment consists of oral analgesics and local injection of anesthetic.

Pneumothorax

Pneumothorax is common in pediatric chest trauma and results in serious respiratory compromise. Although a pneumothorax can be caused by laceration from a rib fracture, over one-half of all pneumothoraces in children with chest trauma occur without a concomitant rib fracture.

Hemothorax

Intrathoracic hemorrhage has three potential sources: pulmonary vessels, intercostal vessels, and major intrathoracic vessels. Pulmonary lacerations rarely lead to significant accumulation of intrathoracic blood, whereas injury to major vessels can result in life-threatening massive hemothorax. Penetrating trauma is the predominant mechanism of major vessel injury, which is therefore rare in children.

The symptoms of hemothorax and pneumothorax are similar. Patients exhibit respiratory distress with decreased breath sounds on the affected side. Percussion of the chest, however, elicits dullness in patients with hemothorax and hyperresonance in patients with pneumothorax. Shock occurs before respiratory failure in a patient with a large hemothorax, whereas the order is reversed during a tension pneumothorax. Hypovolemia and shock may result from blood loss into the chest cavity because of the relatively small blood volume in the young child. An upright chest film often reveals a layer of blood or blunting of the costophrenic angle; radiographs in the lateral decubitus position are helpful in subtle cases.

Management of a hemothorax includes the rapid attainment of venous access and transfusion, as needed, to maintain blood volume. Thoracostomy is performed in the seventh or eighth intercostal space in the posterior axillary line. Persistent bleeding at a rate greater than

10 cc/kg/hr is considered an indication for surgery.

Cardiac Injuries

Cardiac injury is rare in pediatric chest trauma. Commotio cordis or cardiac concussion, is a very rare but fatal injury in children as the result of blunt chest trauma, and is reported to cause several deaths a year in youth baseball and hockey. It appears to be a functional injury with immediate and dire consequences rather than a structural injury.

A traumatic pericardial effusion or hemopericardium, which may result from blunt or penetrating trauma, has been reported in adolescent football players struck in the chest by the helmet of a charging opponent. This injury should be suspected when a direct blow is delivered to the sternal area with moderate to severe force and the patient complains of substernal chest pain. The cardiac examination concentrates on the presence of muffled heart sounds or a friction rub. A chest radiograph may show an enlarged heart shadow; however, normal heart size does not rule out the presence of blood in the pericardial sac. An echocardiogram is necessary for definitive diagnosis. Hemopericardium has the potential to progress to cardiac tamponade. A stable patient may be treated conservatively with hospitalization and close monitoring.

Cardiac tamponade should be considered in the child with hypotension, distended neck veins, and distant heart sounds or in the child with hypotension unresponsive to fluid resuscitation. Pulsus paradoxus may be present but often is difficult to document. Again, a chest radiograph may not demonstrate cardiomegaly, because tamponade may occur with only a small volume of blood in the minimally distensible pericardial sac.

Volume resuscitation results in temporary improvement of the circulation through an increase in venous pressure and cardiac filling. Pericardiocentesis is both diagnostic and therapeutic in the case of tamponade. Improvement is typically immediate and profound. Because reaccumulation of blood may occur, maintenance of a draining catheter within the pericardial sac is recommended.

Chest pain, the most consistent symptom of myocardial contusion, is often attributed mistakenly to overlying chest wall injury. Patients are at risk for developing cardiac dysrhythmias and require hospitalization with close monitoring. The diagnosis is made clinically and is supported by abnormalities on electrocardiogram or echocardiogram as well as by abnormal levels of creatinine phosphokinase (CPK) or CPK isoenzyme.

Intrathoracic injuries associated with extreme force or penetrating trauma are unlikely to present to the general practitioner for evaluation. Such entities include aortic rupture, esophageal rupture, and tracheobronchial tree disruption.

CONCLUSION

Traumatic chest injuries are uncommon in childhood but potentially quite serious, with a high rate of associated mortality. The unique features of the pediatric chest make the diagnosis of thoracic injuries difficult. Accurate detection requires a careful determination of the mechanism of injury and degree of force, a thorough search for physical findings, and a high level of suspicion. A high-quality upright chest radiograph is the most helpful diagnostic test. Assessment and management emphasize the ABCs of basic life support. Only the most severe injuries require surgical intervention.

SUGGESTED READING

1. American College of Surgeons Committee on Trauma: Advanced Trauma Life Support. Chicago, IL, American College of Surgeons, 1989, pp 89–100.
2. Bonadio WA, Hellmich T: Post-traumatic pulmonary contusion in children. Ann Emerg Med 18:1050–1052, 1989.
3. Corso PJ: Chest trauma. Primary Care Clinics in Office Practice 5:543–555, 1978.
4. Eichelberger M: Pediatric Trauma. St. Louis, Mosby, 1993, pp 437–450.
5. Eichelberger MR, Randolph JG: Thoracic trauma in children. Surg Clin North Am 61:1181–1197, 1981.
6. Garcia VF, Gottschall CS, Eichelberger MR, Bowman LM: Rib fractures in children: A marker of severe trauma. J Trauma 30:695–700, 1990.
7. Nakayama DK, Ramenofsky ML, Rowe MI: Chest injuries in children. Ann Surg 210:770–775, 1989.
8. Smyth BT: Chest trauma in children. J Pediatr Surg 14:41–47, 1979.
9. Templeton JM: Thoracic Trauma. In Fleisher GR, Ludwig S (eds): Textbook of Pediatric Emergency Medicine. Baltimore, Williams & Wilkins, 1993, pp 1143–1166.
10. Williams RD, Patton R: Athletic injuries to the abdomen and thorax. Am J Surg 98:447–450, 1959.

25

NEAR-DROWNING

Mark Joffe, M.D.

Drowning is second only to motor vehicle accidents as a cause of injury-related deaths in childhood. Near-drowning, or submersion injury, is defined as survival for more than 24 hours after injury. Once the injury has occurred, prompt and appropriate respiratory management is the single most important factor in minimizing morbidity.

Knowledge of the epidemiology of submersion injuries is helpful in preparing for the management of patients. Two-thirds of victims are pediatric patients under the age of 20. Almost one-half of all victims are less than 4 years old. Injuries are more common in warm climates and during the summer months because of the popularity of outdoor and water-related activities. The majority of drownings are in fresh water. Boys are at greater risk than girls. Bath tubs, large pails, and other household containers pose a risk to young children that may be unappreciated by their caretakers. **Clinicians must consider the possibility of child abuse or neglect when submersion injuries in young children are not clearly explained by the history.**

Older children may have associated injuries to the cervical spine, which can occur when they dive into shallow water. Alcohol abuse is a contributing factor in about 50% of adolescent drownings. Over two-thirds of drowning victims cannot swim. Submersion injuries have a particularly high morbidity and mortality rate. No management strategy can hope to approach the impact of effective prevention (Table 1). In many cases, however, proper respiratory care can make a difference.

PATHOPHYSIOLOGY

Submersion injuries usually begin with a period of panic as the victim struggles to remain at the surface. Gasping can lead to some degree of aspiration, but also important is the tendency to swallow large volumes of water. As the victim becomes submerged, a period of breath-holding and/or laryngospasm is common. Hypoxemia develops, and victims lose consciousness or have a seizure. Most victims gasp while underwater and thus aspirate varying volumes of fluid. In 10–15% of cases, laryngospasm persists until respiratory effort ceases. Such victims asphyxiate without appreciable aspiration of water, a so-called "dry drowning."

The duration of anoxia, which includes the period of submersion plus the time until effective cardiopulmonary resuscitation is begun, is the most important predictor of outcome. Differences among individuals and circumstances account for varying outcomes after periods of anoxia, but morbidity and mortality rates increase abruptly after 4–6 minutes of complete submersion (Table 2).

Small volumes of aspirated fluid may have profound effects on pulmonary function, especially oxygenation. In animal studies, aspiration of 2.2 ml/kg of water results in a fall of arterial PO_2 to 60 mmHg, without significant hypercarbia. Several mechanisms explain this phenomenon. Fresh water washes out surfactant from the lung, whereas salt water inactivates it. The deficiency of functional surfactant leads to alveolar collapse, loss of functional residual capacity, and mismatch of ventilation and perfusion.

TABLE 1. Prevention of Near-Drowning

Enclose pools with fences with self-locking gates.
Teach older children to swim.
Teach parents that no toddler is "water-safe."
Teach parents the risk to young children of bathtubs and large pails.
Teach adolescents the risk of swimming while intoxicated.

Edema, intraalveolar exudate, and fibrin deposition with hyaline membrane formation resemble respiratory distress syndrome of the newborn infant. Pulmonary compliance is greatly decreased, whereas airway resistance and pulmonary artery pressures are greatly increased. Persistent hypoxemia may complicate resuscitation despite the aspiration of only small amounts of water.

Research in the 1950s focused on the effects of fresh water and salt water on serum electrolyte concentrations and the cardiovascular system. Large volumes of aspirated fresh water theoretically may cause hyponatremia, hemolysis, and fluid overload. Salt water (509 mEq/L) in the lung may cause pulmonary edema and intravascular volume depletion. The volume of fluid aspirated during drownings is usually not large. Abnormalities of intravascular volume and electrolytes are rarely of clinical significance in persons who have drowned. Chlorination of fresh water does not significantly change the pulmonary problems associated with drowning. The type of water rarely affects management decisions.

Respiratory problems after near-drowning may become manifest after a relatively symptom-free period. With current technology for monitoring and respiratory support, deaths due to pulmonary insufficiency after resuscitation are infrequent. Adult respiratory distress syndrome (ARDS) often manifests hours after presentation.

TABLE 2. Indicators of Poor Prognosis

Age <3 years
Fixed, dilated pupils
History of submersion $>$ 5 min
Cardiopulmonary resuscitation required in the emergency department
Coma

Pneumonia, especially in victims who aspirate highly contaminated water, may develop after 24–72 hours.

Cold-water drownings have received special attention because of the ability of children to survive after prolonged submersion. The "diving reflex," which is most active during childhood, is activated when cold water ($<20°C$) stimulates the trigeminal and laryngeal nerves. The heart rate and respiratory rate drop precipitously. Perfusion of the brain and heart is maintained, with decreased flow to the muscles, kidneys, and gastrointestinal tract. Hypothermia occurs rapidly in children after immersion in cold water because of the high ratio of surface area to mass. Reductions in metabolic rate and oxygen demand at low body temperatures protect the brain from anoxic injury. Survival without sequelae has occurred in children submerged in ice-cold water for up to 40 minutes.

MANAGEMENT

(Table 3)

Prompt reversal of hypoxemia is the primary goal of therapy for victims of submersion injury. Respiratory management should attempt to expand the lungs and to fill them with 100% oxygen. The volume of fluid aspirated by the patient can usually be absorbed by the lung quite rapidly, once effective ventilation and perfusion are reestablished. **Attempts to remove water from the lungs are unnecessary.**

First aid for the drowning victim should include mouth-to-mouth ventilation at the earliest possible moment. Breaths delivered while

TABLE 3. Management Tips

- Clear the airway, avoiding abdominal thrusts.
- Ventilate with 100% oxygen.
- Intubate for coma, severe respiratory distress, significant hypoxemia, or hypercapnea.
- Use positive end-expiratory pressure (PEEP) if the patient is intubated (5–10 cm H_2O).
- Immobilize the neck if a fall or diving injury is suspected.
- Decompress the stomach with a nasogastric tube once the airway is protected.
- Continue resuscitation of victims of cold-water drowning until they are rewarmed.
- Use antibiotics for documented infections only.

the child is still in the water can be life-saving. Debris that may obstruct the airway must be cleared. A finger sweep is preferable to the Heimlich maneuver, which may induce emesis and aspiration. Basic life support, including chest compressions if the patient is pulseless, must continue as emergency medical systems are mobilized. Many patients regain consciousness at the scene, and the outcome in such children is excellent. They may have asymptomatic hypoxemia and delayed onset of respiratory deterioration, however, and should be taken to a hospital for further care.

Other patients remain unconscious, and many suffer cardiac arrest after the prolonged period of anoxia. Children whose pupils are fixed and dilated and who require resuscitation after arrival in an emergency department rarely survive with intact neurologic function. Case reports of unexpected recoveries, however, and difficulty in clearly establishing a prognosis at the moment of arrival at a hospital justify continued attempts at resuscitation.

The initial hospital management focuses on the airway, breathing, and circulation (ABCs—the basics of any resuscitation). If a diving injury is suspected or if the circumstances are unclear, proper head position must be constantly maintained until cervical spine injury is ruled out. Suctioning of the oropharynx is important for removing water and secretions, which may result from a vagal response to submersion. The awake patient with spontaneous respirations should receive 100% oxygen by nonrebreather bag. If the respiratory effort is poor or absent, hand ventilation with an anesthesia bag and mask is necessary. Cricoid pressure (Selleck maneuver) is useful during bag-valve-mask ventilation to prevent gaseous distention of the stomach and regurgitation. Tracheal intubation is required if a patient does not regain consciousness quickly or if the airway is difficult to maintain.

Careful observation of chest expansion and auscultation of the lung fields are the first steps in evaluating the victim's breathing. Pulse oximetry and arterial blood gas sampling are much more sensitive than visible cyanosis in detecting oxygen desaturation. Patients with hypercapnea ($PCO_2 > 45$) or significant hypoxemia ($PO_2 < 60$ on 50% oxygen) should be mechanically ventilated. Some awake patients with significant hypoxemia have been managed successfully with continuous positive airway pressure (CPAP) delivered by mask or nasal prongs. Ongoing monitoring for hypoxemia with pulse oximetry and periodic determinations of arterial blood gases are important for the prompt identification of respiratory deteriorations. A chest radiograph may be useful, although 25% of patients who develop significant pulmonary problems have an initially normal radiograph.

Pulmonary aspiration of gastric contents is a great risk for victims of near-drowning. Acidic, particulate matter has more deleterious effects on pulmonary function than water alone. High inflating pressures with bag-valve-mask ventilation can distend the stomach, which is already full of swallowed water, making regurgitation more likely. Passage of a nasogastric tube decompresses the stomach and prevents aspiration of gastric contents. It has the additional benefit of reducing the restriction on diaphragmatic excursion caused by a large stomach. The nasogastric tube may induce emesis, and insertion should be attempted only after the airway is secured. In patients who do not require intubation, assessment of the level of consciousness and gag reflex are important to ensure that airway protective responses will prevent aspiration if emesis occurs.

Circulatory problems are usually the result of prolonged hypoxemia and depressed myocardial function. Chest compressions are necessary for the pulseless patient while the airway and breathing are being managed. Vascular access should be obtained rapidly to administer medications for resuscitation, fluids, and pressor support, as needed. Fluid overload from absorption of ingested and aspirated water occasionally may complicate both circulatory and respiratory management, but in critically ill patients circulatory collapse requires fluid therapy to maintain perfusion. Measurement of serum electrolytes, blood urea nitrogen (BUN), and creatinine as well as a complete blood cell count are useful laboratory tests (Table 4).

Attention should focus on respiratory management once the initial phase of resuscitation is completed. Continuous positive airway pressure (CPAP) or positive end-expiratory pressure (PEEP) is extremely effective in reversing hypoxemia in the drowning victim. The opening

TABLE 4. Useful Diagnostic Tests

Chest roentgenogram
Cervical spine roentgenogram
Arterial blood gas determination
Complete blood cell count
Electrolyte, blood urea nitrogen (BUN), creatinine, and glucose measurements
Alcohol level (adolescents)

of collapsed alveoli decreases mismatching of ventilation and perfusion and restores functional residual capacity. Excessive positive intrathoracic pressure, however, may impair venous return and cardiac output. Adjustments in PEEP and fluid therapy should be directed at finding the optimal PEEP, which minimizes barotrauma and oxygen toxicity while maintaining oxygenation and circulation.

Bronchospasm may occur after near-drowning in patients with or without a prior history of reactive airway disease. Inhaled beta-adrenergic agents (albuterol or metaproterenol) are the first choice for therapy. Theophylline may be used when bronchospasm persists. Chest physiotherapy and suctioning may further improve pulmonary function, although frequent interruption of the positive airway pressure should be avoided in the early stages.

ARDS frequently complicates near-drowning. Hypoxemia, dyspnea, tachypnea, and diffuse crackles on auscultation herald its onset, which may occur from a few hours to days after the initial resuscitation. There is no specific therapy other than supportive care. High-dose corticosteroid therapy does not seem to reduce the incidence or severity of ARDS. The prolonged management in an intensive care unit is beyond the scope of this chapter.

Bacterial pneumonias usually become apparent with fever, respiratory deterioration, and new infiltrates on chest radiographs. Prophylactic antibiotics are not generally recommended. When bacterial pneumonia is suspected, broad-spectrum antibiotics should be administered, taking into consideration the potential contaminants in the water that was aspirated.

Patients resuscitated after prolonged periods of anoxia develop cytotoxic cerebral edema and elevations of intracranial pressure (ICP). Elevations of ICP are a poor prognostic sign, but aggressive attempts at cerebral resuscitation to control ICP have not led to significant improvements in outcome. Considerable controversy exists over whether such measures are advisable.

Unfortunately, some survivors of near-drowning have severe encephalopathy and/or chronic lung disease that requires prolonged respiratory care. This result is usually attributable to the initial period of anoxia and not to the specifics of resuscitation or intensive care management.

All health care providers have a role in reducing the number and severity of near-drownings. **Primary care physicians must emphasize water safety with the parents of their patients and in the community.** The dissemination of basic life support skills to the general public is a worthwhile endeavor. Emergency physicians who treat pediatric victims need to maintain their knowledge and skills in managing pediatric patients. And all medical personnel must provide support to the families while they care for the patients.

SUGGESTED READING

1. Allman FD, et al: Outcome following CPR in severe pediatric near-drowning. Am J Dis Child 140:571, 1986.
2. Fandel I, Bancalari E: Near-drowning in children: Clinical aspects. Pediatrics 58:573, 1976.
3. Lavelle JM, Shaw KN: Near-drowning: Is emergency department cardiopulmonary resuscitation or intensive care unit cerebral resuscitation indicated? Crit Care Med 21:368, 1993.
4. Modell JH, et al: Clinical course of 91 consecutive near-drowning victims. Chest 70:231, 1976.
5. Nussbaum E: Prognostic variables in nearly drowned, comatose children. Am J Dis Child 139:1058, 1985.
6. Orlowski JP: Drowning, near-drowning, and ice-water submersions. Pediatr Clin North Am 34:75–92, 1987.
7. Pearn JH: The management of near-drowning. BMJ 291:1447, 1985.
8. Spyker DA: Submersion injury: Epidemiology, prevention, and management. Pediatr Clin North Am 32:113, 1985.
9. Thompson AF: Environmental emergencies. In Fleischer G, Ludwig S (eds): Textbook of Pediatric Emergency Medicine. Baltimore, Williams & Wilkins, 1983.

26

RESPIRATORY INJURY AFTER HYDROCARBON POISONING

James F. Wiley II, M.D.

Hydrocarbon ingestion frequently causes toxic injury to the lung. Fifty percent of cases occur in children under 6 years of age. Up to one-quarter of patients with hydrocarbon poisoning suffer moderate to severe toxicity that necessitates hospitalization. Fatalities occur in fewer than 1% of all cases. Proper therapy requires correct identification of the ingested compound, careful interpretation of history and physical findings, and timely intervention.

Hydrocarbons are diverse substances that include aliphatic, aromatic, halogenated, and terpene groups. These groups can be divided into hydrocarbons with aspiration potential but few systemic effects (kerosene and mineral seal oil) and hydrocarbons with the potential for major systemic effects as well as possible direct lung toxicity (e.g., benzene, toluene, trichloroethane, gasoline, and turpentine). Tables 1 and 2 list the most important hydrocarbons and their potential toxicities.

PATHOPHYSIOLOGY

The risk of aspiration and pneumonitis after ingestion of a hydrocarbon depends on the intrinsic properties of the ingested substance. High volatility, low viscosity, and low surface tension favor aspiration and dispersal of the petroleum distillate throughout the lung. Of these properties, **the viscosity best predicts the likelihood of pulmonary pathology after hydrocarbon poisoning.** Agents with a low viscosity (<60 Saybolt seconds universal [SSU]) are more likely to produce pneumonitis. Aspirated agents with high viscosity (>100 SSU) may produce a localized lipoid pneumonia but do not cause generalized pneumonitis.

Petroleum distillates produce hypoxemia and pulmonary pathology by displacement of oxygen from the alveoli, disruption of surfactant, and direct disruption of alveolar capillaries. Loss of surface tension leads to alveolar collapse, atelectasis, and ventilation-perfusion mismatch, which may be exacerbated by bronchospasm. Chemical pneumonitis and frank pulmonary edema may follow. Bacterial superinfection occurs in a minority of patients with chemical pneumonitis.

Gastrointestinal absorption of petroleum distillates without aspiration does not cause pneumonitis in the amounts usually ingested by children (generally <30 ml). No direct effects on the central nervous system (CNS) have been shown for the hydrocarbons listed in Table 1. CNS depression after poisoning with these agents should be attributed to hypoxemia or ingestion of some other substance.

Mineral seal oil deserves special mention because of the higher morbidity reported with its ingestion. This substance is notable for its attractive color and odor, which make it doubly dangerous for a child. Whereas children typically swallow only a mouthful of kerosene, they frequently drink a whole cup of mineral seal oil, thereby enhancing the chances of aspiration and pulmonary complications.

TABLE 1. Hydrocarbons with Low Systemic Toxicity

Hydrocarbon	Use
Pneumonitis likely*	
Kerosene	Heater fuel
Mineral seal oil	Furniture polish
Naphtha	Lighter fluid
Petroleum ether (benz*ine*)	Dry cleaning solvent
Mineral spirits (Varsol)	Paint thinner, dry cleaning solvent
Gasoline†	Automobile fuel
Turpentine†	Paint thinner
Pneumonitis unlikely‡	
Fuel oil	Furnace heating oil
Lubricating oil	Household oil
Mineral oil	Laxative
Paraffin wax	Candles

* Viscosity <60 SSU.
† Seizures may occur with very large ingestions.
‡ Viscosity <100 SSU.

CLINICAL MANIFESTATIONS

Nontoxic hydrocarbons irritate the mouth, pharynx, and stomach immediately after ingestion. Nausea, vomiting, coughing, or choking may ensue. Hydrocarbon pneumonitis follows aspiration that occurs during ingestion, after vomiting, or after misguided attempts at gastric emptying by medical personnel. Patients with pneumonitis may develop tachypnea, retractions, cough, fever, and cyanosis. Physical examination may reveal inspiratory crackles, expiratory wheezing, decreased breath sounds, or dullness to percussion. Leukocytosis is frequently present. Chest radiographs are abnormal within 2 hours in up to 90% of patients with pneumonitis (Fig. 1). Occasionally a patient may have a normal chest radiograph but appear significantly distressed.

On rare occasions, patients may develop pneumothorax, pneumomediastinum, and pleural effusions within 24-48 hours of ingestion. Pneumatoceles may appear 1-4 weeks after ingestion and may persist (Fig. 2). Long-term changes in pulmonary function—most commonly, increased volume of isoflow related to small airway obstruction—have been reported in children as long as 14 years after aspiration of kerosene.

Common findings after ingestion of a nontoxic hydrocabon include odor on the breath and clothes, spontaneous vomiting, somnolence (related to hypoxemia), and fever. Hepatosplenomegaly and myocardial dysrhythmias are seen rarely. Cardiac dysrhythmias may be precipitated by epinephrine, which is thus contraindicated for treatment of bronchospasm in this setting. Various systemic effects may follow ingestion of toxic hydrocarbons (see Table 2).

TABLE 2. Hydrocarbons with High Systemic Toxicity

Hydrocarbon	Use	Effects
Aromatic		
Benzene	Industrial solvent	Aplastic anemia, leukemia
Toluene	Glue, paint solvent	Acute: sudden death from cardiac dysrhythmias Chronic: peripheral neuropathy, renal tubular necrosis
Xylene	As above	As above
Halogenated		
Trichloroethane	Typewriter correction fluid, fabric cleaners	Cardiac dysrhythmais, sudden death
Trichloroethylene	As above	As above
Chlordane, lindane	Insecticides	Coma, seizures
Carbon tetrachloride	Solvent	Severe hepatotoxicity
Methylene chloride	Paint stripper	Lethargy, carbon monoxide poisoning, pulmonary edema
Aliphatic		
Propane	Fuel for stoves	Sudden death, cardiac dysrhythmias
Butane	Cigarette lighter fuel	As above
Terpenes		
Camphor	Over-the-counter analgesic	Agitation, seizures
Pine oil	Household cleaners	Lethargy, coma

Other poisons are manufactured with hydrocarbons as a solvent, including rodenticides and herbicides containing organophosphates, heavy metals, and strychnine.

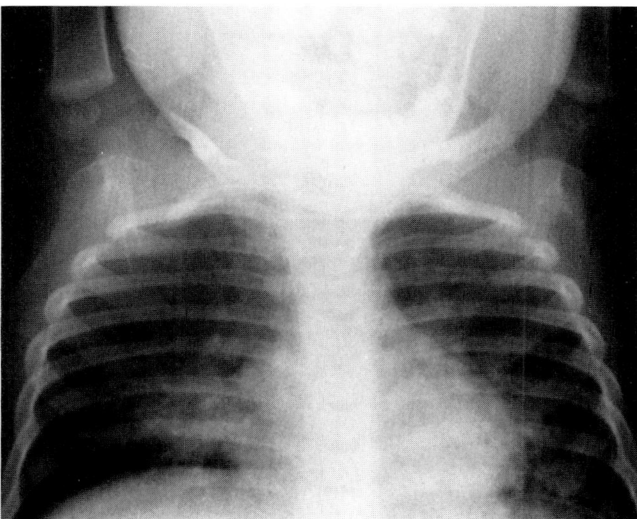

FIGURE 1. Chest radiograph of a girl who developed pneumonitis after ingestion of kerosene. Note the bilateral diffuse infiltrates.

MANAGEMENT

Proper treatment depends on the ingested agent and the clinical presentation. A child who has no symptoms after ingestion of a nontoxic hydrocarbon may be followed at home, provided that the parents are reliable and can rapidly bring the child to medical attention if symptoms develop. The physician must call back frequently to ensure that the child remains asymptomatic. **Any child with a history of coughing, gagging, vomiting, or persistent symptoms after ingestion of a nontoxic hydrocarbon should be evaluated emergently, as should any child after ingestion of a toxic hydrocarbon.**

Patients who are poisoned with nontoxic hydrocarbons (see Table 1) **should receive no gastric-empyting procedures, because ipecac-induced vomiting and gastric lavage increase the likelihood of aspiration and pneumonitis.** Activated charcoal is ineffective, because it

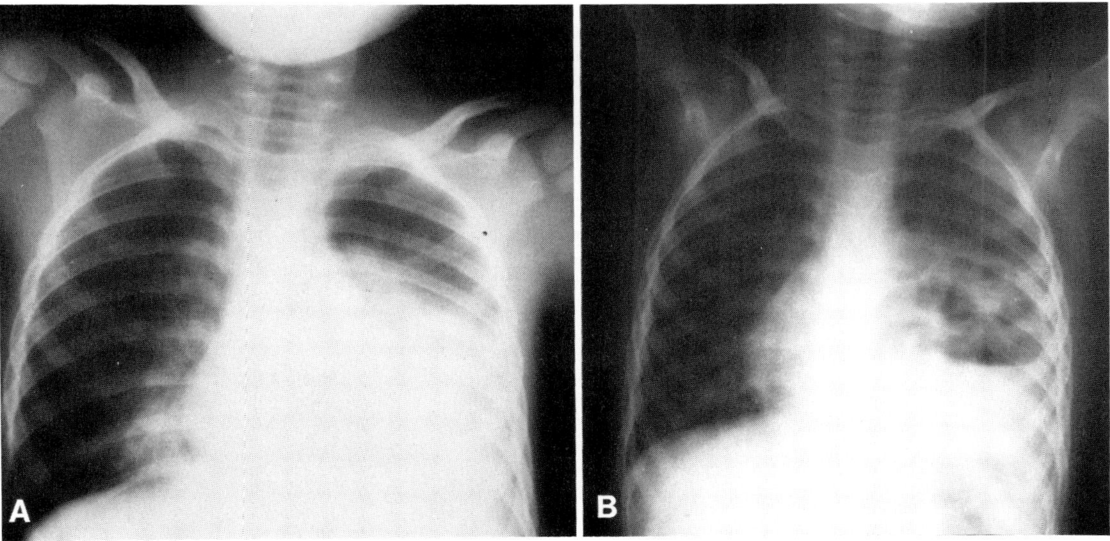

FIGURE 2. *A*, Left lingular and left lower lobe opacification after ingestion of a hydrocarbon. *B*, Same patient, 1 week later. Note pneumatocele formation in the previously affected area.

does not bind to hydrocarbons. Conversely, patients who have ingested toxic hydrocarbons (see Table 2) should receive gastric emptying with ipecac if they ingested enough to cause systemic symptoms and if they exhibit no altered mental status. The exceptions to this treatment are agents that cause seizures or coma (e.g, lindane, large overdose of terpene, camphor). Nasogastric lavage is the preferred method of gastric empyting with these substances. Any patient with a poor gag reflex, altered mental status, or severe respiratory distress should not receive ipecac but should be endotracheally intubated before lavage.

Patients who become asymptomatic before arrival in the emergency department require observation for at least 2 hours after ingestion. At that time, a chest radiograph may be obtained. If the radiograph shows no pneumonitis, the patient may be discharged as long as the vital signs and examination of the lungs are normal. If the radiograph is positive, the child should be admitted for observation of further respiratory effects. Alternatively, the patient can be watched for 6 hours in the emergency department and then discharged if no symptoms develop. **All patients discharged from the emergency department need to be reevaluated by a physician at 24 hours after ingestion.**

Symptomatic children deserve careful evaluation for the presence of hypoxemia and respiratory failure. In addition to vital signs, examination of the lungs, and a chest radiograph, patients require monitoring with pulse oximetry and determination of arterial blood gases. Most require supplemental oxygen. Bronchospasm should be treated with aerosolized beta$_2$-agonists (e.g., albuterol, 0.5% [0.01–0.03 ml/kg]), rather than agents with alpha-adrenergic effects to avoid triggering cardiac dysrhythmias. Endotracheal intubation and mechanical ventilation are indicated for patients with respiratory failure (hypoxemia or hypercarbia) or altered mental status.

All symptomatic patients require hosptial admission for observation and further supportive care. Prophylactic administration of corticosteroids does not help hydrocarbon pneumonitis and may promote bacterial colonization. Similarly, antibiotics serve only to select for resistant organisms if bacterial superinfection occurs. Antibiotics should be reserved for patients with bacterial pneumonia, which is suggested by fever that lasts more than 3 days after ingestion and sputum cultures that display polymorphonuclear cells and a predominant organism. Most patients recover fully from hydrocarbon pneumonitis if given careful respiratory support.

SUGGESTED READING

1. Anas N, Namasonthi V, Ginsburg CM: Criteria for hospitalizing children who have ingested products containing hydrocarbons. JAMA 246:840–843, 1981.
2. Ellenhorn MJ, Barceloux DG: Hydrocarbon products. In Ellenhorn MJ, Barceloux DG (eds): Medical Toxicology: Diagnosis and Treatment of Human Poisoning. New York, Elsevier, 1988, pp 940–993.
3. Klein BL, Simon JE: Hydrocarbon poisonings. Pediatr Clin North Am 33:411–419, 1986.
4. Kulberg AG, Goldfrank LR, Bresnitz EA: Hydrocarbons. In Goldfrank LR, Flomenbaum NE, Lewin NA, et al (eds): Goldfrank's Toxicologic Emergencies, 4th ed. Norwalk, CT, Appleton-Century-Crofts, 1986, pp 672–685.
5. Litovitz T, Greene AE: Health implications of petroleum distillate ingestion. Occup Med State Art Rev 3:555–567, 1988.
6. Litovitz T: Hydrocarbon ingestions. Ear Nose Throat J 62:45–55, 1983.

27

RESPIRATORY COMPLICATIONS OF BURNS AND SMOKE INHALATION

Brian P. O'Sullivan, M.D.

Inhalation injury occurs in one-third of all patients with major burns and is responsible for more than 50% of all burn-related deaths. Inhalation injury has been shown to be more important as a determinant of mortality than age or extent of the burn.

GENERAL CONSIDERATIONS

The evaluation of a child exposed to fire begins with a full history of the events surrounding the incident (Table 1). **The severity and outcome of acute lung injury are determined, to a great extent, by the circumstances of the accident.** A victim of a closed-space fire who has facial burns and is unconscious is at much greater risk of developing serious respiratory complications than the victim of an open-space fire who has no facial burns and is alert and conversant. Therefore, it is essential to obtain a detailed account of the accident, including facts such as where the exposure took place, how long the child was in the smoke-filled environment, and whether the child was exposed directly to the heat source or to smoke only (Table 2). One must also be aware of any underlying health problem or use of medication. For instance, a child with asthma who is exposed to smoke is much more likely to develop significant bronchospasm than a well child.

A careful physical examination to rule out fire-related trauma is crucial. Abdominal injuries and long-bone fractures may occur in fire victims who have jumped from buildings or have been injured in automobile accidents before suffering burns.

Drug or alcohol ingestion must also be considered in the emergency evaluation of burn victims. One report has labeled alcohol as the "hidden toxin" behind inhalation injury, because patients who are inebriated are unable to escape from dangerous environments and suffer more serious smoke intoxication than patients who are sober and competent at the time of the fire. Drinking or use of recreational drugs is not readily admitted by teenagers; thus the physician caring for them must have a high index of suspicion.

Infants and the debilitated elderly are not able to extricate themselves from a burning building and are more frequently the victims of fire than healthy young adults.

PATHOPHYSIOLOGY

Pyrolysis and combustion of household materials produce a number of potentially toxic gases that contribute to the pathogenesis of inhalation injury (Table 3). These noxious gases are generally categorized as asphyxiants, irritants, or systemic toxins.

The clinically most important product of combustion of wood and other cellulosic materials is carbon monoxide (CO), a clear, odorless

TABLE 1. Approach to the Pediatric Burn Victim

History
- Closed- vs. open-space fire
- Type of fire materials
- Initially conscious or unconscious
- Direct exposure to flame or exposure to smoke only
- Spontaneous respirations at the fire scene
- Past medical history
  - Respiratory illness
  - Medications

Physical examination
- Percent of body surface area of burns
- Involvement of respiratory area (see Table 5)
- Lung examination (rales, wheezes, retractions)
- Neurologic status—? hypoxic ischemia
- Associated trauma
  - Acute abdomen
  - Long-bone fractures

Laboratory studies
- Level of carboxyhemoglobin (COHb)
- Arterial blood gas
- Electrolytes
- Complete blood cell count

Therapy
- 100% oxygen until COHb <10%
- Appropriate fluid resuscitation—avoid bolus therapy or overhydration
- Early intubation if signs of respiratory distress occur
- Aggressive use of positive end-expiratory pressure (PEEP) for intubated patients
- Withhold antibiotics and steroids unless indicated for burn care

gas that results from the incomplete combustion of carbonaceous materials. CO, which is responsible for up to 80% of smoke inhalation fatalities, binds to hemoglobin with an affinity 250 times that of oxygen, thereby displacing oxygen from the heme moiety and decreasing tissue delivery of oxygen. Tissue hypoxia is worsened by the fact that the presence of CO increases the affinity between oxygen and hemoglobin, thereby decreasing release of oxygen at the tissue level. Furthermore, CO binds to intracellular cytochrome a_3, producing a depression in cellular respiration, which also exacerbates tissue hypoxia.

The usual blood level of carboxyhemoglobin (COHb) is <1%. Cigarette smokers may have levels in excess of 10%. Clinical symptoms of CO poisoning are directly related to the degree of exposure and correlate well with the measured level of COHb (Table 4). Levels of COHb under 10% are unlikely to produce symptoms in adults; at levels of 10–20% exertional dyspnea occurs. Moderate intoxication (20–40% COHb) cause headache, nausea, dizziness, irritability, and impaired judgment. More severe intoxication leads to syncope, hallucinations, and collapse. Extremely high levels of COHb (60–80%) cause coma, convulsions, and death. End-organ involvement is myriad and includes arrythmias, myocardial ischemia, pulmonary edema, myonecrosis, acute renal failure, and retinal hemorrhages.

Young infants may show signs and symptoms of CO intoxication at lower levels of COHb than adults. Two factors account for this increased susceptibility:

1. Young infants have a higher metabolic rate than adults and an increased oxygen demand at the tissue level. Thus, any intoxicant that decreases tissue delivery of oxygen has a more pronounced effect in children than in adults.

2. Infants in the first few months of life still have significant levels of fetal hemoglobin, which binds oxygen more tightly than hemoglobin A. As a result, they have decreased release

TABLE 2. Factors Influencing the Incidence and Severity of Postburn Respiratory Injury and Carbon Monoxide Intoxication

Factor	Unfavorable	Favorable
Location (environmental)	Enclosed (room, building, automobile)	Open
Anatomic location	Respiratory area involved (mouth, pharynx, nose, nasal hairs, eyebrows, forehead, frontal hair)	Respiratory area spared
Physical finding	Conjunctivitis, rhinitis, laryngitis, stridor, cough	Absent
Type of burn	Flame	Liquid, chemical, irradiation
Heavy smoke products of incomplete combustion	Present	Absent
Steam, high humidity	Present	Absent

of oxygen from hemoglobin to tissue, a shift to the left of the oxyhemoglobin dissociation curve. CO magnifies this shift to the left, producing a marked decrease in the amount of oxygen passed on to the tissue at any given PaO_2.

For these two reasons, modest exposure to smoke may produce significantly greater symptoms in infants than one would expect solely on the basis of COHb level.

In any patient who has been exposed to smoke, COHb should be measured by co-oximetry, which directly measures the percent of hemoglobin saturated with oxygen, CO, and methemoglobin. Co-oximetry must be used in all burn victims. The standard methods of determining oxygen saturation, such as arterial blood gas and pulse oximetry, yield inaccurate results in the presence of CO. The percent saturation of hemoglobin listed on the blood gas panel is calculated from the PaO_2 (which is unaffected by CO) rather than measured directly and does not represent the true oxyhemoglobin saturation. Pulse oximeters poorly discriminate oxyhemoglobin from COHb; thus, if a patient presents with a COHb level of 30% and an oxygen saturation of 65%, the pulse oximeter will read >90% saturation. In contrast, the co-oximeter accurately determines the levels of oxy- and deoxyhemoglobin as well as COHb and methemoglobin.

TABLE 3. Effects of Toxic Components of Smoke

Irritant Gas	Clinical Symptoms of Toxicity
Hydrogen chloride	Dyspnea, burning mucous membranes, chest pain, light-headedness, laryngeal and pulmonary edema
Ammonia	Conjunctivitis, burning mucous membranes, laryngeal and pulmonary edema
Phosgene	Dyspnea, cough, wheeze, pulmonary edema
Styrene	Dyspnea, cough, wheeze, central nervous system syndrome
Aldehydes	Pulmonary edema, wheeze, decreased ciliary activity, decreased macrophage activity
Sulfur dioxide	Conjunctivitis, laryngitis, rhinitis
Nitrogen dioxide	Chest tightness, cough, wheeze, pulmonary edema, fibrosing alveolitis

TABLE 4. Clinical Effects of Varying Concentrations of COHb in Carbon Monoxide Intoxication

COHb (%)	Severity	Symptoms
20	Mild	Headaches, mild dyspnea, visual changes, confusion
20–40	Moderate	Irritability, diminished judgment, dim vision, nausea, easy fatigability
40–50	Severe	Hallucinations, confusion, ataxia, collapse, coma
60	Fatal	

Treatment of CO intoxication consists of supplying supplemental oxygen at the highest concentration possible. Administration of 100% oxygen should start at the fire site with the use of a close-fitting face mask and continued until the COHb level is below 10%. Supplemental oxygen must be started as soon as possible to prevent or minimize tissue hypoxia.

Oxygen therapy shortens the half-life of COHb dramatically from approximately 4 hours in 21% oxygen (room air) to 40–60 minutes in 100% inspired oxygen. The half-life falls to 20–25 minutes when 100% oxygen is inspired at two atmospheres of pressure (hyperbaric chamber). As CO is displaced from hemoglobin, more oxygen can be carried and tissue hypoxia is reversed. The role of hyperbaric oxygen in the therapy of the fire victim with CO poisoning is somewhat controversial. Its use has been recommended by some investigators because it more rapidly displaces CO from hemoglobin and from cytochrome a_3. At two atmospheres of pressure enough oxygen is dissolved in the plasma to provide adequate tissue oxygenation even in the absence of functional hemoglobin. The indications for hyperbaric oxygen vary somewhat from site to site.

Cyanide, which is generated by the combustion of wool, silk, nylon, and polyurethane, is responsible for asphyxia in some fire victims. Cyanide binds to cytochrome oxidase to inhibit respiration at the cellular level, acting in synergy with CO. Inhaled cyanide has a rapid onset of action and theoretically can cause many symptoms similar to those of CO poisoning (e.g., acidemia, end-organ failure).

Persistent acidosis after normalization of COHb levels and cardiac output should make one suspect cyanide poisoning. Because cyanide is so lethal, however, it is unlikely that it plays a major role in the clinical course of patients who survive to reach the hospital. An antidote kit is available (Eli Lilly, Indianapolis, IN); however, it induces formation of methemoglobin, which further diminishes the oxygen-carrying capacity of blood in patients already suffering from CO intoxication. Thus, it is not used routinely.

The act of combustion consumes oxygen and lowers the fraction of inspired oxygen in the air breathed by the victim. Typically, the fraction of inspired oxygen (FiO_2) in a room in which there is a fire is 10–18%; at the source of the fire it may be as low as 5%. Thus, anyone trapped in such an environment will show signs and symptoms of hypoxemia, regardless of CO or cyanide poisoning. Delivery of a high concentration of inspired oxygen at the scene of the fire rapidly reverses hypoxemia of this etiology.

Irritant gases are found most frequently in smoke resulting from combustion of synthetic materials (see Table 3). The effects of these gases are most commonly seen in victims of house and closed-space fires (including automobile fires) in which synthetic materials are burned.

Aldehydes (particularly acrolein), ammonia, chlorine, hydrogen chloride, and sulfur dioxide are soluble in biologic fluids and dissolve in the water of the upper airway. Intense exposure or carriage by soot particles may deliver these gases to the lower airways, where they cause edema and bronchospasm. Conjunctival irritation and oral erythema are good markers of exposure to these gases.

Phosgene and oxides of nitrogen are water-insoluble gases found in smoke. The water-insoluble gases pass directly into the lower airways and alveoli without being adsorbed to the mucous membranes of the upper airway: thus pulmonary edema develops in the lower airways several hours after exposure. Water-insoluble gases are infrequently present in residential fires but play a critical role in victims of welding accidents or fires resulting from nitrogen fuels, which rarely involve children. Patients require long-term observation for development of delayed-onset pulmonary edema.

TABLE 5. Warning Signs of Repiratory Injury

Singed nasal hair	Soot in sputum
Cough	Labored respiration
Hoarseness	Cyanosis
Stridor	Wheezing
Hemoptysis	Abnormal chest radiograph

Systemic toxins (arsenic, heavy metals) have been found in soot and may be of importance in patients with refractory hypoxemia or severe neurologic symptoms. Thermal injury to the lower airways is uncommon in burn victims, because the upper airway acts as a "buffer zone" that cools the air.

Of patients with inhalation injury, 20–30% develop upper airway obstruction due to edema of the glottic and supraglottic structures within 4 hours after inhalation. Chemical irritation from smoke also contributes to the development of this complication.

The degree of edema correlates with the extent of burns and the rate of infusion of intravenous fluids. One must be aware of the potential delay in onset of edema. Normal voice quality and breath sounds on initial examination should not be construed as proof of airway stability.

Facial burns, singed nasal vibrissae, soot in the nares or sputum, hoarseness or stridor are highly worrisome findings (Table 5). Intubation is particularly difficult in patients with marked facial burns who develop massive edema and distortion of facial features. Any patient suspected of having thermal injury to the airway, especially patients with large burns, must be observed closely over 18–24 hours for the development of upper airway obstruction. **It is best to proceed with early prophylactic intubation in such patients rather than to attempt technically difficult intubation through edematous structures later on.**

Upper airway obstruction may occur in the absence of facial burns. The presence of burns in this area is not always indicative of airway involvement; each patient must be evaluated individually. Direct visualization of the airway by means of fiberoptic bronchoscopy allows the most accurate diagnosis of upper airway edema. Personnel capable of performing this procedure in children on a serial basis are rarely available outside major pediatric centers. **Therefore, outside such centers, early prophylactic**

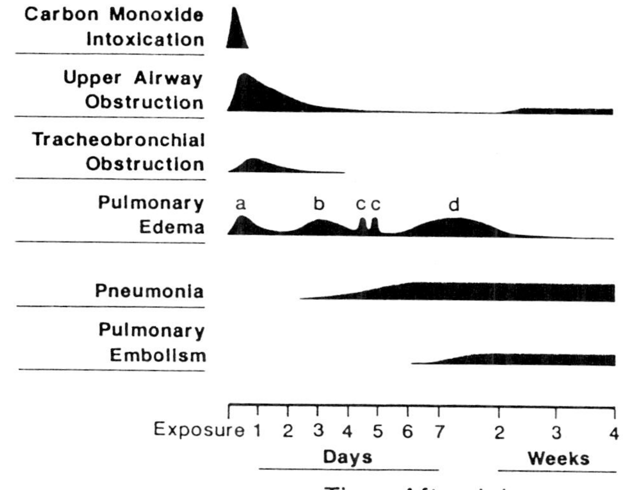

FIGURE 1. Time course of onset of respiratory injury after smoke inhalation. (From Haponik J, Summer WR: Respiratory complications in burned patients: Diagnosis and management of inhalation injury. J Crit Care 2:121, 1987, with permission.)

intubation of burn victims is the safest approach. Tracheostomy early in the course of burn care increases the risk of airway scarring and should be avoided.

Lower airway burns may occur after inhalation of steam or volatile gases that ignite in the airway. In addition, particulate matter may cause punctuate burns of the tracheobronchial tree.

Damage to the lower airways usually results from inhalation of toxic fumes. Reflex laryngospasms and voluntary breath-holding minimize exposure of the lower airways to these irritants as long as the fire victim is alert. Once the victim is overcome by anoxia and loses consciousness, these protective mechanisms are lost—and chemical irritants are inhaled. Thus, the patient with a history of loss of consciousness must be considered to be at high risk for lower airway injury.

Lower airway injury in children progresses in the following sequence: (1) bronchospasm 1–12 hours after the burn; (2) pulmonary edema 6–72 hours after the burn; and (3) bronchopneumonia >60 hours after the burn (Fig. 1).

Bronchospasm is secondary to direct stimulation of irritant receptors within the airways and occurs in most victims of smoke inhalation. Inhaled beta-agonist is the treatment of choice for acute bronchospasm in such situations.

We prefer aerosolized bronchodilators to theophylline because of their wider therapeutic window. Corticosteroid therapy is contraindicated in burn patients because of the associated increase in risk of infection. Despite adequate bronchodilation, wheezing may persist because of airway edema, bronchorrhea, and sloughing of airway epithelium.

Pulmonary edema occurs usually about 6 hours after inhalation, but it may occur as late as 4–6 days later. The absence of rales or significant radiographic findings on initial presentation does not rule out lower airway damage.

Persistent hypoxemia despite administration of supplemental oxygen, which is often seen in burn victims, is generally due to atelectasis and pulmonary edema.

Fluid therapy must balance the need for a large volume of fluid with the need to limit fluid administration to decrease pulmonary edema. Fluid must be given at a steady infusion rate; bolus therapy should be avoided whenever possible. The type of fluid does not influence the formation of pulmonary edema; there is no advantage to the use of colloids as the initial resuscitative fluids.

Patients developing hypoxia, hyperventilation, or an increasing alveolar-arterial gradient require endotracheal intubation and mechanical ventilation. Early and aggressive institution of positive end-expiratory pressure (PEEP) is beneficial. Pneumonia frequently develops 48–72 hours after the initial injury. Prophylactic antimicrobial therapy on presentation, however, is *not* indicated.

Long-term sequelae even to intense smoke exposure are uncommon. Most patients who recover from smoke inhalation return to near-normal pulmonary function within months of injury.

Upper airway sequelae depend on the degree of thermal injury to this area. Laryngeal damage with alteration in voice quality in survivors of fire accidents may be due to severe upper airway injury or to its treatment (e.g., tracheostomy). **The upper airway of any patient with a history of burn injury who presents with stridor, hoarseness, or marked snoring requires careful evaluation.**

Prolonged reactive airways disease rarely develops after a single exposure to smoke, although wheezing is common in the acute setting. Bronchiectasis, bronchiolitis obliterans, airway polyps, and chronic bronchitis have been reported in fire victims, but they are rare.

All children suffering from smoke inhalation experience psychological trauma. The fear inherent in surviving a fire can be devastating for children. The added stresses of loss of family members and property and feelings of guilt or responsibility for the event necessitate long-term psychosocial support.

CHRONIC SMOKE INHALATION

Children are vulnerable to insidious forms of chronic smoke inhalation, such as involuntary cigarette smoking and exposure to home heating devices that burn carbonaceous fuels (wood stoves, coal stoves, kerosene space heaters).

Children with a history of exposure to cigarette smoke have more episodes of airways obstruction, more frequent hospitalizations for respiratory complaints, onset of asthma at an earlier age, and more frequent episodes of otitis media than nonexposed children. Symptoms are dose-related and are significant even when the caretaker smokes as few as 10 cigarettes per day.

Wood stoves emit a large amount of particulate matter in addition to carcinogens, CO, and other noxious gases. Exposure to wood stoves has been shown to impair pulmonary function and to increase the number of episodes of lower respiratory tract illnesses in children from various cultures and socioeconomic backgrounds.

Finally, poorly ventilated or malfunctioning kerosene heaters and natural gas water heaters may be responsible for occult CO poisoning. A moderate increase in COHb in a young infant may cause nausea, vomiting, and listlessness. We and others have documented mild CO intoxication in afebrile children with flulike symptoms who have been exposed to inadequately ventilated heating devices. These reports underscore the importance of considering CO poisoning outside the routine setting of a house fire and known smoke inhalation. When CO poisoning is suspected, a blood sample must be obtained for co-oximetry. Treatment consists of removing the child from the hazardous environment and correcting the underlying cause of CO build-up in the household.

SUGGESTED READING

1. Deitch EA: The management of burns. N Engl J Med 323:1249–1253, 1990.
2. Haponik EF, Munster AM: Respiratory Injury: Smoke Inhalation and Burns. New York, McGraw-Hill, 1990.
3. Haponik EF, Summer WR: Respiratory complications in burned patients: Pathogenesis and spectrum of inhalation injury. J Crit Care 2:49–74, 1987.
4. Haponik EF, Summer WR: Respiratory complications in burned patients: Diagnosis and management of inhalation injury. J Crit Care 2:121–143, 1987.
5. Ilano AL, Raffin TA: Management of carbon monoxide poisoning. Chest 97:165–169, 1990.
6. Ruddy RM: Smoke inhalation injury. Pediatr Clin North Am 41:317–336, 1994.
7. Stone HH: Pulmonary burns in children. J Pediatr Surg 14:48–52, 1979.
8. Terrill JB, Montgomery RR, Reinhardt CF: Toxic gases from fires. Science 200:1343–1347, 1978.
9. Zimmerman SS, Truxal B: Carbon monoxide poisoning. Pediatrics 68:215–224, 1981.

28

PULMONARY MANIFESTATIONS OF PEDIATRIC MALIGNANCIES

Edwin C. Douglass, M.D.

Malignant disease is an infrequent cause of pulmonary pathology in infants and children, but when it occurs, early recognition is of exceeding importance. This chapter discusses the major manifestations of childhood cancer in the thoracic cavity, first from primary and secondary malignant disease, then as side effects of cancer therapy.

PRIMARY AND SECONDARY MALIGNANT DISEASE

Primary Tumors Involving the Lung. Primary tumors of pulmonary parenchymal or bronchogenic origin are exceptionally rare in childhood; however, primary tumors of the mediastinum or chest wall are relatively common (see below). The rare malignancies that originate in the lung or bronchi include pleuropulmonary blastoma (lung) and carcinoid tumors, mucoepidermoid carcinoma, or tumors of squamous cell origin (bronchi). Patients who are long-term survivors of Fanconi anemia may be particularly prone to squamous cell malignancies. The primary treatment for these tumors is surgery; some response to chemotherapy has been noted in pleuropulmonary blastomas.

Primary Tumors Involving the Mediastinum. The mediastinum is conventionally divided into anterior, middle, and posterior compartments. Because few tumors are localized solely to the middle compartment, only anterior and posterior tumors are discussed here (Table 1).

The most important tumors of the anterior mediastinum in the pediatric age group are lymphomas and germ-cell tumors. Patients may present with symptoms of airway compression such as cough, stridor, or localized wheezing. Patients with very large lymphomas may present with a superior vena caval syndrome, including venous congestion of head, neck, and arms. **Patients presenting with anterior mediastinal or hilar masses should be evaluated for possible infectious causes, but when infectious causes are ruled out, bone marrow aspirate and biopsy should be done before thoracotomy.** Lymphoma involves the bone marrow in 15–20% of cases, and examination of the marrow may provide diagnostic material without the need for more invasive procedures.

Posterior tumors such as neuroblastoma are frequently asymptomatic but may be associated with neurologic symptoms. These tumors are frequently dumbbell-shaped with a large intraspinal component in addition to the intrathoracic tumor. Neuroblastomas usually respond rapidly to cytoreductive chemotherapy and seldom require laminectomy or radiation therapy for relief of early neurologic symptoms. Patients presenting with hemiparesis, however, require surgical intervention to prevent permanent neurologic damage.

Primary Tumors of the Chest Wall. The small round-cell tumors of childhood, such as Ewing sarcoma, peripheral neuroectodermal tumor (PNET, Askin tumor), and rhabdomyosarcoma, frequently present with very large masses arising from the ribs or chest wall. The

TABLE 1. Tumors Originating in the Mediastinum

Anterior	Posterior
Malignant (or potentially malignant)	
Lymphomas (thymic masses): T-cell lymphoma, Hodgkin's disease	Neuroblastoma
Germ-cell tumors, teratomas, dermoid	Neurogenic tumors (nerve sheath tumors, schwannoma)
Thyroid tumors (rare)	Ewing sarcoma/PNET
Thymomas (rare)	Rhabdomyosarcoma
Benign	
Bronchogenic cysts	Bronchogenic cysts
Hygromas	Thoracic meningocele
Lipomas	
Lymphangiomas	

PNET = peripheral neuroectodermal tumor.

masses may grow large enough to cause dyspnea or cough. Combined modality treatment with surgery, chemotherapy, and radiation therapy is necessary for treatment.

Tumors Metastatic to the Lungs. Malignant tumors arising elsewhere in the body may present with pulmonary metastases that are sufficiently widespread to be symptomatic at diagnosis. **The most common childhood tumor to present in this fashion is Wilms' tumor; pulmonary tumors may be numerous enough to give the appearance of pulmonary consolidation.**

TABLE 2. Pediatric Tumors that Metastasize to the Lungs

Primary Site	Tumors
Bone	Osteosarcoma Ewing sarcoma Chondrosarcoma (rare) Ameloblastoma (very rare)
Musculoskeletal System	Rhabdomyosarcoma Soft-tissue sarcomas, e.g., synovial sarcoma, malignant fibrous histiocytoma
Gastrointestinal Tract	Hepatoblastoma/hepatocellular carcinoma Embryonal sarcoma of liver Leiomyosarcoma Adenocarcinoma of colon
Genitourinary Tract	Wilms' tumor Malignant rhabdoid tumor of the kidney Clear-cell sarcoma of the kidney Gonadal germ-cell tumor Trophoblastic choriocarcinoma

Cure may be possible, however, with radiation therapy and chemotherapy. Adolescents with thyroid carcinoma may develop a miliary picture of pulmonary metastases that may remain stable for years. In female adolescents, a picture of multiple pulmonary nodules without an obvious primary site may indicate trophoblastic (gestational) choriocarcinoma. Treatment may be complicated by pulmonary hemorrhage. Other pediatric solid tumors that commonly metastasize to the lung are listed by primary site in Table 2. Although 70% of patients with neuroblastoma present with stage IV (metastatic) disease to bone and bone marrow, neuroblastoma only rarely metastasizes to the lung.

Patients with acute myeloid leukemia or chronic myelocytic leukemia who present with white blood cell counts >100,000 are at risk for pulmonary leukostasis. This is a medical emergency that requires early institution of cytoreductive therapy, including chemotherapy and leukapheresis.

SIDE EFFECTS OF TREATMENT

Infectious Complications. Patients who are immunosuppressed by chemotherapy are at high risk for pulmonary infections. The most likely etiology varies according to patient status (Table 3).

Patients with septic shock secondary to gram-negative organisms of Group A *Streptococcus* may develop severe adult respiratory distress syndrome (ARDS) even after control of the bacteremia. Diffuse interstitial pneumonia

TABLE 3. Infectious Complications of Chemotherapy

Patient Status	Differential Diagnosis
Nonneutropenic, diffuse infiltrate	*Pneumocystis carinii* Varicella-zoster, cytomegalovirus
Nonneutropenic, localized infiltrate	Mycoplasma Histoplasma Respiratory syncytial virus (RSV) *Streptococcus*
Neutropenic, diffuse infiltrate	Any bacteria *Candida, Aspergillus,* etc. Herpes, varicella-zoster RSV, etc.
Neutropenic, localized infiltrate	Any bacteria *Candida, Aspergillus,* etc.

associated with cytomegalovirus infection is particularly devastating in patients recovering from allogeneic bone marrow transplant.

Pulmonary Complications of Radiation Therapy. Radiation therapy to the lungs is associated with some degree of fibrosis in as many as 50–100% of patients if highly sensitive measures of pulmonary function are used; however, symptomatic radiation pneumonitis occurs in only 5–15% of patients. Patients who receive >30 Gy to 50% or more of the lungs are at highest risk. Radiation fibrosis may develop more frequently when children receive radiation therapy at a younger age, such as treatment for metastatic Wilms' tumor.

Pulmonary Complications of Chemotherapy. The most common chemotherapeutic agent implicated in the development of pulmonary fibrosis is bleomycin. Its use, especially in a cumulative dose >400 units, is associated with a 10% chance of symptomatic fibrosis. Other chemotherapy agents, especially methotrexate, vinblastine, and alkylating agents such as 1,3-bis-(2-chloroethyl)-1-nitrosourea (BCNU), cyclophosphamide, melphalan, and busulfan, are associated with a low incidence of pulmonary fibrosis.

SUMMARY

In the child with malignant disease, pulmonary complications may ensue from primary or metastatic tumors that compromise respiration, from opportunistic infections arising in the immunosuppressed host, and from long-term complications of therapy. Care of the child with cancer requires an interdisciplinary approach with the combined efforts of pediatric oncologists, surgeons, and radiation oncologists in a setting in which subspecialty consultation (infectious disease, pulmonology, cardiology) is readily available.

SUGGESTED READING

Pizzo PA, Poplack DG (eds): Principles and Practice of Pediatric Oncology, 2nd ed. Philadelphia, J.B. Lippincott, 1993.

29

RESPIRATORY COMPLICATIONS OF SICKLE-CELL DISEASE

Brian P. O'Sullivan, M.D.

Respiratory complications are the second leading cause of hospitalization in patients with sickle-cell disease, ranking behind only acute painful crises. As with other complications of sickle-cell disease, the pulmonary consequences stem from the abnormal hemoglobin that causes red blood cells to take on their typical sickled appearance under conditions of hypoxemia, acidosis, and increased temperature. These abnormally shaped red blood cells have increased viscosity and decreased plasticity compared with normal red blood cells and lodge in small blood vessels, causing vasoocclusion and tissue ischemia. In long bones and muscles this phenomenon leads to the clinical syndrome of acute painful crisis. In the pulmonary vasculature vasoocclusion leads to pulmonary infarction, pulmonary edema, and, over time, cor pulmonale.

In this chapter the term sickle-cell disease (SCD) is used to denote the syndrome secondary to the abnormal shape and mechanical properties of red blood cells resulting from any of the hemoglobinopathies that may cause sickling (e.g., SS, SC, S-thalassemia). Low partial pressure of oxygen and low flow states cause sickling of red blood cells in any of these hemoglobinopathies. Sickling is inhibited by an increase in oxygen tension and by the presence of non-S hemoglobin.

It is important to remember that the spleen is the predominant site of intravascular sickling in young children with SCD. Because of splenic infarction and the resultant loss in splenic function after repeated episodes of intravascular sickling, children with SCD are at increased risk for infection, particularly with the encapsulated organisms *Streptococcus pneumoniae* and *Hemophilus influenzae*. Historically, bacterial pneumonia and overwhelming sepsis with these organisms have been the leading cause of death in patients with SCD. Although the routine use of polyvalent pneumococcal vaccine and daily penicillin prophylaxis has decreased this risk significantly, infection remains the leading cause of death in patients with SCD. Therefore, all patients with SCD must be carefully evaluated and aggressively managed whenever they have a febrile illness.

ACUTE CHEST SYNDROME

Acute chest syndrome (ACS) is defined as chest pain, fever, dyspnea, cough, and radiographic signs of a pulmonary process in a patient with SCD. It is the most common pulmonary manifestation of SCD and may be caused by infarction of lung tissue or by any of numerous infectious agents. Unfortunately, **differentiating acute bacterial pneumonia from infarction in ACS is almost impossible on clinical grounds alone** (Table 1). Patients with bacterial infection are generally sicker than patients with viral infection or infarction, but this fact may be evident only in retrospect and is not helpful in the acute setting for evaluating individual patients.

The etiology of ACS in children, as in adults, is most frequently noninfectious. In

TABLE 1. Differential Diagnosis of Acute Chest Syndrome

	Pneumonia	Pulmonary Infarction
Age	Any, younger (1–3 yr)	Any, older (school age)
Fever	+ +	+
Chest pain	+	+ +
Abnormal CXR	+	+
Pleural effusion	+ +	+/–
Elevated WBC	+	+
Hypoxemia	+	+

*The marked overlap between pneumonia and infarction makes it virtually impossible to distinguish the two on clinical grounds. CXR = chest x-ray film; WBC = peripheral white blood cell count.

some clinical series, bacterial infection was proved in fewer than 15% of pediatric patients with ACS; another 10–12% were noted to have serologic evidence of mycoplasma infection, and viral infections were detected in approximately 10% of episodes of ACS. Although other infectious agents (such as *Chlamydia pneumoniae*) may also precipitate ACS, the majority of episodes are secondary to pulmonary infarction. The infarction may be caused by occlusion of vessels by sickled red blood cells, in situ thrombosis, or bone marrow emboli arising from infarcted long bones.

There is no simple, reliable method to differentiate infection from infarction in the clinical setting. History, physical examination, and chest roentgenograms are similar in both situations. Ventilation-perfusion scans are not useful in making a specific diagnosis, because both entities cause abnormalities of air and blood flow throughout the lung. Arteriography is the most accurate way to detect pulmonary thromboembolism, but the hypertonic nature of the dye used in this procedure precipitates sickling of red blood cells. Therefore, routine angiography has been contraindicated in patients with SCD. New-generation angiographic contrast agents may make this important test more feasible in patients with SCD.

The evaluation and initial management of a child with ACS therefore must be all-encompassing. Diagnostic studies that should be obtained on admission include urinalysis for the detection of bacterial antigens, cultures of blood and sputum, and routine blood counts and chemistries as well as specific serologic and microbiologic studies for the detection of mycoplasma and chlamydia infection (Table 2).

Of note is the fact that children with hemoglobin-SS disease often have lower than normal oxygen saturations by pulse oximetry, even when they are well. This is particularly true of children older than 5 years and children with a history of previous episodes of ACS. It is therefore useful to be able to compare pulse oximetry results in the setting of an acute illness with readings obtained when the child was well.

Antibiotic therapy aimed at treating the usual infecting organisms, *S. pneumoniae, H. influenzae*, and *Staphylococcus aureus*, should be started at once. Initial therapy (Table 3) includes a broad-spectrum antibiotic such as cefuroxime, 75–150 mg/kg/day. Antibiotic therapy may then be modified in accordance with the results of the initial studies. Supplemental oxygen treats the hypoxemia caused by pneumonia or infarction and helps to reverse intravascular sickling. Intravenous hydration also should be started at the time of admission.

Evidence of infection with *Mycoplasma pneumoniae* and *Chlamydia pneumoniae* has been found in some children with SCD and acute chest syndrome. Although the significance of chlamydia infection in these patients is yet to be determined, it is well appreciated that mycoplasma infections may cause serious disease in

TABLE 2. Diagnostic Studies in Acute Chest Syndrome

Complete blood count and reticulocyte count
Chest roentgenogram
Blood culture
Sputum culture
Urine for bacterial antigen detection
Nasopharyngeal swab for *Chlamydia pneumoniae*
Bedside cold-agglutinin test
Mycoplasma titers
Arterial blood gas determination (if clinically indicated)

TABLE 3. Therapy for Acute Chest Syndrome

Intravenous fluids (D_5 ½ normal saline)
Intravenous antibiotics (cefuroxime, 75–150 mg/kg/day)
Supplemental oxygen to keep pulse oximetry >92%
Judicious use of narcotic analgesics
Transfusion to get hemoglobin >10 gm/dl
Consider inhaled albuterol
Consider oral erythromycin (40 mg/kg/day)

patients with SCD. If the child does not respond to the initial antibiotic therapy, erythromycin in a dose of 40 mg/kg/day should be added. Mycoplasma infections appear to be especially prevalent in the autumn; therefore, during this season erythromycin should be considered as part of the initial therapy.

Transfusion with packed red blood cells (pRBC) is indicated to elevate the hemoglobin to a level of 10 mg/dl and to decrease the percentage of sickle cells present. We give pRBC to any patient with SCD and acute pulmonary symptoms if the hemoglobin is <8.0 mg/dl. The mechanism of therapeutic action of transfusion is unclear; it does not reverse the sickling of cells already trapped in pulmonary capillaries. Prophylactic transfusion therapy to keep the hemoglobin above 10 mg/dl is known to decrease intravascular sickling and has been reported to decrease the number of episodes of ACS in children with SCD.

Recently, inhaled bronchodilators have been advocated for patients with ACS. Both infection and infarction may cause inflammation of airways leading to bronchial edema and smooth muscle spasm; hence inhaled beta-agonists may be beneficial. A trial of albuterol by metered-dose inhaler or nebulization seems warranted in the child with ACS who is in respiratory distress.

A subset of patients develops delayed onset of respiratory complications of SCD. Such patients are initially admitted with complaints of chest wall pain but without radiographic evidence of pulmonary involvement. Over 48–72 hours they develop respiratory distress, and repeat chest radiographs demonstrate total white-out of one or both lungs. The amount of narcotic analgesia seems to correlate with progression to acute white lung. In patients who are already hypoventilating because of chest wall pain secondary to musculoskeletal crisis, **narcotic agents may induce further reduction in ventilation, sufficient to cause atelectasis. Thus, narcotic agents must be used judiciously in patients with SCD and chest wall pain.** Such patients should be reevaluated for ACS if they develop respiratory symptoms while in the hospital, even if they had no evidence of the syndrome on admission.

Pleural effusion may be present in up to 30% of patients with ACS. Therapy for this complication is the same as in the child without SCD; that is, small effusions are monitored clinically and radiographically, whereas large effusions should be drained. Initial drainage may be done by needle aspiration. However, if the pleural fluid has the characteristics of an empyema, closed-chest tube drainage is required.

CHRONIC LUNG DISEASE

Recurrent episodes of the acute chest syndrome described above lead to pulmonary scarring and restrictive lung disease over time. Pulmonary function tests in children with SCD infrequently demonstrate such abnormalities; in adults with SCD, however, decreased total lung capacity, decreased vital capacity, and increased shunt fraction have been documented.

The progression from normal pulmonary function in childhood to restrictive lung disease in adulthood has been documented to occur in a predictable fashion. The stages associated with chronic lung disease progress from minimal dysfunction with only mild radiographic abnormalities (stage 1) to hypoxemia at rest and an inability to perform pulmonary function tests (stage 4). Most patients are in the third decade of life at the onset of clinically apparent chronic lung disease, but some children in their first decade already have evidence of restrictive changes.

The changes in pulmonary function seen in SCD chronic lung disease are directly correlated with the severity and frequency of episodes of ACS experienced by the patient. We recommend that children with frequent episodes of ACS be monitored yearly with pulmonary function tests to detect early signs of chronic lung disease. Children with recurrent episodes of ACS should be considered for chronic transfusion therapy as a means of reducing the number of episodes of red cell sickling. Aggressive treatment of episodes of ACS is of paramount importance to minimize cumulative lung damage.

OBSTRUCTIVE SLEEP APNEA

Obstructive sleep apnea (OSA) causes hypoxemia during sleep; such episodes may precipitate acute sickling crises in patients with

SCD. Unfortunately, patients with SCD are at increased risk for OSA because of enlargement of tonsillar and adenoidal tissue as part of a generalized hypertrophy of lymphatic tissue.

This phenomenon may explain why some patients with SCD experience painful crises late at night or in the early morning hours when they are at highest risk for obstructive events.

A careful history regarding snoring, sleep disturbance, hypersomnolence, and other signs of OSA should be obtained in children with SCD and painful crises of increasing frequency. Particular interest should be paid to the time of onset of painful crises to look for a clustering of symptoms around sleep time. Any patient with SCD and symptoms of sleep disturbance should be evaluated for OSA (see chapter 22). We have seen one patient with SCD and obstructive apnea secondary to hypertrophy of the lingual tonsils. The tonsillar tissue regressed and symptoms improved after oral corticosteroid therapy.

RESPIRATORY COMPLICATIONS OF SICKLE-CELL TRAIT

Children who are heterozygous for SCD—that is, who have sickle-cell trait—are generally not at risk for developing intravascular sickling and vasoocclusive crises. There is some concern that under extreme conditions of hypoxemia and lactic acidosis, sickling may occur. Although recent studies have further fueled this concern, accumulated experience with intercollegiate and Olympic athletes indicates that hypothetical risks do not warrant exclusion of children with sickle-cell trait from participation in interscholastic sports. Nevertheless, patients with sickle-cell trait should be aware of the small but real risk of developing sickling at high altitudes, where the partial pressure of oxygen is decreased. Although travel on commercial airlines should not be a problem, it is wise to advise patients to avoid avocations that involve chronic exposure to a low ambient partial pressure of oxygen, such as aviation and mountaineering.

CONCLUSION

Acute chest syndrome remains one of the most common causes of hospitalization in children with SCD. Children with ACS should be managed aggressively for hypoxemia and possible infection. Repeated episodes lead to chronic lung changes with corresponding changes in pulmonary function studies.

It should not be forgotten that children with SCD are at the same risk for other pulmonary diseases as patients without SCD. Cystic fibrosis, asthma, and foreign body aspiration must be considered in any child who presents with recurrent pneumonias, chronic cough, and pulmonary infiltrates, whether or not he or she has SCD.

SUGGESTED READING

1. Barrett-Connor E: Acute pulmonary disease and sickle cell anemia. Am Rev Respir Dis 104:159–165, 1971.
2. Craft JA, Alessandrini E, Kenney LB, et al: Comparison of oxygenation measurements in pediatric patients during sickle cell crises. J Pediatr 124:93–95, 1994.
3. Handelsman E, Voulalas D: Albuterol inhalations in acute chest syndrome. Am J Dis Child 145:603–604, 1991.
4. Maddern BR, Ohene-Frempong K, Reed H, Beckerman RC: Obstructive sleep apnea syndrome in sickle cell disease. Ann Otol Rhinol Laryngol 98:174–178, 1989.
5. Pianois P, D'Souza SJA, Dic Charge T, et al: Pulmonary function abnormalities in childhood sickle cell disease. J Pediatr 122:366–371, 1993.
6. Ponz M, Kane E, Gill FM: Acute chest syndrome in sickle cell disease: Etiology and clinical correlates. J Pediatr 107:861–866, 1985.
7. Powars D, Weidman JA, Odom-Maryon T, et al: Sickle cell chronic lung disease: Prior morbidity and risk of pulmonary failure. Medicine 67:66–76, 1988.
8. Rackoff WR, Kunkel N, Silber JH, et al: Pulse oximetry and factors associated with hemoglobin oxygen desaturation in children with sickle cell disease. Blood 81:3422–3427, 1993.
9. Sprinkle RH, Cole T, Smith S, Buchanan GR: Acute chest syndrome in children with sickle cell disease. Am J Pediatr Hematol Oncol 8:105–110, 1986.
10. Weil JV, Castro O, Malik AB, et al: Pathogenesis of lung disease in sickle hemoglobinopathies. Am Rev Respir Dis 148:249–256, 1993.

COMMENTARY

by Carlton Dampier, M.D.

The pathophysiology of acute chest syndrome (ACS) in patients with sickle-cell disease (SCD) remains poorly understood. Current management recommendations represent the clinical experience of large pediatric and adult sickle-cell programs. A large multiinstitutional trial examining the role of transfusion therapy in ACS began in late 1993 and may provide more definitive recommendations in the future.

ACS Treatment Recommendations. Because distinguishing between infarction and infection is difficult, supportive therapy must be directed at both problems. Primary therapy with a parenteral cephalosporin or ampicillin is universal. However, in patients with SCD and a high degree of compliance with prophylactic penicillin therapy, the incidence of bacterial infections from encapsulated organisms is low. I also use oral erythromycin in all febrile patients with ACS, because the respiratory effects of mycoplasma infections can be very severe.

Because an acute pain crisis is a frequent precursor, patients are often treated with aggressive parenteral fluid regimens (1½–2 times maintenance rates) when ACS develops. This excessive fluid administration should be reduced once an ACS has been identified. Otherwise, the areas of damaged pulmonary tissue will leak intravascular fluid and contribute to worsening pulmonary edema, which will cause a vicious cycle of hypoxia and further sickling. Therapy for such complications ranges from judicious use of diuretics to mechanical ventilation. Pleural effusions are relatively common, but the likelihood that they represent empyemas is low; thus diagnostic thoracocentesis has little if any role. I use thoracocentesis only as a therapeutic procedure with large effusions that contribute to respiratory compromise.

Transfusion therapy for ACS remains controversial and is potentially complicated by the risks of transfusion-related infections and red blood cell alloimmunization. However, I currently transfuse patients with ACS who have significant tachypnea and hypoxia, because this combination often results in rapid clinical improvement. Simple transfusions (5–10 ml/kg of packed red blood cells) are adequate in most situations; many patients with clinically significant ACS have a worsening anemia, often as low as 6–7 gm/dl. For patients who are critically ill with a rapidly progressive course toward adult respiratory distress syndrome, I resort to a partial exchange transfusion. However, no controlled evidence indicates that such therapy is more beneficial than simple transfusion.

Many patients who develop ACS have concurrent vasoocclusive pain treated with narcotic analgesics, which may cause sedation and potential hypoventilation. Splinting from sternal or rib pain may be an equally serious risk factor for the development of ACS; thus adequate analgesia is also important. Because the pharmacokinetics of narcotic analgesics in these patients is as yet poorly characterized, prudence dictates a balance between excessive sedation and inadequate analgesia.

What Is the Meaning of Chronic Hypoxia? Routine monitoring of oxygen saturation identifies patients with SCD who have some degree of reduced oxygen saturation. Some have a history of recurrent vasoocclusive symptoms, whereas others are largely asymptomatic. Studies show a positive correlation between lower baseline hemoglobin levels and lower baseline oxygen saturations; however, no studies have yet shown an association between low baseline oxygen saturations and frequent or nocturnal vasoocclusive pain. Sickling is probably only one component of a multifactorial event that leads to vasoocclusion.

Some patients with borderline oxygen saturations may be at risk for nocturnal hypoxia, particularly if they have coexistent upper airway obstruction. This chronic or intermittent hypoxia may put them at increased risk for long-term pulmonary or cardiac complications as older adults. However, the role of supplemental oxygen remains controversial, because oxygen therapy has been shown to reduce erythropoiesis in patients with SCD and to increase the need for transfusion therapy. Patients also may be at greater risk for vasoocclusive symptoms after discontinuing a course of supplemental oxygen.

SCD and Upper Airway Obstruction. Upper airway obstruction from tonsilar and adenoidal hypertrophy is recognized as a common problem in children with SCD. Symptoms of obstructive sleep apnea and sleep disturbances should be carefully sought. When symptoms are related to or exacerbated by intercurrent upper respiratory infections or allergies, a short course of nasal corticosteroids and/or decongestants may be helpful. Patients with chronic symptoms are best managed with tonsillectomy and/or adenoidectomy after a short course of preoperative transfusion therapy to reduce intra- and postoperative risk.

SCD and Asthma. It is not unusual for patients to have asthma and sickle-cell disease; both are common in the African-American population. Poorly controlled asthma is a potentially serious problem for patients with SCD. I personally have seen many children in whom an asthma attack precipitated a painful crisis or ACS, and many of my most symptomatic patients with SCD also have significant reactive airway disease. Thus optimal management for asthma is extremely important to prevent or ameliorate complications of sickle-cell disease.

30

RESPIRATORY COMPLICATIONS OF CONGENITAL HEART DISEASE

Daniel V. Schidlow, M.D.

Respiratory symptoms occur commonly in children with congenital heart disease, particularly in infants under 1 year of age. The close proximity of the airways and the increases in pulmonary blood flow and vascular pressures associated with cardiac malformations are the most important predisposing factors for the complications described below.

Increased pulmonary blood flow and pulmonary artery pressure at or above systemic pressures result in significant decreases in lung compliance. The network of hypertensive blood vessels acts like a wire mesh that stiffens the lung, decreasing its distensibility. This phenomenon occurs in patent ductus arteriosus, ventricular septal defect, and, in general, any defect with significant shunting from the systemic to the pulmonary circuit. Such decrease in compliance results in tachypnea and breathing difficulty even in the absence of associated respiratory infections. Surgical repair, undertaken before development of irreversible damage to the vascular bed, usually restores normal compliance to the lungs.

Passive congestion of the lung due to left ventricular failure causes edema of the airway wall, airway obstruction, and increased mucus secretion; it also predisposes the patient to the development of frequent respiratory infections. Acute episodes of heart failure and congestion manifest with wheezing and respiratory distress, tachypnea, and hypoxemia (so-called cardiac asthma). Treatment with cardiotonic and diuretic drugs is necessary. Bronchodilators may bring about some relief, but treatment must be directed to unloading the retained fluid and improving myocardial function.

Respiratory infections, particularly pneumonia and bronchitis, further reduce lung compliance and increase the severity of respiratory distress. Hypoxemia in a patient with noncyanotic congenital heart disease should alert the practitioner to the presence of a pulmonary complication or decompensated heart failure. Reversal of the direction of the blood flow across the foramen ovale and right-to-left shunt may occur if the pressure in the pulmonary circuit equals or exceeds that of the systemic circuit because of pulmonary hypertension. Although the latter is usually due to heart disease in patients with large pulmonary blood flow, intrinsic lung disease may generate areas of ventilation-perfusion mismatch and hypoxemia, and also contribute to the elevation of pressure in the pulmonary vessels.

A rather frequent respiratory complication of congenital heart disease is the extrinsic obstruction of large airways by enlarged, hypertensive blood vessels. Great vessels normally compress slightly or come in very close contact with the airways in several areas of the respiratory tree.

Under normal circumstances, the aorta causes a small indentation in the left side of the trachea. When pulmonary hypertension is present, the left pulmonary artery pushes the aorta against the trachea, accentuating the normal compression. In complex heart diseases, the aorta may be enlarged and have an aberrant shape or course (right aortic arch, truncus arteriosus).

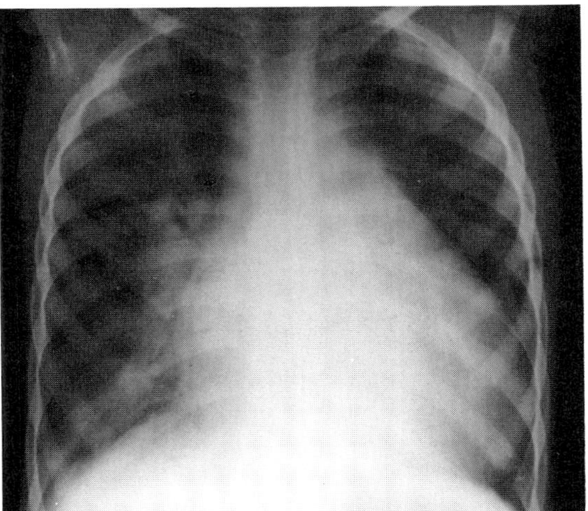

FIGURE 1. Atelectasis of the left lower lobe due to compression of the corresponding bronchus in an infant with ventricular septal defect.

Persistent compression of the trachea (probably already present during intrauterine life) results in areas of localized cartilage deficiency and airway obstruction. Some patients with complex cardiac anomalies also have concomitant airway anomalies, such as complete cartilaginous rings or aberrant anatomy, all of which may cause signs and symptoms of airway obstruction. Thus, severe indentation of the trachea by the aorta is indicative of pulmonary hypertension.

Enlargement of the left atrium results in upward compression of the main bronchi. The angle of bifurcation of the trachea increases, particularly because of upward deflection of the left main bronchus, which sits on the left atrium. The left pulmonary artery is located anterior to the main left bronchus in its upward course, arches behind the left upper bronchus, and then begins its descent, basically hooking the left upper bronchus from behind and anchoring it. Enlargement of the left atrium and left pulmonary vein pushes the main left bronchus and left lower bronchus upward. A very enlarged left atrium can compress the left lower bronchus, with subsequent atelectasis (Fig. 1). This complication is quite characteristic of ventricular septal defects and endocardial cushion defects with large flows. In the presence of massive atrial enlargement, the entire main left bronchus may become flattened and obliterated, causing atelectasis of the entire left lung (Fig. 2). **If treatment of heart failure does not result in resolution of the obstruction, endoscopy of the airway may be necessary to assess the severity of the compression and to detect associated abnormalities.** Radiographic assessment of cardiomegaly also may be helpful in the diagnosis.

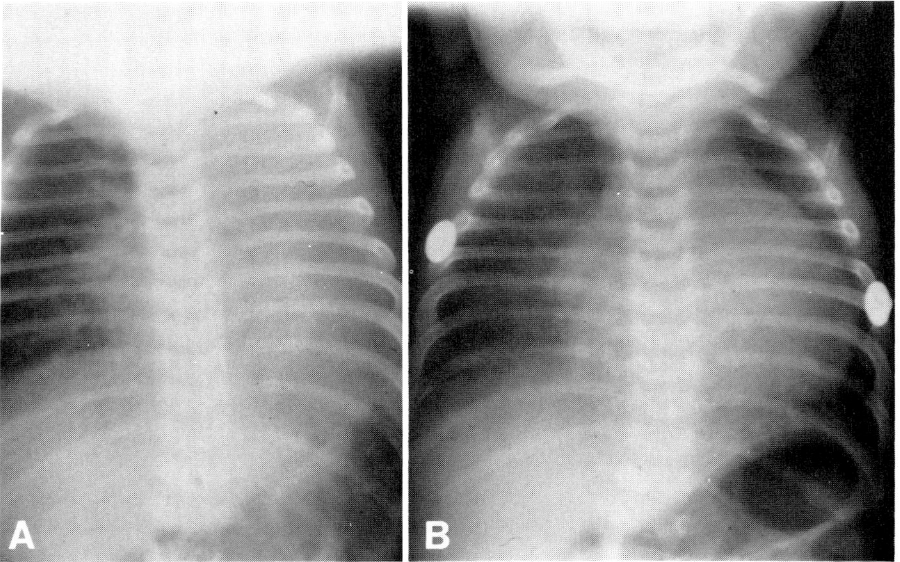

FIGURE 2. Complete atelectasis of the left lung *(A)*, which resolved after control of cardiac failure *(B)*, in an infant with endocardial cushion defect.

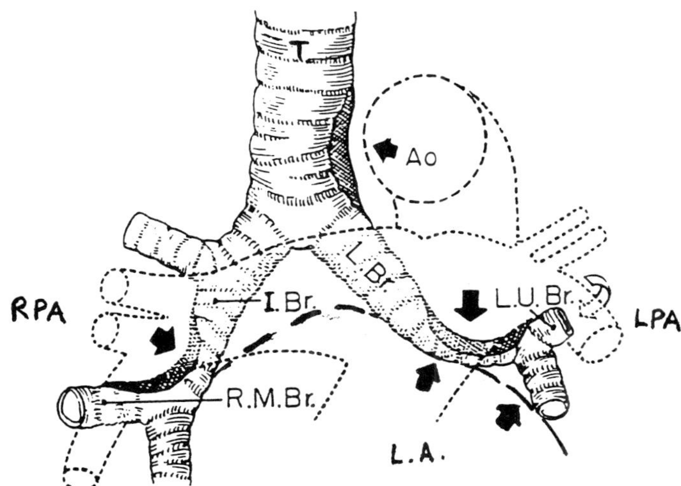

FIGURE 3. Front view of the tracheobronchial tree. The pulmonary arteries are in front of the airways. The arrows point to the potential areas of compression. Ao = aorta; IBr = bronchus intermedius; R,M,Br = right middle lobe bronchus; L,U,Br = left upper lobe bronchus; LBr = left main stem bronchus; T = trachea; LA = left atrium; RPA = right pulmonary artery; LPA = left pulmonary artery. (Modified from Stanger P, Lucas RV, Edwards JE: Anatomic factors causing respiratory distress in acyanotic congenital cardiac disease. Special reference to bronchial obstruction. Pediatrics 43:760–769, 1969, with permission.)

Gross cardiomegaly may cause atelectasis of the left lower lobe through direct compression of the lung by a massively enlarged left ventricle. This phenomenon can be seen in myocardiopathies, for instance, those due to storage diseases.

Another common site of compression is the junction of the right middle lobe bronchus and the bronchus intermedius. Enlargement of the right pulmonary artery and its branches is responsible for this phenomenon.

An uncommon complication of congestive heart failure in patients with severe cardiac malformations is the so-called cardiovocal syndrome. Traction and compression of the left recurrent laryngeal nerve by an enlarged pulmonary artery between the trachea and the aorta cause paralysis of the left vocal cord, mild stridor, and chronic hoarseness. Restoration of normal vocal cord function requires surgical correction of the underlying heart disease.

Figure 3 illustrates the anatomic relationship among the heart, great vessels, and the airways and indicates the sites of compression.

Hemoptysis may occur in older children with pulmonary vascular obstruction, Eisenmenger complex, and increased collateral bronchial circulation (usually tetralogy of Fallot or truncus arteriosus). Pulmonary venous congestion also may result in hemoptysis. This complication occurs most commonly in older children and is unusual in infants, because the abnormalities listed above develop over time.

SUGGESTED READING

1. Capitanio MA, Wolfson BJ, Faerber EN, et al: Obstruction of the airway by the aorta: An observation of infants with congenital heart disease. AJR 140:675–679, 1983.
2. Cochran ST, Gyepes MT, Smith LE: Obstruction of the airways by the heart and pulmonary vessels in infants. Pediatr Radiol 6:81–87, 1977.
3. Condon LM, Katkov H, Singh A, Helseth HK: Cardiovocal syndrome in infancy. Pediatrics 76:22–25, 1985.
4. Haroutunian LM, Neill CA: Pulmonary complications of congenital heart disease: Hemoptysis. Am Heart J 84:540–559, 1972.
5. Stanger P, Lucas RV, Edwards JE: Anatomic factors causing respiratory distress in acyanotic congenital cardiac disease. Special reference to bronchial obstruction. Pediatrics 43:760–769, 1969.

31

RESPIRATORY MANIFESTATIONS OF PEDIATRIC RHEUMATIC DISORDERS

Donald P. Goldsmith, M.D.

Many childhood rheumatic disorders have multisystem involvement; hence, respiratory manifestations may occur. Aside from the uncommon vasculitis syndromes, most of these disorders seldom present with significant respiratory signs and symptoms. Some medications used to treat rheumatic disorders also have the potential for pulmonary toxicity.

SPECIFIC DISORDERS

Juvenile rheumatoid arthritis is the most common rheumatic disorder of childhood. The three major presentations are the systemic, polyarticular, and pauciarticular varieties. The systemic variety is a multisystem disease with a characteristic rash, pericarditis, growth retardation, lymphadenopathy, and hepatosplenomegaly.

Pulmonary involvement is most common in systemic disease. Pleuritis occurs in association with pericarditis in about 1-2% of all affected children. Acute diffuse interstitial pulmonary fibrosis occurs rarely. Subclinical decreases in air flow and lung volumes and abnormal matching of ventilation and perfusion after exercise also have been reported.

Juvenile spondyloarthropathy is an entity that includes several related disorders, such as ankylosing spondylitis, Reiter syndrome, reactive arthritis, arthritis associated with inflammatory bowel disease, and psoriatic arthritis. These entities are characterized by asymmetric peripheral arthritis of the lower extremities, followed years later by sacroiliac and spinal involvement. Inflammation at sites of insertion of tendons to bone enthesis is characteristic. Pulmonary parenchymal disease is rare. Thoracic spine stiffness may cause diminished chest expansion and decreased vital capacity. Pleural effusion occurs rarely in children with Reiter syndrome. In adults with ankylosing spondylitis, apical pleural thickening is seen rarely.

Systemic lupus erythematosus (SLE) is the second most common rheumatic disorder of childhood. Inflammatory changes in various organs are mediated by the deposition of circulating immune complexes and subsequent complement activation. **Cough, pleuritic chest pain, or dyspnea may be presenting symptoms of children with SLE. The most frequent complications are pleuritis and pleural effusion, followed by acute and chronic interstitial pneumonitis and "shrinking lung syndrome"** (loss of lung volume with elevation of the diaphragm and shortness of breath). Defects in lung diffusions and decreased lung volumes occur in up to two-thirds of children with SLE. Acute pulmonary hemorrhage also may occur in this disease and is associated with a high rate of mortality. Radiographic infiltrates that result from SLE are difficult to differentiate from those caused by infection. Definitive diagnosis may require a lung biopsy and histologic examination. Increased susceptibility to respiratory infections is also related to hypocomplementemia, leukopenia, and relative hyposplenism. Unexplained episodes of dyspnea and cyanosis may be a clue to pulmonary thromboembolism, which is seen particularly in association with anticardiolipin antibodies.

Juvenile dermatomyositis is a multisystem disorder expressed primarily by both acute and chronic inflammatory changes of skin and striated muscle. In contrast to the adult form, juvenile dermatomyositis is not associated with pulmonary parenchymal or mediastinal malignancy. **The majority of children with severe disease present with impaired respiratory muscle movement and restrictive pulmonary disease.** Interstitial pneumonitis is rare. Approximately 10% of affected children develop hypopharyngeal or palatal muscle weakness with difficulty in swallowing and altered esophageal motility. Such abnormalities predispose to aspiration pneumonia.

Progressive systemic sclerosis (PSS) is a disorder characterized by symmetric fibrous thickening of the skin (sclerosis) and abnormalities of many visceral organs. Fibrous degenerative changes occur in the digital arteries, esophagus, intestinal tract, kidneys, heart, and lungs. Onset of PSS in childhood is very rare. **Pulmonary parenchymal disease is seen in almost all patients with PSS.** Bibasilar fibrosis is one of the minor criteria for the diagnosis. Involvement of the pulmonary vasculature, pulmonary hypertension, and rapidly progressive right ventricular failure are common. Restrictive lung disease and decreased carbon monoxide diffusion are usually detected in pulmonary function tests. Obstructive disease of the small airways occurs occasionally. The earliest symptom of pulmonary involvement is a dry, hacking, nonproductive cough with progression to dyspnea on exertion.

Mixed connective tissue disease is a syndrome with clinical features of SLE, dermatomyositis, and PSS as well as high titers of antiribonuclear protein antibodies. Early in the course of the disease, pleuritis and pleural effusions are relatively common, in keeping with symptoms suggestive of SLE. Over time—usually years—fever, arthritis, and myositis become less severe, and sclerodermatous changes predominate. **Over one-half of affected children eventually develop pulmonary involvement.** Restrictive lung disease is most common; pulmonary hypertension has also been recognized. Pulmonary function studies show reduced lung volumes and abnormal diffusion.

Goodpasture syndrome is a rare disorder in which severe inflammatory changes occur as a result of cross reactivity of antibodies with basement membrane constituents in the lungs and glomeruli of the kidney. **Most patients present with acute pulmonary hemorrhage and crescentic glomerulonephritis.**

VASCULITIS OF CHILDHOOD

Vasculitis in childhood includes various conditions of which inflammation of blood vessels is the hallmark. **Pulmonary involvement may be quite severe and occasionally is the primary presentation.**

Kawasaki disease, the most common vasculitis of childhood, is a necrotizing arteritis involving small and medium-sized arteries. Its incidence is highest between the ages of 1–3 years. Cough and coryza often occur early in the course of the disease, occasionally accompanied by pulmonary infiltration.

Schönlein-Henoch purpura, the second most comon vasculitis of childhood, is characterized by nonthrombocytopenic purpura, abdominal pain, gastrointestinal hemorrhage, nephritis, and arthritis. Leukocytoclastic vasculitis is the common pathologic lesion. Pulmonary involvement is very rare, but when it occurs, severe pulmonary hemorrhage results.

Polyarteritis nodosa primarily affects small and medium-sized muscular arteries. Severe necrotizing arteritis of pulmonary vessels occurs rarely and may cause hemoptysis and migratory pulmonary infiltrates.

Churg-Strauss vasculitis is characterized by granulomatous inflammatory changes in medium-sized and small muscular arteries and often presents with significant pulmonary symptoms. Most children with this disease have a past history of frequent and severe episodes of asthma and recurrent infiltrates. Other signs and symptoms include marked eosinophilia, prominent involvement of the skin, peripheral neuropathy, and often significant changes in gastrointestinal and coronary vessels.

Wegener granulomatosis, which is rare in childhood, is a necrotizing granulomatous vasculitis of the small veins and small and medium-sized arterioles. **Both the upper and lower respiratory tracts are involved; manifestations**

include epistaxis, otitis media, sinusitis, rhinorrhea, cough, and fever. Kidney damage is also typical of the disease.

ANTIRHEUMATIC DRUGS

Several medications currently used in the treatment of rheumatic disorders have potential pulmonary side effects. Gold salts, used primarily in children with polyarticular juvenile arthritis that is unresponsive to other antiinflammatory agents, has been reported to cause dyspnea, cough, pleuritic pain, and cutaneous eruption in adults. D-penicillamine is the drug of choice for children with PSS and on rare occasions may cause an SLE-like illness or Goodpasture syndrome. Methotrexate is often used as a remissive drug for children with juvenile rheumatoid arthritis and also as a secondary drug in juvenile dermatomyositis and SLE. Approximately 1% of adults treated with methotrexate develop interstitial pneumonitis and pleural effusion. The experience to date in children, however, has not demonstrated similar pulmonary toxicity.

SUGGESTED READING

1. Athreya BH, Doughty RA, Bookspau M, et al: Pulmonary manifestations of juvenile rheumatoid arthritis. Clin Chest 1: 361–374, 1980.
2. Falcini F, Pignono A, Matucci-Cerinic G, et al: Clinical utility of noninvasive methods in the evaluation of scleroderma lung in pediatric age. Scand J Rheumatol 21:82–84, 1992.
3. Fink CW: Vasculitis. Pediatr Clin North Am 33:1203–1219, 1986.
4. Garty BZ, Athreya BH, Wilmott R, et al: Pulmonary functions in children with progressive systemic sclerosis. Pediatrics 88:1161–1167, 1991.
5. Lang BA, Silverman ED: A clinical overview of systemic lupus erythematosus in childhood. Pediatr Rev 14:194–201, 1993.
6. Wegener JS, Taussig LM, DeBenedetti C, et al: Pulmonary function in juvenile rheumatoid arthritis. J Pediatr 99:108–110, 1981.

COMMENTARY

by Daniel V. Schidlow, M.D.

The most common respiratory manifestations of connective tissue disorders in children (as well as adults) include restrictive lung disease due to interstitial inflammation, pleuritis, and lung hemorrhage.

A more difficult diagnostic issue is when to suspect a rheumatic disorder in a patient with any of the above conditions. Helpful clinical features include joint involvement, vasculitic rashes, blood in urine and stools, and, of course, iridocyclitis, pericarditis, and other signs of polyserositis.

A simple but helpful laboratory test that can be done in any physician's office or obtained with a routine blood cell count is the erythrocyte sedimentation rate. Conditions that cause sedimentation rates in excess of 100 mm/hr can be counted on the fingers of one hand—as an experienced professor of internal medicine used to say—and collagen vascular diseases account for one of the fingers. Thus, in a patient afflicted by an unusual pulmonary disease, an abnormal sedimentation rate may be the first *laboratory* clue to a rheumatic disorder.

Infections with viruses, *Rickettsia* sp., and *Mycoplasma pneumoniae* may resemble the clinical picture of the rheumatic diseases and their respiratory manifestations. Serology, cultures, and microscopic examination of tissues may be necessary to arrive at a definitive diagnosis.

32

RESPIRATORY COMPLICATIONS OF NEUROMUSCULAR DISEASES

Raj Padman, M.D.

Neuromuscular diseases are associated with respiratory difficulties ranging from mild elevation of respiratory rate to severe respiratory failure, depending on the severity of muscle dysfunction. The integrity of the respiratory pump is essential for normal respiration. This system consists of the chest wall, its muscles and nerves, and central control mechanisms. The diaphragm, which is the principal muscle of inspiration, is like a piston that moves downward, enlarging the thorax and generating the negative pressure necessary for inspiration to occur. The primary function of the intercostal muscles is to stabilize the chest wall during changes in intrathoracic pressure.

Most pathologic processes of the neuromuscular system affect primarily the ability to perform an effective inspiratory effort. During quiet breathing, exhalation is passive secondary to the elastic recoil forces of the lungs. As breathing becomes more vigorous, as with respiratory infections, exhalation is not passive; intercostal muscles and rectus abdominis muscles contract to increase pleural pressure during exhalation.

In patients with neuromuscular diseases, the three most important derangements that contribute to abnormalities in gas exchange are (1) lack of muscle tone, (2) decreased inspiratory force, and (3) lack of effective cough mechanism. Lack of muscle tone leaves the recoil pressure of the lung relatively unopposed. Thus, resting lung volumes are smaller (decreased functional residual capacity). This deficiency causes stiffening of the lungs and impairment in gas exchange.

Patients with neuromuscular diseases become unable to generate normal inspiratory efforts. **Patients are able to take only smaller breaths (lower tidal volumes) and therefore must increase their respiratory rate to maintain adequate alveolar ventilation.** This pattern of rapid, shallow breathing leads to shortening and stiffening of elastic fibers and a decrease in lung compliance, thus increasing the work of breathing and decreasing reserves. A decline in reserve leads to exercise intolerance; affected patients, however, do not complain of shortness of breath on exertion, because they are wheelchair-bound early in the disease. In a system that functions suboptimally with minimal reserve, a minor respiratory infection may precipitate respiratory failure.

Another major factor in respiratory impairment is lack of an effective cough mechanism. Coughing is a form of forced exhalation against a closed glottis. The diaphragm and accessory muscles of the neck, as well as intercostal muscles and muscles of the abdominal wall and pelvic floor, contribute to generating the high intrathoracic pressures and flows required for an effective cough. The generated pressure is a direct function of muscle contraction. Retention of secretions secondary to depressed cough mechanism is a hallmark of respiratory failure secondary to neuromuscular diseases.

Neuromuscular impairment of respiratory mechanisms causes the following abnormalities:

1. Hypoxemia due to ventilation-perfusion mismatch and intrapulmonary shunting;
2. Hypoventilation and CO_2 retention due to progressive muscle weakness; and

3. Inadequate handling of secretions and aspiration pneumonia secondary to loss of cough and gag reflexes due to myopathic involvement of palatopharyngeal muscles and bulbar neuropathy.

In the terminal phases of these diseases, pulmonary hypertension, right ventricular dysfunction, and cor pulmonale supervene as a result of severe fibrosis, chronic hypoxia, hypercarbia, and polycythemia.

Ventilatory failure in association with pneumonia is a frequent cause of death in many patients with neuromuscular disease. It may occur at the onset of diseases such as myasthenia, Guillain-Barré syndrome, and botulism or in the later stages of diseases such as muscular dystrophy and motor neuron diseases.

EVALUATION

History

Dyspnea at rest or with exertion and recurrent respiratory infections with pneumonia are indicative of low respiratory reserve. **Difficulty in breathing in the supine as opposed to the sitting position is indicative of diaphragmatic weakness.** Restless sleep, excessive sweating during sleep, early morning headaches, daytime somnolence, and poor school performance are suggestive of nocturnal hypoventilation. Shortness of breath, chest pain, palpitations, cyanosis, and ankle swelling are suggestive of cor pulmonale or congestive heart failure.

Examination

Simple inspection and palpation of the chest wall yield important information about the movement of the chest wall and the function of the respiratory muscles. The patient must be observed during spontaneous breaths in various positions. During normal respiratory excursion, the chest and abdomen move out on inspiration. In patients with diaphragmatic paralysis or weakness, the falling pleural pressure during inspiration is transmitted across the flaccid hemidiaphragm; thus the abdominal wall moves paradoxically inward on inspiration. **Patients with paralysis of one hemidiaphragm (i.e., phrenic nerve injury) exhibit an inspiratory shift of the umbilicus cephalad toward the side of the paralyzed diaphragm ("belly dancer" sign).**

The onset of diaphragmatic fatigue is indicated first by tachypnea, then by paradoxical inward motion of the diaphragm on inspiration, and finally by respiratory alternans, in which the intercostal muscles and the diaphragm alternate in supporting ventilation.

In patients with spinal cord injury that spares the diaphragm (lesions below C5), spinal muscular atrophy and intercostal muscle weakness, or Duchenne muscular dystrophy (before diaphragmatic weakness sets in), the rib cage paradoxically caves in with decreasing pleural pressures created by the diaphragm during inspiration.

Visible and palpable use of the accessory muscles of respiration (sternocleidomastoid, scalene, and trapezius) may be seen in patients with neuromuscular diseases in whom diaphragmatic activity is not sufficient to maintain adequate gas exchange.

Tests of Respiratory Muscle Function

Tests of respiratory muscle function are simple to perform and can be done in any community medical center.

Inspiratory and Expiratory Pressures. A good index of respiratory muscle strength is the maximal inspiratory pressure measured after a complete exhalation and exhalatory mouth pressures measured at full inspiration. Low measurements reflect a decrease in strength. A drop in these pressures is the earliest detectable abnormality even in asymptomatic individuals. The tests are highly sensitive and reproducible with good effort. Normal inspiratory and expiratory pressures are between 60–100 cm of water. In patients with significant neuromuscular weakness the pressures fall to 35 cm or less.

Pulmonary Function Testing. Provided that the patient performs maximally, a decrease in total lung capacity, an increase in residual volume, or a decrease in vital capacity is suggestive of respiratory muscle weakness (Fig. 1). A decrease in the strength of the inspiratory muscles results in a decrease in total lung capacity, whereas a similar decrease in strength of the exhalatory muscles results in increased

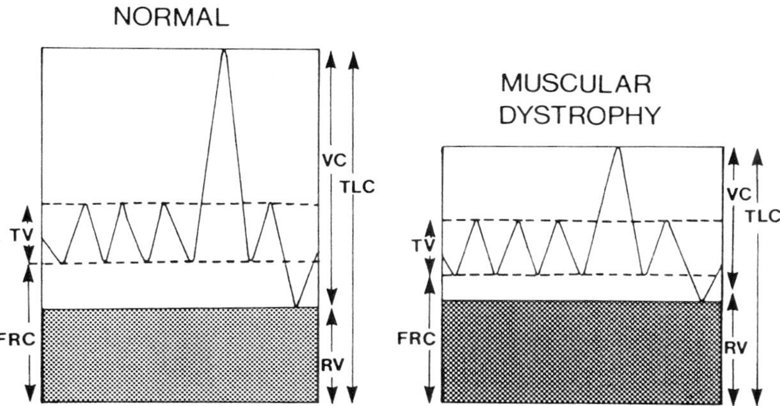

FIGURE 1. Pulmonary function abnormalities in neuromuscular diseases: maximal inspiratory pressure (PI max) decreases; maximal expiratory pressure (PE max) decreases; total lung capacity (TLC) decreases; residual volume (RV) increases; vital capacity (VC) decreases; PaO_2 decreases; and $PaCO_2$ increases.

residual volume. The decline in flow rates is proportional to the decline in lung volumes (see chapter 41).

Radiologic Studies. An elevated hemidiaphragm, fixed in position in chest radiographs obtained during inspiration and expiration, suggests diaphragm weakness or paralysis. Restrictive lung disease results in underaeration of the chest. A bell-shaped thoracic cage is obvious in patients with intercostal muscle weakness or hypotonia.

Fluoroscopy. Fluoroscopy is useful in evaluating the function of the diaphragm. During quiet breathing, the normal diaphragm moves smoothly up and down like a piston, with the dome preserving an evenly rounded contour. A paralyzed diaphragm is usually immobile during quiet breathing; in some cases, it moves paradoxically. The "sniff" test is used to diagnose diaphragmatic paralysis. The diaphragm is observed fluoroscopically during a sudden sniff; if paralysis is present, the other respiratory muscles produce a decrease in intrapleural pressure, which draws the paralyzed diaphragm into the chest. The paradoxical movements should be >2 cm and involve the whole diaphragm to establish the diagnosis.

Specialized Tests. Specialized tests include electromyography and magnetometry. Electromyogram of the diaphragm with needle or surface electrodes is helpful in distinguishing between neuropathic and myopathic diaphragmatic dysfunction as well as in detecting fatigue. Magnetometry is an investigational tool used to measure the relationships between the dimensions of the rib cage and the abdomen.

RECOGNITION OF RESPIRATORY FAILURE

Early diagnosis and management of respiratory failure are essential to improve survival and quality of life. **Speech difficulties, pooling of secretions, vital capacity <10–15 ml/kg, and maximal inspiratory force <25 cm of water are indications for an artificial airway and assisted ventilation.** In acute respiratory failure, such as occurs with botulism, Guillain-Barré syndrome, myasthenia, and high spinal cord lesions, vital capacity is a good indicator of pulmonary impairment and helps to guide the level of intervention. When vital capacity decreases to 2–3 times the tidal volume, the ability to sigh is compromised and atelectasis and hypoxemia ensue. The onset of pharyngeal paresis and aspiration is an indication for intubation, independently of measurements of vital capacity. The patient needs to be observed for signs and symptoms of hypoxia and hypercarbia.

Confusion, restlessness, and dyspnea are indicative of hypoxemia. In severe hypoxemia, a decrease in sympathetic tone produces bradycardia and hypotension. Cyanosis is an unreliable index of hypoxemia.

Impending carbon dioxide narcosis leads to nonspecific symptoms similar to those seen after general anesthesia: headache, drowsiness, coma, peripheral vasodilatation, and increases in sympathetic tone, including hypertension and tachycardia. All these signs and symptoms are indicative of serious derangement and necessitate mechanical ventilation.

Blood gas analysis and oximetry are important to confirm clinical suspicions of hypoxemia and hypercarbia. In patients with chronic

CO_2 retention, oxygen supplementation may promote further hypoventilation. A slight increase in PCO_2 may indicate severe ventilatory impairment and the imminent need for intubation and ventilation.

The most important clinical characteristic of neuromuscular respiratory failure is its insidious onset. **Patients may progress from slight dyspnea to life-threatening respiratory arrest within minutes.**

Other problems affecting the respiratory system in patients with neuromuscular diseases include (1) trauma and infection related to artificial airway; (2) nosocomial respiratory and urinary tract infections; (3) malnutrition; (4) decubitus ulcers; and (5) development of contractures. Meticulous attention must be paid to nutritional support and early physical therapy with range-of-motion exercises. Other significant complications, especially in patients with high spinal cord injury, include autonomic instability with wide swings in blood pressure and dysrhythmia.

MANAGEMENT OF SPECIFIC NEUROMUSCULAR DISEASES

Duchenne Muscular Dystrophy

Duchenne muscular dystrophy, a multisystem disease affecting the skeletal muscles, heart, and brain, is inherited as a sex-linked, recessive trait. Patients present with muscle weakness at 2–4 years of age. The disease progresses rapidly, and patients become wheelchair-bound by 10–12 years of age. With a decline in ambulation, pulmonary function declines progressively, especially during adolescence. Sleep hypoventilation out of proportion to pulmonary function may result from a weak diaphragm, reduction in inspiratory capacity, and weak tone of accessory neck muscles during rapid eye movement (REM) sleep. More than 80% of patients die from respiratory failure by age 30 years.

Multidisciplinary management involves physical therapy, surgery, and rehabilitation. Pulmonary function tests should be monitored every 6 months to 1 year in ambulatory patients and every 3–4 months in wheelchair-bound patients. Intermittent positive pressure breathing (IPPB) should be given with intercurrent infections if vital capacity drops below 80% of the predicted normal value, and routinely 3 times/day if it decreases to 50% or less. When vital capacity decreases to 30% or less, patients need to be monitored for sleep hypoventilation and hypoxemia. Nocturnal hypoventilation predisposes the patient to daytime hypercarbia and chronic increase in bicarbonate concentrations. If measurements of PCO_2 during sleep exceed 55 mmHg, ventilatory support should be offered.

Periodic orthopedic evaluations are important. Posterior spinal fusion with instrumentation should be offered to patients with a Cobb angle of 30° or more and before vital capacity decreases to 35% of normal. Cardiac evaluation should be obtained to assess myocardial involvement and detect dysrhythmias.

Surgical risk is identified by preoperative measurements of vital capacity. Postoperative ventilatory support can be predicted if preoperative vital capacity is $<$30%. Ventilatory support with a noninvasive nasal mask allows adequate care in the postoperative period without the need for an indwelling artificial airway over an extended period of time.

Early mobilization, assisted coughing, deep breathing, and tracheal toilet are essential elements of postoperative care. Spinal fusion may not arrest the decline in pulmonary function tests with age, but it may improve sitting comfort and appearance.

Patients should be protected with influenza vaccine every winter. Pneumococcal vaccine is also given, along with other routine immunizations, because all patients have low respiratory reserve.

Myotonic Dystrophy

In myotonic dystrophy, an autosomal dominant disease, myotonia and muscle weakness are the prominent clinical features. Involvement of the respiratory system is a major factor contributing to morbidity and mortality. Poor development of pharyngeal and diaphragmatic muscles has been found in infants who die at birth.

Congenital myotonic dystrophy presents in the neonatal period. The mother is invariably the affected parent. Mildly affected infants have hypotonia, problems with sucking and swallowing, usually facial diplegia, and possibly limb contractures. More severely affected infants suffer asphyxia at birth and require assisted ventilation. Because of intrauterine decrease in fetal breathing, patients have associated pulmonary hypoplasia. The need for prolonged ventilation is associated with poor prognosis.

Withdrawal of ventilatory support should be considered if no progress is seen over a 1-month period and if there are no indications for surgical corrections, such as plication for a paradoxically moving diaphragm.

Aminophylline therapy may be tried in an effort to stimulate central respiratory drive and to increase the strength of muscle contractions.

Spinal muscular atrophy—type I (Werdnig-Hoffmann disease) is an autosomal recessive disorder that causes mucle weakness, wasting, hypotonia, and absent tendon reflexes. About 65% of affected children develop symptoms before 6 months of age. They may appear normal during the first 2–3 months of life but gradually lose control of the head and trunk and show decreased movements of the extremities. Tongue fasciculations are virtually pathognomonic for the disorder. The thorax is bell-shaped with appropriate diaphragmatic excursion; the abdomen rises during inspiration, but the thoracic cage sinks inward because of the lack of muscle tone and weak intercostal muscles. Werdnig-Hoffmann disease in its most severe form has a grave prognosis and poor survival beyond infancy. Chronic ventilatory support is the only option for survival.

About one-third of patients with spinal muscular atrophy have a more benign variant called **spinal muscular atrophy—type II**. Symptoms do not appear until later in infancy, and patients may survive until adulthood. Patients can sit, and a few remain ambulatory for many years.

Kugelberg-Welander syndrome, an even milder juvenile variant of anterior horn cell disease, is an autosomal recessive disorder that exhibits slower progression of weakness with no loss of ambulation until the second or third decade of life and relative sparing of pulmonary functions.

All patients have restrictive pulmonary disease. Some patients may have a component of airway reactivity and exacerbations with infection and should be treated with antiinflammatory agents as well as bronchodilator therapy.

Progressive reduction in pulmonary function leads to respiratory failure. Patients with chronic respiratory acidosis should be offered assisted mechanical ventilation to avoid further complications and death.

Nocturnal ventilatory support may be provided noninvasively with a nasal mask and a portable volume ventilator or bilevel support system for positive airway pressure. Patients who continue to have difficulty handling secretions need the conventional tracheostomy and positive pressure ventilation for 12–24 hours/day, depending on the degree of respiratory insufficiency. Special devices facilitate communication in patients with a tracheostomy.

Our experience with a total of 8 patients (6 with noninvasive ventilation and 2 with tracheostomy and conventional positive pressure ventilation) has been rewarding. All are attending regular schools; two have graduated from high school and one from college. We have been able to document a 10–20% improvement in vital capacity after initiation of ventilatory support, perhaps as a result of full passive expansion of the lungs or of resting fatigued ventilatory muscles at night.

SUGGESTED READING

1. Derenne JP, Macklem PT, Roussous CH: The respiratory muscles: Mechanics control and pathophysiology. Am Rev Respir Dis 118:119–133, 1978.
2. De Troyer A, Deisser P: The effects of intermittent positive pressure breathing on patients with respiratory muscle weakness. Am Rev Respir Dis 124:132–137, 1981.
3. Ellis ER, Bye PT, Bruderer JW, Sullivan CE: Treatment of respiratory failure during sleep in patients with neuromuscular disease. Positive-pressure ventilation through a nose mask. Am Rev Respir Dis 135:148–152, 1987.
4. Fraser RG, Pare JAP: Diseases of the diaphragm and chest wall. In Diagnosis of Diseases of the Chest. Philadelphia, W.B. Saunders, 1970, pp 1217–1219.
5. Gilgoff JG, Kahlstrom E, MacLaughlin E, Keens TG: Long-term ventilatory support in spinal muscular atrophy. J Pediatr 115:904–909, 1989.
6. Jenkins JG, Bohn D, Edmonds JF, et al: Evaluation of pulmonary function in muscular dystrophy patients requiring spinal surgery. Crit Care Med 10:645–649, 1982.
7. Miller RG, Chalmers AC, Dao H, et al: The effect of spine fusion on respiratory function in Duchenne muscular dystrophy. Neurology 41:38–40, 1991.
8. Roussos C, Macklem PT: The respiratory muscles. N Engl J Med 307:786–797, 1982.
9. Shelbourne P, Davies J, Bruxton J, et al: Direct diagnosis of myotonic dystrophy with a disease-specific DNA marker. N Engl J Med 328:471–475, 1993.
10. Siegal IM: Pulmonary problems in Duchenne muscular dystrophy: Diagnosis, prophylaxis, and treatment. Phys Ther 55:160–162, 1975.
11. Smith PE, Calverley PM, Edwards RH, et al: Practical problems in the respiratory care of patients with muscular dystrophy. N Engl J Med 316:1197–1205, 1987.

33

RESPIRATORY COMPLICATIONS OF SCOLIOSIS AND SPINAL DEFORMITIES

Raj Padman, M.D.

Clinicians have known for centuries that deformities of the thoracic cage cause deleterious effects on the heart and lungs. Hippocrates first noted that hunchbacks had breathing difficulties. He also mentioned that patients with kyphoscoliosis in whom the curvature was above the diaphragm commonly had dyspnea and seldom lived to be 60 years old.

Scoliosis results from a pathologic process leading to lateral curvature of the spine. This lateral rotation of the spine (Fig. 1) causes the ribs to protrude posteriorly, forming a hump; in addition, the angle of articulation of the ribs and the spine is grossly distorted. The severity of the lateral curvature is easily measured, but the rotation, which is probably a more important contributor to respiratory failure and cor pulmonale, cannot be easily ascertained.

Scoliosis is a common deformity. The incidence of spinal curvature >35° is 1 per 1,000; of curvature >70°, 0.1 per 1,000. Structural scoliosis is characterized by the presence of a fixed rotational prominence on the convex side of the curve, which is best seen with the patient in the forward-bending position. The vertebrae are rotated into the convexity of the curve (see Fig. 1).

KYPHOSIS AND LORDOSIS

Kyphosis is increased posterior or decreased anterior angulation of the spine, whereas lordosis is an increased anterior or decreased posterior angulation of the spine. A curvature >40° is considered abnormal kyphosis in the thoracic spine and abnormal lordosis in the lumbar spine. Kyphoscoliosis, the rare combination of kyphosis and scoliosis, is usually a congenital abnormality seen in progressive infantile scoliosis. **Scheuermann juvenile kyphosis** is a fixed kyphosis that develops around the time of puberty. Because no rotation of vertebrae is involved, lung function is not affected, in contrast to scoliosis. Kyphosis of 35–40° is treated only for pain or cosmetic reasons. Progressive severe deformity may be treated with exercise, orthosis, or, on rare occasions, surgery.

The severity of scoliosis is usually defined by the degree of deformity, as measured by drawing (1) parallel lines between the upper border of the highest vertebral body and the lower border of the lowest vertebral body of the curve and (2) perpendicular intersecting lines. The angle of curvature (Cobb angle) consists of the cephalad or caudad angles. The more severe the scoliosis, the larger the angle. For many reasons, thoracic scoliosis may result in respiratory and cardiac problems. **A curve of <70° is usually associated with asymptomatic cardiorespiratory status at rest. Patients with curves of about 100° experience symptoms such as dyspnea on exertion. A curve of >120° leads to alveolar hypoventilation** (Table 1). Long-term studies of patients with untreated severe idiopathic scoliosis have demonstrated a mortality rate twice that of the general population. In one study, average age of death was 46.6 years. Respiratory or right-heart failure accounted for 60% of deaths. Of living patients with a mean age of 62 years, about one-half were incapacitated.

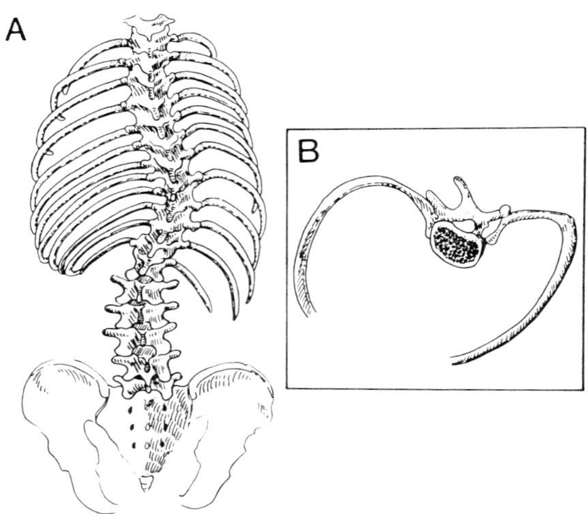

FIGURE 1. Deformity of vertebrae and rib cage in scoliosis illustrating the lateral curvature and rotation of vertebrae.

PULMONARY FUNCTION AND SCOLIOSIS

Spinal curvatures >90° predispose the scoliotic individual to cardiorespiratory failure. Restrictive pulmonary function is seen with a 50–60° curve. The degree of restrictive lung disease is related to the severity of the scoliosis. The greatest reduction is in vital capacity. Residual volume remains more or less within the predicted normal values (Fig. 2). This relative increase in residual volume is not indicative of obstructive airways disease. The rates of expiratory air flow fall in proportion to the restricted lung volumes. Chest deformity and stiffness, inspiratory muscles that work at a mechanical disadvantage, and impaired lung growth contribute to the negative effect on lung function (see chapter 41).

At any given Cobb angle, patients with congenital scoliosis have at least 15% less vital capacity than patients with idiopathic scoliosis. Because the loss of vital capacity in both groups increases progressively with the Cobb angle, **the lungs of patients with congenital disease are always at a functional disadvantage.** Patients with congenital scoliosis also have varying degrees of pulmonary hypoplasia, with reduced bronchial generations due to a developmental defect before 16 weeks of gestational age. The role played by rib anomalies in congenital scoliosis may be an important factor that contributes to a greater loss in vital capacity. Congenital scoliosis seems to involve failure of alveolar multiplication. In idiopathic scoliosis, the alveoli do not increase in size.

A clinician must be alert especially to the possibility of diaphragm weakness, which may

TABLE 1. Respiratory and Cardiovascular Impairment in Scoliosis

Curve <70°:	asymptomatic at rest
Curve >100°:	dyspnea with exertion
Curve >120°:	alveolar hypoventilation
Pulmonary impairment	
Restrictive lung disease	
Lung hypoplasia	
Decreased lung compliance	
Decreased chest wall compliance	
Increased elastic work of breathing	
Reduced diffusion capacity—hypoxemia	
Increased ventilation-perfusion mismatch—hypoxemia	
Hypoventilation (increased volume dead space/tidal volume)	
Reduced respiratory drive	
Respiratory failure	
Cardiovascular impairment	
Pulmonary arterial hypertension	
Cor pulmonale	
Cardiomegaly	

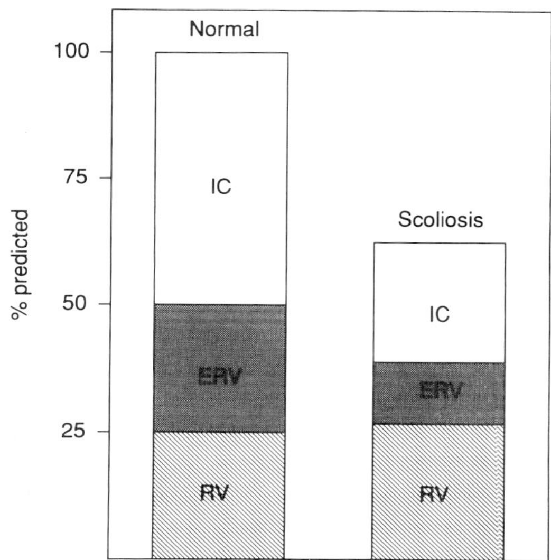

FIGURE 2. Comparison of lung volumes in normal patients and in patients with scoliosis. ERV = expiratory reserve volume; IC = inspiratory capacity; RV = residual volume.

be signaled by severe orthopnea and confirmed by a drop of about 50% in vital capacity when the patient goes from the upright to the supine position.

The elastic work and energy cost of mobilizing the deformed chest are increased by severe deformity. A stiff chest cage with small lungs results in abnormal mechanics of breathing. The predominant abnormality is the increased elastic resistance of the chest wall, which leads to a pattern of rapid, shallow breathing and increased dead-space ventilation. Increase in the alveolar arterial gradient for oxygen also results from ventilation-perfusion mismatch and reduction in diffusion capacity.

In asymptomatic adolescents with idiopathic scoliosis, diffusion capacity may be reduced as low as 70% of predicted values. Patients who already have dyspnea and cor pulmonale have drops in diffusion capacity, as measured during pulmonary function testing, to under 50% of predicted values.

In summary, hypoxemia in scoliosis is related to alveolar hypoventilation, decreased diffusion, and ventilation-perfusion mismatch. The ventilation-perfusion mismatch is due to compression of the lungs with loss of volume; airway closure; unilateral, localized underventilation; or microatelectasis. **The lung in the convex hemithorax has the slowest flow rate and the smallest volume; it is poorly ventilated but well perfused. The lung on the concave side has increased perfusion without an associated increase in ventilation.** Thus, both lungs contribute to ventilation-perfusion mismatch.

The respiratory drive in such patients is often below normal and impairs the ventilatory response to stress and injury. This abnormality is proportional to the defect in vital capacity and the stiffness of the chest wall and lungs, as previously described.

Respiratory failure in severe scoliosis occurs initially at night, especially during rapid eye movement (REM) sleep. Nocturnal hypoxemia is highly important in the development of pulmonary hypertension, cor pulmonale, and right-heart failure. Hypoxic cardiac arrhythmias during sleep are a common cause of death.

Patients also have a limited ability to exercise because of ventilatory limitation and commonly develop steep rises in pulmonary artery pressure during activity, which predisposes to the development of cor pulmonale.

All patients with kyphoscoliosis appear to have small lungs. The cross-sectional area of the vascular bed is also diminished through compression, distortion of vessels, and decreased distensibility. Eventually, a functional increase in pulmonary vascular resistance, imposed by hypoxemia, complicates the previously described anatomic changes. Anatomic changes in pulmonary vessels eventually lead to irreversible pulmonary hypertension.

MANAGEMENT OF IDIOPATHIC SCOLIOSIS

The management of idiopathic scoliosis depends on two critical questions: (1) whether the curve is likely to progress before cessation of growth and (2) whether further progression is expected in the mature patient.

The risk of progression of the curve is increased in premenarchal girls, individuals with large curves, and individuals with thoracic rather than lumbar deformities. Current treatment modalities include bracing and surgical intervention. **Bracing for thoracic scoliosis decreases lung volumes by approximately 15–20%.** Bracing may have deleterious effects on lung growth and impose an additional risk factor in the presence of disorders such as asthma and diaphragmatic weakness. When scoliosis progresses with thoracic lordosis, most surgeons elect to perform spinal fusion.

Spinal surgery with instrumentation provides good cosmetic correction, particularly of rib hump deformities, and is recommended for progressive curves >45° in skeletally immature patients. Immediately after surgery, pulmonay function usually declines. All volumes decrease with changes in posture from the upright or seated to the supine position because of the mass effect of abdominal contents. Abnormalities in pulmonary function also occur as an immediate effect of surgery because of changes in the configuration and properties of the rib cage and the lung as well as other factors that alter neuromotor control of the diaphragm and intercostal muscles. It takes up to 2 years after surgery for pulmonary function to recover to presurgery values.

MANAGEMENT OF KYPHOSCOLIOSIS

Most individuals with kyphoscoliosis—particularly children—do not develop respiratory failure. Measurements of vital capacity must be repeated on a yearly basis during growth to detect children at risk of developing cardiorespiratory failure in adulthood due to progressive chest deformity. When vital capacity declines to <50%, intermittent positive pressure breathing (IPPB) should be instituted. The chronically decreased lung compliance increases an average of 70% and is maintained for as long as 3 hours after the administration of one such treatment. The resistance of lung tissue decreases and lung compliance increases after positive pressure treatment. Collapsed air spaces expand, and the work of breathing decreases.

When vital capacity declines to 30% or less, patients must be referred to a pulmonary specialist for evaluation to rule out nocturnal hypoxemia and hypoventilation with sleep studies. Oxygen supplementation to delay the onset of cor pulmonale and assistive ventilation during acute illnesses and sleep may be required to prevent severe hypoxemia and its complications. Mechanical devices used to achieve these goals include iron lungs, tracheostomy and intermittent positive pressure breathing, rocking beds, and Cuirass shells. Noninvasive nocturnal ventilation with volume ventilators or bilevel positive airway pressure (Bi-PAP) devices with a nasal mask may improve respiratory failure as well as right-heart failure in patients with severe kyphoscoliosis. Treatment with diuretics, normalization of acid-base balance, and avoidance of hypokalemic alkalosis are important in therapy at the advanced stage. Respiratory stimulants such as theophylline also have been used as coadjuvant therapy.

In summary, physicians treating patients with thoracic and spinal deformities need to anticipate potential complications and to intervene early to avoid serious consequences. Team work with orthopedists, pulmonary specialists, orthotic specialists, physical therapists, and other professionals provides the best care for patients.

SUGGESTED READING

1. Baydur A, Swank SM, Stiles CM, Sassoon CS: Respiratory mechanics in anesthetized young patients with kyphoscoliosis: Immediate and delayed effects of corrective spinal surgery. Chest 97:1157–1164, 1990.
2. Bergofsky EH: Respiratory failure in disorders of the thoracic cage. Am Rev Respir Dis 119:643–669, 1979.
3. Cooper DM, Rojas JV, Mellins RB, et al: Respiratory mechanics in adolescents with idiopathic scoliosis. Am Rev Respir Dis 130:16–22, 1984.
4. Davies G, Reid L: Effect of scoliosis on growth of alveoli and pulmonary arteries and on right ventricle. Arch Dis Child 46:623–632, 1971.
5. Kafer ER: Respiratory and cardiovascular functions in scoliosis and the principles of anesthetic management. Anesthesiology 52:339–351, 1980.
6. Kennedy JD, Robertson CF, Hudson I, Phelan PD: Effect of bracing on respiratory mechanics in mild idiopathic scoliosis. Thorax 44:548–553, 1989.
7. Mezon BL, West P, Israels J, Kryger M: Sleep breathing abnormalities in kyphoscoliosis. Am Rev Respir Dis 122:617–621, 1980.
8. Owange-Iraka JW, Harrison A, Warner JO: Lung function in congenital and idiopathic scoliosis. Eur J Pediatr 142:198–200, 1984.
9. Pehrsson K, Bake B, Larsson S, Nachemson A: Lung function in adult idiopathic scoliosis: A 20 year follow up. Thorax 46:474–478, 1991.
10. Smyth RJ, Chapman KR, Wright TA, et al: Ventilatory patterns during hypoxia, hypercapnia, and exercise in adolescents with mild scoliosis. Pediatrics 77:692–697, 1986.

34

CHEST WALL DEFORMITIES

Charles Vinocur, M.D., and Daniel V. Schidlow, M.D.

The chest wall is an asymmetric structure. Minor deformities of little consequence are common. Some children, however, have noticeable congenital abnormalities of the chest wall, which may be placed into five categories: (1) pectus excavatum or funnel chest; (2) pectus carinatum or pigeon breast, (3) Poland syndrome, (4) sternal defects, and (5) thoracic deformities seen in diffuse skeletal disorders.

PECTUS EXCAVATUM

Pectus excavatum is the most common chest wall deformity. The sternum is angled posteriorly toward the spine. The lower costal cartilages flair dorsally to create the depression. The bending is greatest in the lowermost cartilages. The ribs themselves are entirely normal. Most defects are asymmetric with the greatest concavity to the right side. In some female patients, the right breast is less well developed. In addition to the depressed sternum, children with pectus excavatum have rounded shoulders, a slight dorsal kyphosis, abnormal retraction of the sternum on deep inspiration, and a prominent pot belly.

The defect is usually present at birth, with variable progression in different children as they grow. Mild forms of pectus excavatum may develop in infants with upper airway obstruction and persistent retractions (i.e., children with bronchopulmonary dysplasia). The male-to-female ratio for congenital pectus excavatum is 3:1.

Although the etiology is unknown, the deformity is probably due to an unbalanced overgrowth of the costal cartilages, which results in downward displacement of the sternum. Often other family members are affected. In addition, about 15% of the patients have concomitant scoliosis, and 2% have coexistent heart disease. Severe pectus excavatum with scoliosis may be associated with Marfan syndrome, especially in male patients; an echocardiogram and an ophthalmologic examination are required for confirmation.

The majority of patients with pectus excavatum are asymptomatic. Therefore, most physicians believe that surgery is done only for cosmetic or psychological reasons. Children with a very deep deformity may develop large airway compression and tracheobronchomalacia with bronchoscopically demonstrated airway collapse that manifests with wheezing. Children with a moderately severe or severe defect may present with intolerance to exercise, dyspnea, and decreased cardiovascular performance during exercise testing. Surgical correction results in functional improvement of these abnormalities. The current surgical management of children and adolescents with significant abnormality aims at relief of the structural compression of the chest to allow for normal growth. Other aims of surgery include possible prevention of cardiorespiratory dysfunction during adult life and avoidance of the psychological impact of the cosmetic defect on the child's self-image.

Children with mild pectus excavatum need not be referred for evaluation. Those with a more severe defect should undergo evaluation, particularly if they appear to have symptoms attributable to the defect or significantly diminished self-image. Patients and families in whom the nature or appearance of the defect has generated concern and anxiety benefit from a detailed evaluation and explanation of the nature and prognosis of the defect. Children with pectus excavatum also may benefit from postural and breathing exercises.

Referral for surgery ideally should occur no later than the age of 4 years; time must be allowed for evaluation of the patient, education of the parents, and development of the relationship between the surgeon and the family. It is our practice to perform surgery between the ages of 4 and 6 years so that it is completed before school begins. The best long-term results, furthermore, are seen in patients who undergo surgery at a younger age.

No discussion of pectus excavatum is complete without addressing the psychological impact of the abnormality on the child's self-image. Although some children ignore the defect, usually when the parents are quite comfortable with it, others have poor self-image regardless of parental tolerance and avoid sporting activities and exposure of the chest at any cost. Thus, a good assessment of the psychological impact of the deformity is very important.

The diagnosis of pectus excavatum is easily made on physical examination; chest radiographs help to document the defect and the secondary mediastinal displacement. Various criteria have been suggested for selecting patients for corrective surgery, including the ratio of transverse to narrowest anteroposterior diameter on chest tomography and pulmonary function and cardiovascular studies during exercise. In the absence of symptoms or abnormalities in cardiopulmonary performance, the psychological impact of the deformity may be the most important indication. No long-term longitudinal studies have followed patients with pectus excavatum into adulthood to determine whether patients with mild or asymptomatic deformity will develop cardiopulmonary decompensation later in life.

In general, it is best to refer patients to centers with ample experience in the surgical correction of pectus excavatum. The operative repair differs from center to center. All operative techniques, however, involve the removal of malformed cartilages and freeing the sternum from its depressed position to be brought forward. A substernal strut may or may not be used for stabilization of the chest. Children are admitted the day of surgery and usually need to remain in the hospital for 4–5 days. If a repair is delayed until the teenage years, longer hospitalization may be anticipated. Patient-controlled analgesia has greatly improved pain management, allowing early postoperative mobilization. Need for blood transfusions and complications such as pneumothorax are quite unusual. Fluid collections in the chest or wound are no longer a concern with the use of mediastinal and wound drains. Superficial wound infections occur occasionally and are easily treated.

Some surgeons use an external protector of rigid plastic fitted to the patient's chest for 6–12 weeks after surgery. If a substernal strut is placed during surgery, it is removed 6–12 months later during a limited outpatient procedure. Good to excellent results, including patient and family satisfaction, normal chest configuration, inconspicuous scar, and resolution of symptoms, are seen in the vast majority of patients.

PECTUS CARINATUM

Pectus carinatum is a protrusion deformity of the chest; it is substantially less common than the depression deformities. The spectrum of presentation includes protrusion of part or all of the sternum and unilateral and bilateral involvement of the cartilages. As in pectus excavatum, male predominance is 3:1. Similarly, a familial incidence is found in about one-fourth of the patients. Concomitant scoliosis (seen in about 15% of patients) should raise the suspicion of Marfan syndrome; homocystinuria and Morquio or Noonan syndrome also may be associated. This defect is rarely apparent before the age of 3–4 years and often goes unnoticed until adolescence.

No cardiovascular changes have been documented in patients with pectus carinatum. **The major indication for surgical intervention is cosmetic.** If the defect is relatively minor, surgery is unnecessary. Surgical correction is indicated in children with a bizarre chest configuration. The repair is similar to the one for pectus excavatum, although individual modifications may be necessary in children with unusual defects. Operative complications also are similar to those for pectus excavatum. Results are excellent, but if the procedure is done before chest growth is nearly complete, recurrence is common. Thus, most patients should undergo corrective surgery during the adolescent years.

POLAND SYNDROME

Poland syndrome is a sporadic and uncommon defect (1 in 30,000 live births) that includes a constellation of abnormalities due to hypoplasia of various components of the chest wall; the most common finding is partial or complete absence of the pectoralis major muscle. In the most severe form, partial agenesis of the ribs and the sternum, mammary aplasia, absence of the latissimus dorsi and serratus anterior muscles, brachysyndactyly, and scoliosis may be present. Certain leukemias, Möbius syndrome, and renal hypoplasia have been described in association with Poland syndrome.

Varying elements of the constellation are seen in each patient. Sex distribution is unclear. Surprisingly, even in its most severe form, patients have little or no associated disability. Therefore, **surgery is indicated for cosmetic reasons and only in patients with a major depression defect and aplasia of the ribs.** It is especially indicated in girls with breast maldevelopment, which further accentuates the appearance of hypoplasia.

STERNAL DEFECTS

Sternal defects include cleft or bifid sternum and thoracic, cervical, or thoracoabdominal ectopia cordis.

In patients with a cleft sternum the heart is normal and skin covers the defect, which usually involves the manubrium and the upper sternum. This defect is easily correctable, particularly in the newborn period when the chest wall is pliable and the sternal elements are easily approximated.

Thoracic ectopia cordis is an almost uniformly fatal defect in which the heart is totally uncovered and visible to the naked eye. The heart is displaced anteriorly and cephalad. Patients die because the heart, which is usually abnormal, does not tolerate return to an intrathoracic position.

Cervical ectopia cordis, which is similar to the thoracic form, involves a more superior displacement of the heart, often with fusion of the heart to the mouth. This defect is uniformly fatal.

Thoracoabdominal ectopia cordis or pentalogy of Cantrell is a constellation of defects, including coverage of the heart with an omphalocele, sternal cleft, and defects of the diaphragm and pericardium, often in association with pulmonary hypoplasia. Mild defects are correctable; many patients, however, also have intrinsic heart disease. Personal experience with 8 patients suggests that in the most severe form, poor outcome is likely to result from small chest size and attendant pulmonary hypoplasia.

THORACIC DEFORMITIES AND DIFFUSE SKELETAL DISORDERS (SMALL CHEST)

Poor development of the chest cage is usually associated with generalized dysfunction of osseous and cartilaginous growth; the chest is only one of the affected areas. Conditions that cause such syndromes include various forms of dwarfism, such as achondroplasia, and certain forms of spondyloepiphyseal dysplasia. Jeune syndrome or asphyxiating thoracic dystrophy is a condition in which the chest fails to grow appropriately. Respiratory failure is common; associated problems include renal failure and pelvic abnormalities. The syndrome is inherited in an autosomal recessive fashion.

In such syndromes, the ribs are typically very short and horizontal. The chest has an increased anteroposterior diameter and decreased mobility; it is frequently bell-shaped, with flaring of the lower edges (Fig. 1). The abdomen is protuberant. The rigidity and small size of the chest cause restrictive lung disease. Because each breath is smaller, affected children are forced to breathe faster to maintain adequate ventilation, much like other patients with restrictive lung disease. **In children with severe deformities, even minor respiratory infections may cause significant distress and respiratory failure.** The magnitude of the respiratory embarrassment is proportional to the severity of the deformity of the chest and of associated defects, such as oropharyngeal and nasopharyngeal narrowing. The

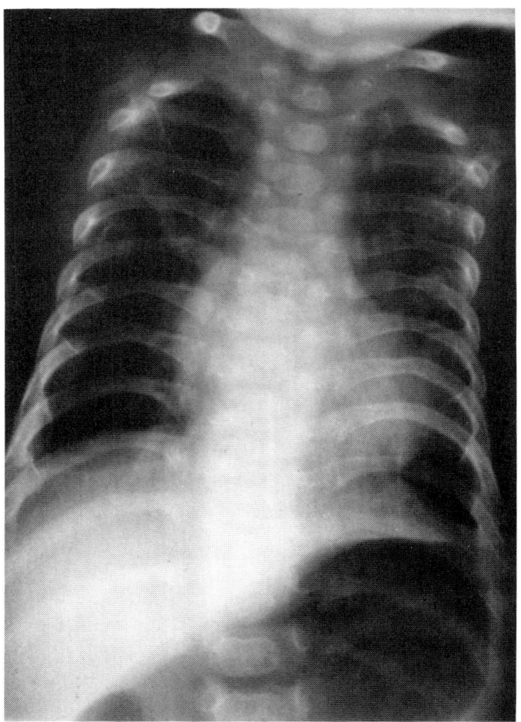

FIGURE 1. Chest radiograph of an infant with asphyxiating thoracic dystrophy (Jeune syndrome). The chest is bell-shaped, and the ribs are horizontal. Infiltration is present in the right upper and left lower lobe.

spectrum of presentation is quite varied, ranging from minimal symptoms to life-threatening disease.

Health professionals caring for such children must keep them under close surveillance. Resting respiratory rate (during sleep) as well as breath count during activity must be obtained as a baseline during periods of well-being. **Increases in respiratory rate may be the first sign of increased restriction and should never be dismissed as unimportant.** Blood gas determinations are particularly important, given the difficulty of clinical assessment of oxygenation and ventilation. Bronchial toilet is essential, including chest physiotherapy, postural drainage, and suction of secretions when indicated. Oxygen administration to correct hypoxemia is also very important. Antimicrobial agents should be used if bacterial infection is suspected. Children with associated maxillofacial deformities are highly prone to middle-ear disease and upper airway obstruction secondary to edema and secretions. Atelectasis and pneumonia are common. Patients with the most severe deformities will succumb early in life to respiratory complications. Patients with milder forms, however, may live into adulthood. Thus, preventive actions are always warranted.

Surgical expansion of the rib cage has been attempted in patients with severe forms of Jeune syndrome, with varied but limited success. All procedures involve the same concept. The sternum is split longitudinally, and the sternal halves are kept apart to increase the intrathoracic volume. Separation is maintained by various substances, including autologous rib grafts, donor bone grafts, iliac bone with metal plate fixation, sternal struts, and methyl methacrylate prosthesis. Although the increase in intrathoracic volume can be maintained, success or failure is determined by the degree of underlying pulmonary hypoplasia. To date, experience is limited; outcome, therefore, must be assessed on a case-by-case basis.

SUGGESTED READING

1. Andrews TM, Myer CM III, Gray SP: Abnormalities of the bony thorax causing tracheobronchial compression. Int J Pediatr Otorhinolaryngol 19:139–144, 1990.
2. Beiser GD, Epstein SE, Stampfer M, et al: Impairment of cardiac function in patients with pectus excavatum, with improvement after operative correction. N Engl J Med 287:267–272, 1972.
3. Castile RG, Staats BA, Westbrook PR: Symptomatic pectus deformities of the chest. Am Rev Respir Dis 126:564–568, 1982.
4. Ellis DG: Chest wall deformities in children. Pediatr Ann 18:161–165, 1989.
5. Harcke HT, Grissom LE, Lee MS, Mandell GA: Common congenital skeletal anomalies of the thorax. J Thorac Imag 1(4):1–6, 1986.
6. Hull D, Barnes ND: Children with small chests. Arch Dis Child 47:12–19, 1972.
7. Stokes DC, Wohl ME, Weiss RA, et al: The lungs and airways in achondroplasia: Do little people have little lungs? Chest 98:145–152, 1990.

35

RESPIRATORY DISEASE IN THE IMMUNOCOMPROMISED CHILD

Michael R. Bye, M.D.

Recurrent infections, including those of the respiratory tract, are a hallmark of immune deficiency disorders. This chapter discusses pulmonary infections in the child known to have an immune deficiency disorder. The reader is referred to chapter 17 for guidance on when to consider an underlying immune dysfunction in children with chronic or recurrent respiratory disorders.

In the simplest terms, the immune system consists of B-cells, T-cells, and other components. Recurrent bacterial infection may occur as a consequence of B-cell disorders; T-cell disorders predispose to recurrent infections with viruses, fungi, and protozoal organisms; abnormalities of polymorphonuclear cells may result in infections with bacteria; and defects of complement and miscellaneous enzyme deficiencies may lead to a broad variety of recurrent infections. Although overlap among the immune problems is considerable, it is helpful to know the nature of the child's defect in order to anticipate the type of infections likely to be encountered. This information makes it easier to approach the diagnosis in immunocompromised children in an expeditious fashion.

Children with acquired immunodeficiency syndrome (AIDS) develop multiple defects in their immune function. The development of opportunistic infection and general clinical decompression are more likely to occur when counts of CD4+ lymphocytes fall. Although children with AIDS often have hypergammaglobulinemia, their B-cell function is depressed. The circulating immunoglobulins are nonspecific and nonfunctional, and the antibody response to bacterial antigens is markedly diminished. Thus, children with AIDS suffer from recurrent bacterial and severe viral infections in addition to opportunistic infections with organisms such as *Pneumocystis carinii*, cytomegalovirus, tuberculosis, and fungi. In addition, AIDS in children is associated with the development of noninfectious lung disorders, such as lymphocytic interstitial pneumonitis and Kaposi's sarcoma. Intrathoracic non-Hodgkin's lymphoma has been reported in adults infected with the human immunodeficiency virus (HIV) but not in children with AIDS.

Children with B-cell disorders may have a spectrum of abnormalities from agammaglobulinemia to defects in specific antibody production. Bruton agammaglobulinemia predisposes to recurrent bacterial infections in the soft tissues throughout the body, including the lung. Defects in the production of the secretory component of IgA result in altered mucosal immunity and manifest as chronic or recurrent sinopulmonary infections. Decreases in IgG subclasses two and four are associated with "difficult-to-control" asthma and recurrent bacterial pneumonia.

The most common primary T-cell defect is the DiGeorge syndrome, which includes abnormalities in parathyroid function, congenital heart disease, and anomalies of the aortic arch. Similar T-cell abnormalities and abnormalities in T-cell–dependent B-cell function are found in Nezelof syndrome, which does not have the accompanying defects of the third and fourth pharyngeal pouches. An idiopathic T-cell lymphocytopenia with opportunistic infections similar to those in patients with AIDS has been described in adults but not in children. However, we have seen young children with *Pneumocystis carinii* pneumonia (PCP) who are HIV-negative and have low CD4+ counts. Although some patients with cartilage-hair hypoplasia have been found to have low or absent T-cell function, their clinical problems relate mostly to vaccinia or varicella virus; other clinical manifestations of T-cell dysfunction are rare.

Other diseases with combined T- and B-cell defects include combined immunodeficiency disease and Wiskott-Aldrich syndrome. The latter usually includes thrombocytopenia, eczema, and elevated concentrations of serum IgA and IgE. T-cell dysfunction and variably depressed levels of IgG subclasses and/or IgA are found in ataxia-telangiectasia. Patients with chronic mucocutaneous candidiasis have defects of T-cell immunity but also may have some degree of IgA deficiency. Children with deficiencies of adenosine deaminase and nucleoside phosphorylation frequently have alterations in both lines of cellular immunity.

Children with deficiencies of the complement system are at risk for collagen vascular diseases and recurrent severe bacterial infections.

The most common disorder of phagocytic function is chronic granulomatous disease. Because of abnormal oxidative metabolism within the phagocytes, their ability to generate radicals capable of killing ingested organisms is diminished. This results in recurrent soft-tissue infections and abscesses. Defects in phagocytosis are also seen in Chediak-Higashi syndrome, deficiencies of glucose-6-phosphate dehydrogenase and myeloperoxidase, and transiently in states such as malnutrition, Down syndrome, leukemia, overwhelming bacterial and/or viral infections, and burns.

Defective chemotaxis on the part of the phagocytic cells results in poor response to infecting organisms. This abnormality is seen in children with the hypergammaglobulin E syndrome, also known as Job or Buckley-Job syndrome. Affected children have recurrent staphylococcal skin and sinopulmonary infections as a result of the abnormal chemotaxis of neutrophils and/or monocytes.

Lastly, children receiving immunosuppressive therapy have several risk factors for pulmonary disease (see chapter 28). The underlying malignancy may metastasize to the lung, causing either multiple nodular metastases or occasionally a diffuse infiltrative process. Both chemotherapy and radiation therapy may directly cause pulmonary fibrosis. Chemotherapy may cause bone marrow suppression, which results in decreased numbers of lymphocytes and neutrophils and predisposes to infection with any type of organism. Recipients of bone marrow transplantation are at risk for recurrence of disease, infection due to immunosuppression, graft-versus-host disease, and bronchiolitis obliterans. Chronic daily corticosteroid therapy alters lymphocyte function and places the child at risk for infection with tuberculosis, fungi, *Pneumocystis carinii*, viruses, and possibly *Legionella* species.

EVALUATION OF THE IMMUNOSUPPRESSED CHILD WITH RESPIRATORY SYMPTOMS

Immunosuppressed children who develop respiratory symptoms are at risk not only for developing infections with serious or uncommon organisms but also for rapid clinical deterioration. Thus, their respiratory symptoms deserve careful attention. Although overevaluation and overtreatment of a simple upper respiratory infection are possible results, the risks associated with underevaluating and undertreating a serious pneumonia are much greater.

After the history and physical examination, we usually start the evaluation with a chest radiograph, which gives a baseline view of the extent and severity of disease and is the starting point in considering the etiology of the infection. A dense, lobar infiltrate is more likely to be bacterial than viral. A diffuse, interstitial picture is more consistent with viral disease, *Pneumocystis carinii*, some fungal diseases, noncardiogenic pulmonary edema, or a noninfectious, diffuse inflammatory lesion. Nodular lesions raise suspicion of fungal disease, tuberculosis, or noninfectious disease. Because some organisms, particularly *Pneumocystis carinii* and certain viruses, "hide" in the interstitium, the radiograph underestimates the degree of disease.

This latter presentation is highly unusual for bacterial disease. **However, children with PCP and viral infections may have normal chest radiographs. In such cases, measurement of arterial blood gas values and evaluation of the alveolar-arterial oxygen gradient are very helpful, because the interstitial disease causes hypoxemia.** We have noted degrees of hypoxemia in patients with AIDS and PCP that are out of proportion to the physical or radiographic findings.

The next step is to attempt to find the causative infectious agent(s). If an acute bacterial infection is likely, sputum examination, including Gram stain and culture, and blood cultures are indicated. Production of sputum may be induced by mechanically stimulating the posterior pharynx and vocal cords or by having the patient inhale a hypertonic saline solution. In the former procedure, a flexible wire swab is passed through the nose around the pharynx and down to the vocal cords. This procedure initiates a gag and cough reflex, which often yields material from the tracheobronchial tree. An assistant should use a tongue blade and sterile swab to collect the sputum. Gram stain and culture of the sputum are helpful in diagnosing an infecting organism. If pleural effusion is present, thoracentesis with examination of the fluid is important. Fluid should undergo a Gram stain and be cultured for all possible and practical organisms as well as examined for evidence of bacterial antigens by tests such as countercurrent-immunoelectrophoresis or latex agglutination. If such studies are unrewarding, empirical broad-spectrum antibiotic therapy is a reasonable approach. However, if there is no clinical response within 48–72 hours, more invasive studies should be considered.

If the radiograph reveals diffuse interstitial disease or is normal, an acute bacterial process is less likely than PCP, viral infection, tuberculosis, or fungal disease, all of which are more difficult to treat and may cause rapid clinical deterioration. Thus greater efforts should be made to detect the organism. In addition, therapy for some of these entities (e.g., steroids for noninfectious disease or PCP) may be harmful in patients with other infecting organisms (e.g., viruses, fungi). Viruses may be detected by nasopharyngeal swabs, followed by either culture or direct fluorescent antibody techniques, such as those commonly used to detect respiratory syncytial virus. Bronchoscopy with bronchoalveolar lavage (BAL) has been used successfully to find an organism in immunosuppressed children with pneumonia. BAL is most commonly used for the detection of PCP in patients with AIDS, but it also may be useful in detecting organisms in any patient. *Mycobacterium tuberculosis* may be recovered with BAL, but a properly performed early morning gastric aspirate is more effective at recovering the acid-fast bacilli. In diffuse disease, if the organism is not detected by the above techniques and the patient is not improving, an open lung biopsy is indicated. Because the commonly used pediatric bronchoscope does not have a biopsy forceps for its channel, open lung biopsy must be performed.

As much as possible, therapy should be narrowly focused on the infecting organism. Broad-spectrum antibiotics, such as cefuroxime or cefotaxime, are useful if suspicion of acute bacterial disease is strong and sputum and blood cultures are nondiagnostic. If there is a risk of infection with *Pseudomonas aeruginosa*, as in patients with bronchiectasis, therapy should include drugs such as ceftazidime, broad-spectrum semisynthetic penicillins, aminoglycosides, or quinolones. In other instances, broad-spectrum therapy may be a reasonable start, but efforts should be made to detect the organism and to treat specifically. This approach reduces the morbidity of therapy and the likelihood of creating a resistant organism.

Follow-up chest radiographs are an important part of management. It is necesssary to know that the previous pneumonia has cleared radiographically as well as clinically. If a subsequent episode of respiratory symptoms requires a radiograph, one can assess the subsequent films more accurately by comparison with previous abnormalities and thus decide whether the new infiltrate truly represents new infection. A period of 2 months should be adequate for clearing of the previous infiltrate.

SUGGESTED READING

1. Berthit F, Le Deist F, Duliege AM, et al: Clinical consequences and treatment of primary immunodeficiency syndromes characterized by functional T and B lymphocyte anomalies (combined immune deficiency). Pediatrics 93:265–270, 1994.

2. Bye MR, Bernstein LJ, Shah K, et al: Diagnostic bronchoalveolar lavage in children with AIDS. Pediatr Pulmonol 3:425–428, 1987.
3. Bye MR, Bernstein LJ: Identifying pulmonary sequelae in children with AIDS. J Respir Dis 10:27–39, 1989.
4. Bye MR, Bernstein LJ, Glaser J, Kleid D: *Pneumocystis carinii* pneumonia in young children with AIDS. Pediatr Pulmonol 9:251–253, 1990.
5. Falloon J, Eddy J, Wiener L, Pizzo PA: Human immunodeficiency virus infection in children. J Pediatr 114:1–30, 1989.
6. Hauger SB: Approach to the pediatric patient with HIV infection and pulmonary symptoms. J Pediatr 110(Suppl):S25–S32, 1991.
7. Hong R: Update on the immunodeficiency diseases. Am J Dis Child 144:983–992, 1990.
8. Johnston RB: Recurrrent bacterial infections in children. N Engl J Med 310:1237–1243, 1984.
9. Krowka MJ, Rosenow EC, Hoagland HC: Pulmonary complications of bone marrow transplantation. Chest 87:237–246, 1984.
10. Lischner HW, Huang NN: Respiratory complications of primary hypogammaglobulinemia. Pediatr Ann 6:514–525, 1977.
11. Prober CG, Whyte H, Smith CR: Open lung biopsy in immunocompromised children with pulmonary infiltrates. Am J Dis Child 138:60–63, 1984.
12. Stephan JL, Vlekova V, Le Deist F, et al: Severe combined immunodeficiency: A retrospective single center study of clinical presentation and outcome in 117 patients. J Pediatr 123:564–572, 1994.

36

RESPIRATORY COMPLICATIONS OF DOWN SYNDROME

Brian P. O'Sullivan, M.D.

Down syndrome (DS) occurs in approximately 1.5/1,000 live births and is generally recognized by a constellation of associated anomalies, including small ears, oblique palpebral fissures, a single palmar crease, and generalized hypotonia. In addition, many children with DS have abnormalities that affect lung function, such as (1) congenital heart disease, (2) pulmonary hypertension, (3) pulmonary hypoplasia, (4) upper airway obstruction, and (5) immunodeficiency (Table 1). As a consequence, respiratory disease (with or without congenital heart disease) is the leading cause of death in children with DS.

CONGENITAL HEART DISEASE

Of children with DS, 30–40% have congenital heart disease, usually consisting of atrioventricular canal or ventral septal defect. Although often diagnosed at birth, some of these defects may escape detection in the nursery before pulmonary vascular resistance has decreased. Acyanotic lesions, such as patent ductus arteriosus and atrial septal defect, may also go undiagnosed. Over time, the increased pulmonary blood flow caused by any of these lesions may lead to severe, irreversible pulmonary hypertension (Eisenmenger physiology) in any child. Because of a predisposition to pulmonary hypertension, the progression is especially common in children with DS.

The presence of congenital heart disease with or without pulmonary hypertension puts children with DS at risk for severe complications from even ordinary respiratory pathogens. The problems may be due to direct pulmonary infection or secondary to tonsillar and adenoidal hypertrophy, which can exacerbate the tendency toward upper airway obstruction. In a series of 35 patients with DS admitted to St. Christopher's Hospital for Children in Philadelphia with the diagnosis of pneumonia, 27 had accompanying cardiac disease (unpublished data). Because St. Christopher's is a referral center for cardiac surgery, the patient population is skewed toward children with heart defects; nonetheless, these data highlight the considerable risk for pulmonary complications in children with DS and congenital heart defects. Thus, a child with DS and congenital heart disease who develops respiratory tract symptoms must be observed closely. Hospitalization and therapy with supplemental oxygen as well as antimicrobial agents should be considered early in the disease process.

Of particular note for children with congenital heart disease is respiratory syncytial virus (RSV) infection. RSV infection can be life-threatening in any child with cardiopulmonary disease. It begins insidiously with rhinorrhea and low-grade fever but may progress rapidly to severe airways obstruction and acute respiratory failure. The American Academy of Pediatrics considers children with congenital heart defects to be at high risk for severe illness from RSV infection and recommends ribavirin therapy for such patients. This aerosolized antiviral agent has been shown to decrease viral shedding, to shorten hospital stay, and to improve outcome in patients in high-risk groups. Because

TABLE 1. Common Causes of Pulmonary Disease in Down Syndrome

Congenital heart defects
Pulmonary hypertension
Pulmonary hypoplasia
Obstructive sleep apnea
Immunodeficiency

of concerns about environmental contamination, possible teratogenic effects, and high cost, ribavirin should not be given to children without documented RSV infection. This medication and indications for its usage are discussed in greater detail in chapter 20.

PULMONARY HYPERTENSION

Children with DS are at increased risk for development of pulmonary hypertension, both idiopathic and secondary to congenital heart disease. The pathogenesis of this increased incidence is unclear. Some investigators believe that the increased incidence is related to the pulmonary hypoplasia seen in DS. Although some studies indicate that pulmonary hypoplasia is accompanied by a reduction in capillary cross-sectional area that may explain the hypertension, not all investigators agree that it is a key element. Over the last 10 years a greater understanding of the prevalence of obstructive sleep apnea in DS has lead to its consideration as a possible cause of pulmonary hypertension. Obviously, in children with left-to-right cardiac shunts, increased pulmonary blood flow is another contributing factor.

No matter what the cause, the most obvious physiologic effect of elevated pulmonary arterial pressure is its influence on cardiac function. Prolonged pulmonary hypertension leads to dilatation and eventually failure of the right ventricle (cor pulmonale). The accompanying increase in right-sided pressures causes right-to-left shunting in children with structural defects or patent foramen ovale. When pulmonary arterial pressure rises abruptly as a result of the local pulmonary hypoxic vasoconstriction that accompanies an intercurrent respiratory illness, the arterial oxygen saturation of blood may fall precipitously because of increased shunting across such an anatomic defect. Children with pulmonary hypertension present with fatigue, dyspnea on exertion, and syncope. This diagnosis, rarely considered in the usual pediatric population, must be entertained in children with DS and such a constellation of complaints.

The diagnosis of pulmonary hypertension is best made by a pediatric cardiologist with color Doppler echocardiography or cardiac catheterization. Therapy is limited; treatment of other conditions (congenital heart defects, obstructive apnea) that contribute to pulmonary hypertension may alleviate the problem, and supplemental oxygen may promote pulmonary vascular dilation. There are no reports of long-term pharmacotherapy in patients with DS and primary pulmonary hypertension.

PULMONARY HYPOPLASIA

Pulmonary hypoplasia in DS is due to a lack of radial growth of lung tissue after birth. This error in organ growth presumably results from the basic genetic defect. Along with this abnormal development, the alveolar capillary network is disorganized and predisposes the children to pulmonary hypertension. Mild pulmonary hypoplasia has no direct effect on respiration: as long as ventilation and perfusion are matched, oxygenation and excretion of carbon dioxide are normal.

OBSTRUCTIVE APNEA

Children with DS are at particularly high risk for obstructive apnea because of their maxillofacial dysmorphism. These midfacial structural defects include choanal stenosis, mandibular hypoplasia, decreased palatal dimensions, and relative macroglossia. In addition, lymphoid hyperplasia, hypopharyngeal hypotonia, and obesity commonly contribute to airway obstruction (Table 2). Atlantoaxial joint instability may lead to subluxation with spinal cord compression resulting in central apnea.

In many cases a presumptive diagnosis of obstructive apnea can be based on history alone. **The child with daytime hypersomnolence, snoring, nocturnal stridor, enuresis, and fitful sleep probably suffers from obstructive apnea.** Pulse oximetry obtained when the child is asleep

TABLE 2. Factors Predisposing Children with Down Syndrome to Obstructive Sleep Apnea

Choanal stenosis
Mandibular hypoplasia
Relative macroglossia
Lymphoid hyperplasia
Hypotonia
Obesity

supports the diagnosis if hypoxemia is noted. Measurements of serum electrolytes or arterial blood gas values are helpful in detecting carbon dioxide retention, but not all children with periodic hypoxemia during sleep retain CO_2. As with any child suspected of having obstructive apnea, a polysomnogram (sleep study) should be obtained to confirm the diagnosis.

It has been appreciated for many years that children with DS are at increased risk for obstructive sleep apnea; however, the prevalence of obstruction in this patient group has been elucidated only recently. Marcus et al. performed nap polysomnograms on 53 patients with DS, ranging in age from 2 weeks to 51 years, less than one-third of whom were suspected of having obstructive apnea. Of these patients, 70% had obstructive apnea, central apnea, hypoventilation, hypoxemia, or a combination thereof. Most striking was the fact that the nap studies, as abnormal as they were, actually underestimated the scope of the problem. Overnight polysomnograms in 16 children demonstrated even more severe problems than the shorter nap studies. In a study of a cohort of children with DS less than 5 years of age, Stebbens et al. found that 31% had obstructive sleep apnea; the incidence increased with age, presumably because of increased tonsillar size.

These data imply that all children with DS should be suspected of having obstructive apnea or hypopnea. Although routine polysomnographic screening is unwarranted, one should not delay such a study in any child with DS and unexplained cardiopulmonary symptoms. Children with documented obstruction should be referred to an otolaryngologist to ascertain if the obstruction is anatomic in nature and if surgical intervention will be remedial. Often a tonsillectomy and adenoidectomy relieve enough of the upper airway obstruction to allow normal ventilation. If this procedure is not successful in enlarging the airway, palatopharyngeoplasty or tracheotomy may be necessary.

IMMUNODEFICIENCY

Children with DS have an inordinate number of infections, particularly of the respiratory tree. Severe cardiopulmonary compromise may develop from infections with *Streptococcus pneumoniae, Mycoplasma pneumoniae,* or RSV. In addition, children with DS have frequent non-life-threatening infections of the upper and lower respiratory tracts. The predisposition to pneumonia is due not only to the cardiac and pulmonary vascular changes noted above but also to abnormalities in the immune system. The nature of the immune defects in DS are not well understood, but abnormalities in humoral immunity, cell-mediated immunity and phagocytic cell function have been documented (Table 3).

Deficiencies in the number and function of B-, T-, and natural killer (NK) cells and an inversion of the usual helper/suppressor cell ratio have been reported in children with DS. Moreover, because phagocytic cells have decreased superoxide content, intracellular killing of ingested organisms is diminished. **Perhaps most germane to the issue of increased respiratory illnesses is the finding of IgG_2 and IgG_4 subclass deficiencies in children with DS.** These immune globulins play an important role in the host defenses against respiratory pathogens, particularly encapsulated organisms, and their absence undoubtedly predisposes some patients to pneumonia. IgG subclass deficiencies and NK cell dysfunction appear to be age-related; thus a child may develop more rather than fewer problems with age.

TABLE 3. Alterations in Immunity in Patients with Down Syndrome

Thymic deficiency
Decreased T-cell number and function
Inverse T-4/T-8 (helper/suppressor) ratio
Natural killer cell dysfunction
Altered B-cell function
IgG subclass deficiencies
Decreased phagocytic cell chemiluminescence
Poor response to polysaccharide antigens
Decreased interleukin-2 production
Altered adhesion molecule production

Therapy for the immune defects seen in DS is nonspecific. Infection should be suspected and antibiotic therapy begun early in the course of any acute respiratory illness in a child with DS. Routine therapy for immune globulin subclass deficiency consists of replacement with intravenous gammaglobulin and may be of benefit to children with DS and documented subclass hypogammaglobulinemia.

SUMMARY

The number of anatomic and physiologic abnormalities in children with DS obviously places them at increased risk for pulmonary problems. Thus, the approach to any child with DS and chronic or severe acute lung disease must take such factors into consideration. Close observation and monitoring of oxygen saturation are vital for children with DS when they are ill.

Specific infectious agents that are most worrisome include *S. pneumoniae*, RSV, and *M. pneumoniae*. Thus, empirical therapy with erythromycin early in the course of respiratory disease is warranted in a patient with DS.

In children with chronic, lingering lung disease the possibility of obstructive sleep apnea or pulmonary hypertension must be considered. Diagnosis and treatment of these conditions requires consultation with subspecialists familiar with the problems of children with DS.

A host of other respiratory tract problems have been reported in combination with DS, ranging from hydrops fetalis with pleural effusions in newborn infants to cystic fibrosis, airway compression, and thyroid disease in older children and adults. Therefore, one must consider the entire range of pulmonary diseases in evaluating the child with DS; however, in a child with DS who is in respiratory distress the most common problems relate to cardiac disease, infection, and airway obstruction.

SUGGESTED READING

1. Anneren G, Magnusson CG, Lilja G, Nordvall SL: Abnormal serum IgG subclass pattern in children with Down's syndrome. Arch Dis Child 67:628–631, 1992.
2. Clapp S, Perry BL, Farooki ZQ, et al: Down's syndrome, complete atrioventricular canal, and pulmonary vascular obstructive disease. J Thorac Cardiovasc Surg 100:115–121, 1990.
3. Cooney TP, Wentworth PJ, Thurlbeck WM: Diminished radial count is found only postnatally in Down's syndrome. Pediatr Pulmonol 5:204–209, 1988.
4. Crone RK: Case records of the Massachusetts General Hospital, Case 8-1985. N Engl J Med 312:497–506, 1985.
5. Loh RKS, Harth SC, Thong YH, Ferrante A: Immunoglobulin G subclass deficiency and predisposition to infection in Down's syndrome. Pediatr Infect Dis J 9:547–551, 1990.
6. Marcus CL, Keens TG, Bautista DB, et al: Obstructive sleep apnea in children with Down syndrome. Pediatrics 88:132–139, 1991.
7. Schloo BL, Vawter GF, Reid LM: Down syndrome: Patterns of disturbed lung growth. Hum Pathol 22:919–923, 1991.
8. Stebbens VA, Dennis J, Samuels MP, et al: Sleep related upper airway obstruction in a cohort with Down's syndrome. Arch Dis Child 66:1333–1338, 1991.
9. Ugazio AG, Maccario R, Notarangelo LD, Burgio GR: Immunology of Down's syndrome: A review. Am J Med Genet S7:204–212, 1990.
10. Yamaki S, Horiuchi T, Takahashi T: Pulmonary changes in congenital heart disease with Down's syndrome: Their significance as a cause of postoperative respiratory failure. Thorax 40:380–386, 1985.

COMMENTARY

by Daniel V. Schidlow, M.D.

Most trisomy syndromes and chromosomal defects cause handicaps more serious than those usually associated with Down syndrome. Children with chromosomal defects and multiple congenital malformations, particularly those involving the central nervous system, share certain characteristics that predispose them to respiratory complications. Children with unusually small or retropositioned chins (e.g., Pierre-Robin or Treacher-Collins anomalads) are at high risk for obstructive apnea and hypoxemia due to mechanical narrowing of the upper airway. Children with large tongues, midline facial defects, or severe hypotonia also commonly develop obstructive sleep apnea. Swallowing dysfunction, gastroesophageal reflux, and aspiration pneumonia are very common among patients with severe hypotonia or psychomotor retardation.

A diminished cough reflex and thoracic and facial malformations, as well as associated orthopedic complications such as severe scoliosis, contribute to the inability to clear secretions and to fight infection properly. Severe respiratory complications are a frequent cause of mortality in such children.

37

INTERPRETATION OF THE RADIOGRAPH OF THE CHEST AND UPPER AIRWAY

Barbara J. Wolfson, M.D.

The evaluation of any radiograph requires a systemic approach, but this is especially true for the chest film of a child. Most chest radiographs in children are obtained because of respiratory distress. Therefore, it is tempting to look at the lungs first and to ignore the rest of the film. If the lungs are abnormal, most examiners look no further and may miss other important findings on the film.

Observers should look at all other structures before looking at the lungs. The recommended order of observation is (1) bones and soft tissues, (2) abdomen (including diaphragms and costophrenic angles), (3) heart and mediastinum, and, lastly, (4) the lungs.

BONES AND SOFT TISSUES

A great deal of useful information about the patient may be obtained from looking at the bones and soft tissues. In the first place, the patient's nutritional status can be evaluated. Children with cystic fibrosis, for example, frequently have diminished soft tissues on initial presentation. Soft-tissue swelling, on the other hand, may indicate an underlying fracture. Child abuse is very common, and occult rib fractures may indicate that a child is battered (Fig. 1). Metabolic bone disease such as rickets (Fig. 2) may be identified on a chest film, and congenital anomalies of the vertebrae or ribs may indicate a genetic syndrome (Fig. 3).

While checking the bones and soft tissues, one must also check the radiographic technique. The ideal film is rather grey and shows the soft tissues in detail. The film also should be well-penetrated so that the spine and ribs are visible through the heart. Fine detail is not expected for bone—just the outline of the vertebrae and the presence of the pedicles (Fig. 4). If the radiograph is dark, a bright light, which is available in most radiology departments, facilitates examination of the soft tissues.

ABDOMEN

By looking at the abdomen, one can determine the position of the patient—i.e., upright or supine—most easily from the stomach bubble. When the patient is upright, one sees air in the fundus of the stomach, along with an air-fluid level (see Fig. 8). When the patient is supine, the air rises to the body and antrum of the stomach and frequently overlies the midabdomen, but no air-fluid level is visible (see Fig. 1). It is important to note the patient's position because then one knows where to look for a pleural effusion or a pneumothorax. If the patient is upright, a pleural effusion will collect in the costophrenic sulcus; if the patient is supine, a pleural effusion will layer out posteriorly and laterally or collect in the apex of the hemithorax, which is dependent (Fig. 5). In children, even in the upright position, a pleural effusion rarely shows the "meniscus sign" of blunting of the costophrenic angle, as in adults. Instead, the angle remains sharp, but the lung appears to be "pushed away" from the ribs (see chapter 19).

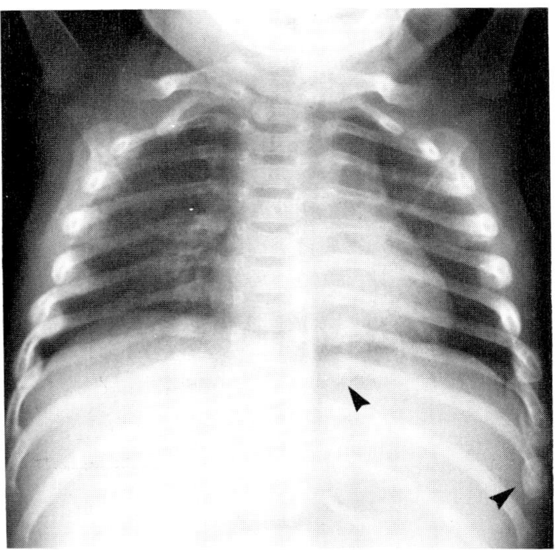

FIGURE 1. **Rib fractures.** Frontal radiograph of a 6-week-old child shows multiple rib fractures in various stages of healing, suggesting that they occurred at different times. The ribs involved include the right lateral sixth and seventh ribs; the right posterior fifth, eighth, ninth, and tenth ribs; the left lateral seventh, eighth, and ninth ribs; and the left posterior eighth and ninth ribs (*arrowheads*). Physical abuse was unsuspected before the film was taken.

Air in the pleural space acts in just the opposite manner from fluid. If the patient is supine, the air rises to the highest point in the chest, which is the anterior and lateral costophrenic sulcus (Fig. 6). Most physicians look for pneumothorax at the apex of the hemithorax, but air localizes to the apex only if the patient is upright. In children, because of their small size, it is less important than in adults to determine whether the exposure of the radiograph was anteroposterior or posteroanterior (AP or PA). These terms refer to the direction of the x-ray beam. If the exposure is AP, the beam goes from anterior to posterior, and the film cassette is against the patient's back. In our institution most children under the age of 10 years are exposed with an AP projection.

Examination of the abdomen also reveals the location of the stomach and helps to determine visceral situs as well as the presence of free air, masses, or calcifications. Free air in the abdomen acts the same as free air in the chest. Free air collects under the diaphragm only if the patient is upright.

HEART AND MEDIASTINUM

The mediastinum of a child is strikingly different from that of an adult because of the size of the thymus. We now know from computed tomographic (CT) scanning that the thymus is present into old age. However, as the patient grows larger, the thymus becomes smaller so that it is less apparent on a plain radiograph. CT scanning also shows that the thymus has a different density from the heart, but plain radiography is not sensitive enough to distinguish the difference. Therefore, on a plain radiograph of the chest it may be very

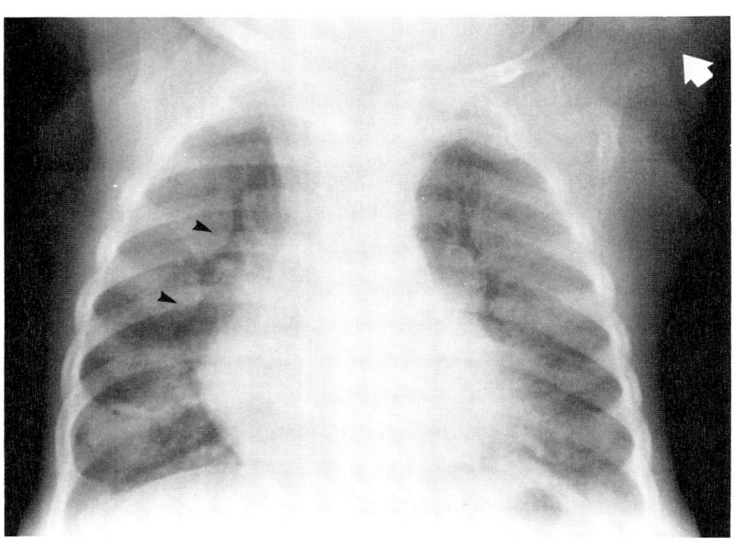

FIGURE 2. **Rickets.** Frontal radiograph shows rachitic changes in the proximal humeri and anterior ribs. The scalloped densities overlying the right lung and left upper lobe represent the soft-tissue swelling of the "rachitic rosary" (*arrowheads*). The proximal humeri show widening of the cartilaginous growth plate, loss of the zone of provisional calcification, and fraying of the metaphysis (*white arrow*).

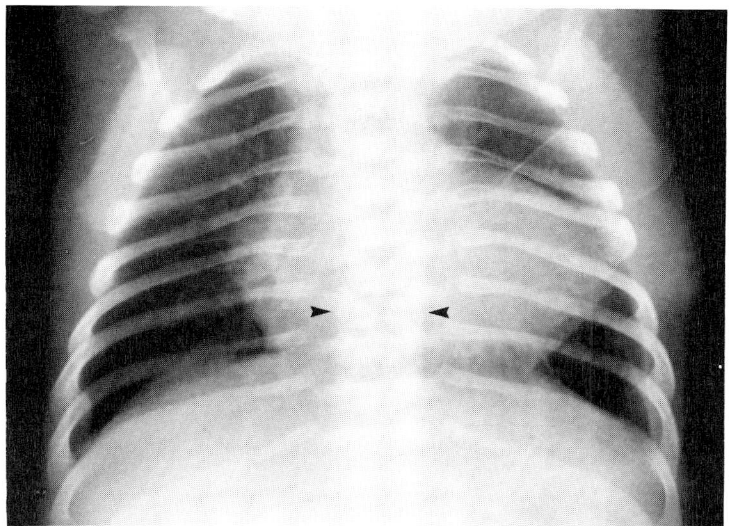

FIGURE 3. **Vertebral anomalies.** Note the butterfly sixth and seventh vertebrae visible through the heart (*arrowheads*). The child also has cardiac disease. The deformity of the left fourth and fifth ribs is due to surgery.

difficult to distinguish the thymus from the heart.

Capitanio[1] stated that the presence of the thymus is probably responsible for the specialty of pediatric radiology. One of the most common questions asked of the pediatric radiologist is, "Is this thymus normal?"—and in 99% of patients the answer is yes. Thymic enlargement alone is rarely a sign of abnormality. In a small child the thymus may be quite large, extending from one side of the chest to the other. Even in a child as old as 9 or 10 years, the thymus may be visible and still normal. The thymus is a soft, fleshy structure indented by the harder structures around it, such as the ribs and trachea. If the airway is narrowed or compromised, the mass is not normal thymus (Fig. 7). The thymus normally is confined to the anterior chest; thus, no matter how big it looks on the anterior projection, on the lateral projection the location of the trachea is normal and the thymus remains anterior. Very rarely a portion

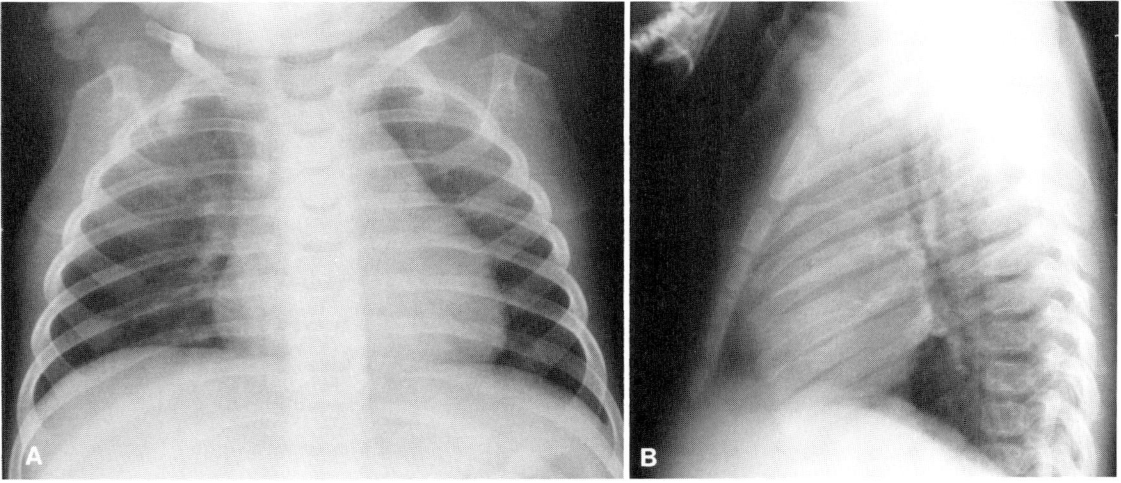

FIGURE 4. **Normal chest.** Frontal (*A*) and lateral (*B*) radiographs of a 4-week-old infant. Note that the patient is supine on the frontal film, because the gastric air is in the body rather than the fundus. The diaphragms are nicely domed, and no lung is visible between the ribs. The pulmonary vasculature branches and tapers from the hilum, with no markings in the outer third of the lung. On the lateral film the hila are not easily outlined. The heart is a uniform gray density on both the frontal and lateral films. Note also how the normal trachea may buckle but is not narrowed.

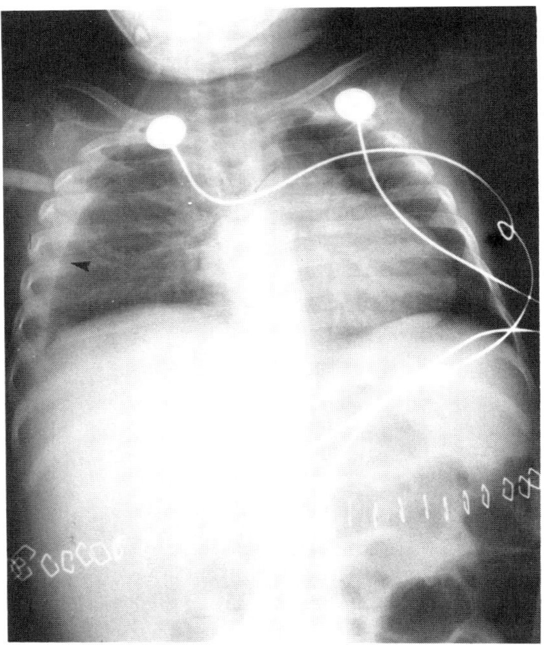

FIGURE 5. **Pleural effusion supine.** The patient had a liver transplant 2 weeks before the study and now has a right pleural effusion. Note how the costophrenic angle remains sharp and the lung is pushed away from the lateral chest wall by the fluid (*arrowhead*). The right lung appears denser than the left, because the fluid is layering posteriorly.

of thymus insinuates itself between or around the great vessels of the superior mediastinum and looks like a mediastinal mass. In the past a patient with such a variant would have undergone thoracotomy, because the diagnosis could not be made preoperatively. Now, however, CT often identifies such an aberrant thymus (see chapter 38).

If the thymus can be huge, how does one recognize the presence of a large heart? The answer is—it is not simple: from circumstantial evidence on the anterior projection and heavy reliance on the lateral film. On the anterior film the major clue to heart size is the shape and angle of the carina. Beyond infancy the angle of the carina is acute. When the heart is enlarged, the left main bronchus is often elevated and the angle of the carina becomes obtuse, especially when the patient has a lesion that causes enlargement of the left atrium, such as a ventricular septal defect. On the lateral film, the thymus is located in the anterior part of the chest and does not displace the heart or airway posteriorly. If the mediastinal structures look large on the lateral film, there is probably a large heart (or other mediastinal mass). In addition, in a normal patient the main bronchi are aligned in a straight line on the lateral film (Fig. 8). In a patient with a large heart, the left main bronchus is not only elevated but also pushed posteriorly. Thus its position on the lateral film also helps to identify the presence of a large heart (Fig. 9).

Important but frequently overlooked structures in the mediastinum are the great vessels. It is useful to know on which side the aortic arch is located because of the high incidence of tetralogy of Fallot in children with right-sided

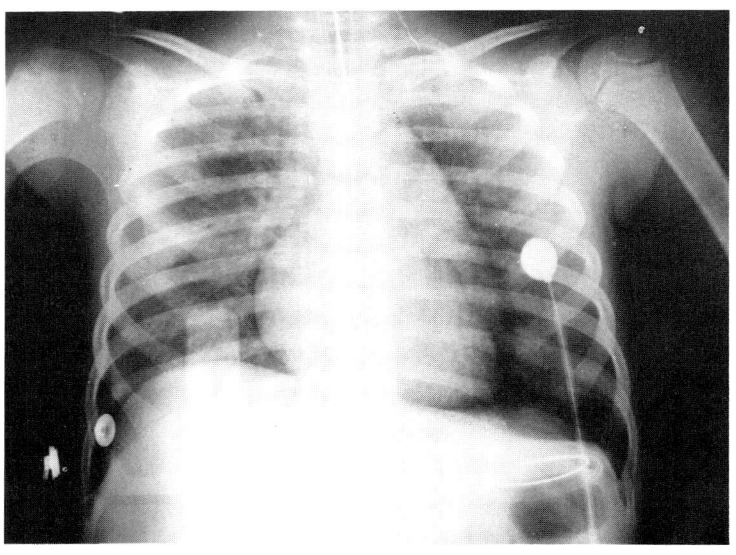

FIGURE 6. **Pneumothorax supine.** Bilateral pneumothoraces in a child hit by a car. Note that the pleural air is identified in the costophrenic angle, not at the apex.

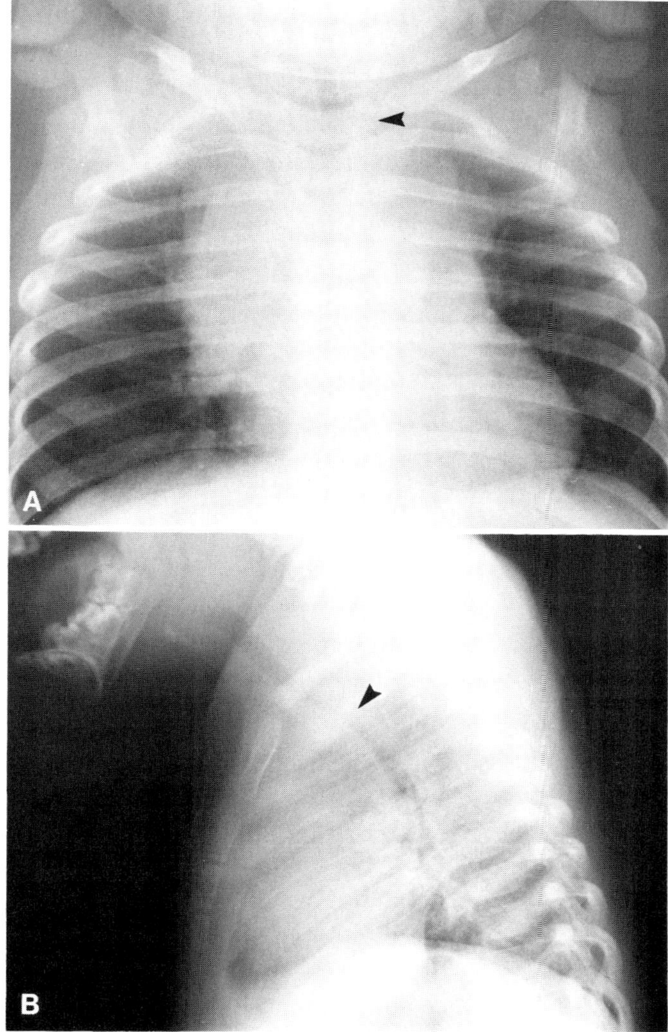

FIGURE 7. **Anterior mediastinal mass compressing the trachea.** Frontal (*A*) and lateral (*B*) chest radiographs of a 15-month-old child presenting with stridor. An anterior mediastinal mass compresses the trachea on the lateral film (*arrowhead*). This mass widens the superior mediastinum on the frontal film and deviates the trachea near the thoracic inlet (*arrowhead*). Histiocytosis was diagnosed by biopsy of a cervical lymph node.

aortic arches (about 90%). Radiologists frequently report that "the trachea is midline," but actually **the trachea in a healthy child is not in a midline position.** The trachea bows away from the side of the aortic arch, and in most patients with normal, left-sided aortic arches, **the trachea bows to the right.** Because the trachea is so compliant in a child, it can bow beyond the pedicles on the right and still be normal. Therefore, if the trachea bows to the left, the aortic arch is probably right-sided (Fig. 10); if the trachea is midline, there may be a vascular ring (Fig. 11).

It is important to look for the main pulmonary artery, but in a small child with a large thymus it may be difficult to see. Absence of a normal pulmonary artery segment suggests the presence of tetralogy of Fallot or transposition of the great vessels. Prominence of the pulmonary artery segment may be seen in children with valvular pulmonic stenosis and left-to-right shunts (see Fig. 9). However, in an older child with chronic respiratory disease, the pulmonary artery segment may be quite prominent without the presence of cardiac disease.

LUNGS

It is finally time to look at the lungs. The first feature to be evaluated is the degree of expansion or inflation, which is important for two reasons:

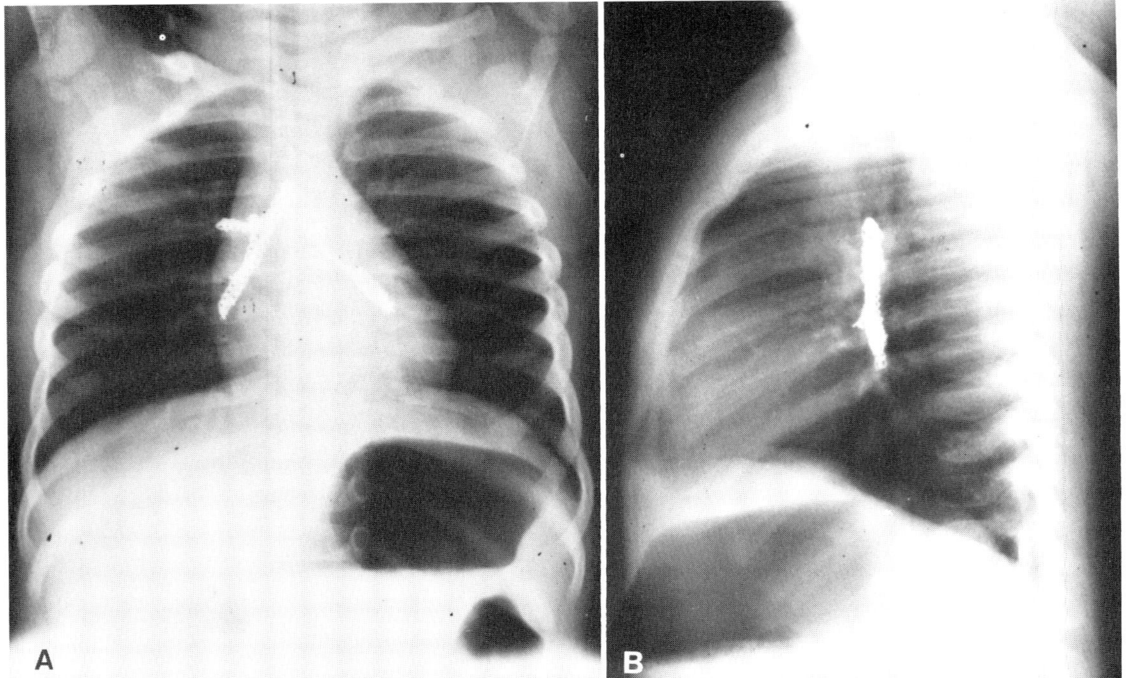

FIGURE 8. **Chain bronchogram.** Frontal (*A*) and lateral (*B*) chest radiographs of a 1-year-old child who aspirated a necklace. The top of the chain is at the carina on the frontal film. Note that the level of the carina on the lateral film is higher than most observers expect. Also note that the airways are superimposed on the lateral film.

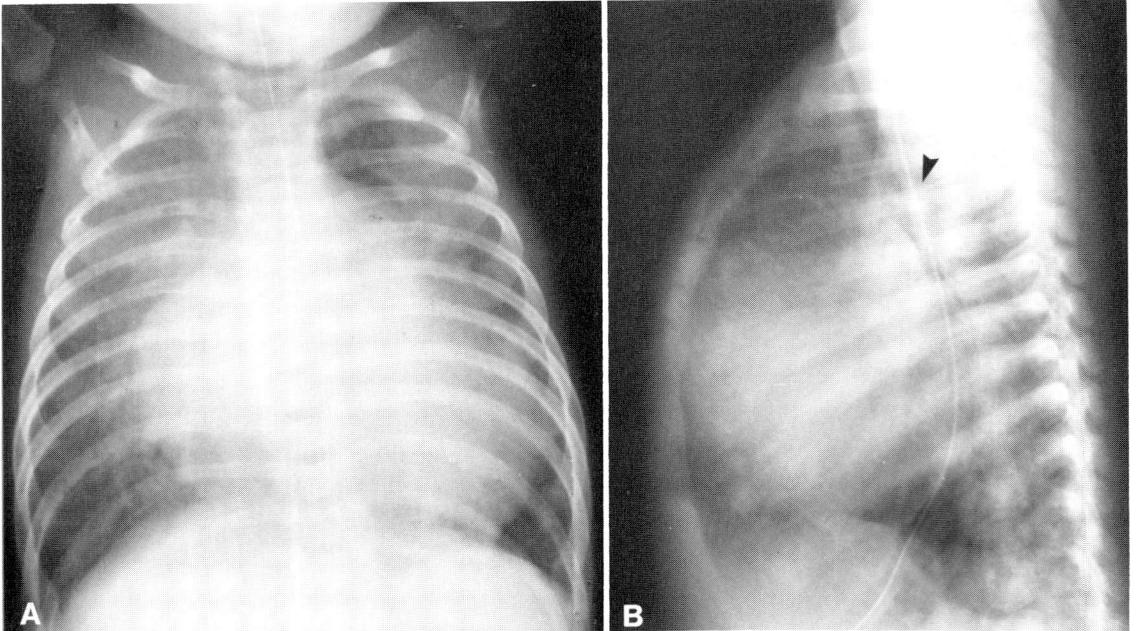

FIGURE 9. **Cardiomegaly.** Frontal (*A*) and lateral (*B*) chest radiographs of a 5-month-old girl with a large ventricular septal defect. The lungs are well expanded, but the heart is large, the main pulmonary artery segment is prominent, and the intrapulmonary vasculature is increased. Note the posterior displacement of the bronchus on the lateral film (*arrowhead*).

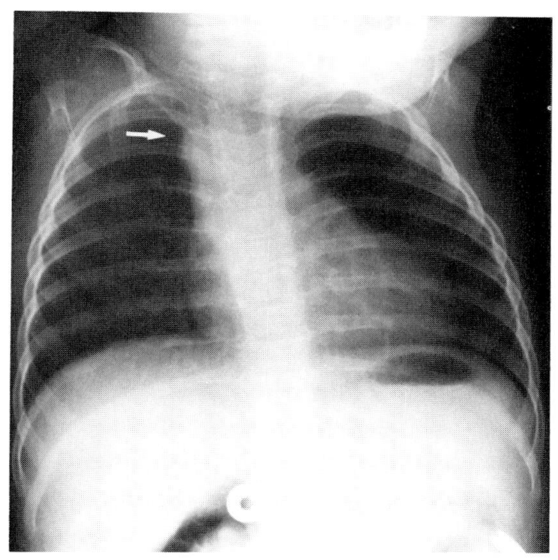

FIGURE 10. **Right aortic arch.** Frontal radiograph shows that the trachea is deviated to the left, indicating that the aortic arch is right-sided (*white arrow*). The descending aorta can also be identified on the right. The patient has tetralogy of Fallot.

1. The markings can be evaluated only after one evaluates the amount of air present in the chest. Because their chests and lungs are usually very compliant, children are able to expel almost all the air on expiration. If one attempts to evaluate an underexpanded chest, one frequently misinterprets the increased density as an infiltrate, congestive failure, or cardiomegaly. On the other hand, if a chest is overinflated, the markings appear diminished and can even seem normal when in fact they are increased (Fig. 12).

2. Hyperinflation is abnormal in a child under the age of 1 year. An older child can voluntarily take a deep breath, but in an infant hyperinflation of the chest frequently implies air-trapping.

The most popular way to evaluate inflation is to count ribs. In children the anterior ribs are counted instead of the posterior ribs. In a child who is normally inflated, the apex of the diaphragm is usually aligned with the anterior fifth rib (see Fig. 4). In a child who is underinflated, the apex of the diaphragm is usually aligned with the third or fourth rib. In a child whose chest is hyperinflated, the apex of the diaphragm is usually aligned with the sixth or seventh rib. Counting ribs works most of the time, but not always; thus one needs to be prepared to use other criteria as well. For example, the shape and configuration of the ribs are also important. When a child is inspiring normally, the ribs slant downward and the anterior

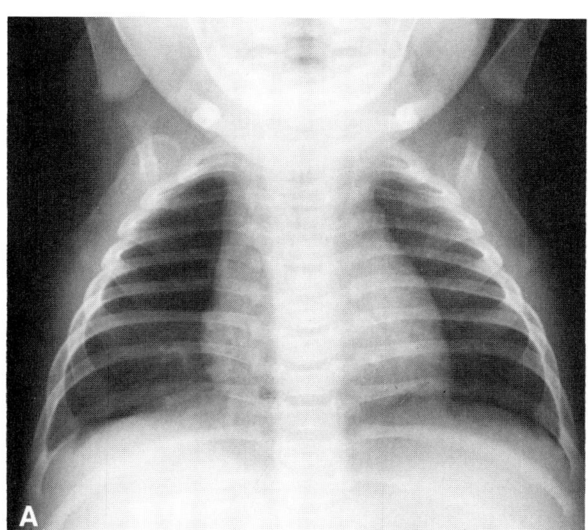

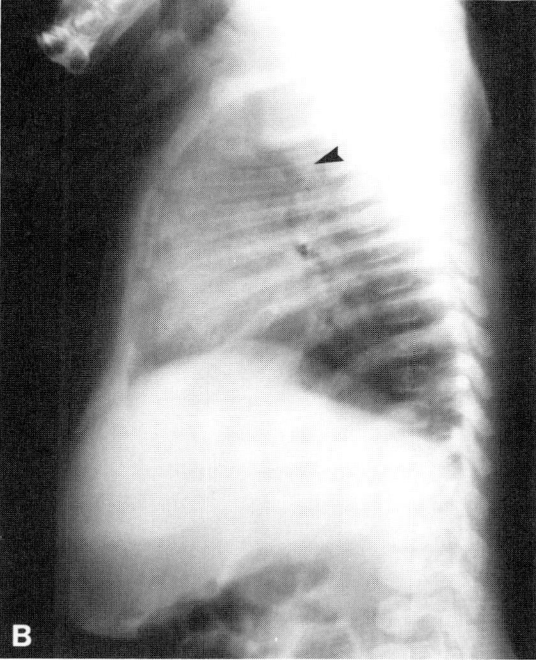

FIGURE 11. **Vascular ring.** *A*, Frontal film shows that the trachea is midline. It is initially deviated to the left but then curves back to the right so that the carina is in the midline. *B*, Lateral radiograph shows that the trachea is S-shaped and has both an anterior and a posterior impression (*arrowhead*).

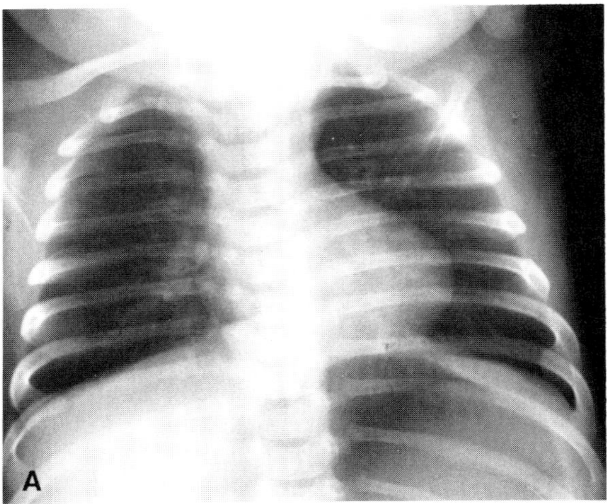

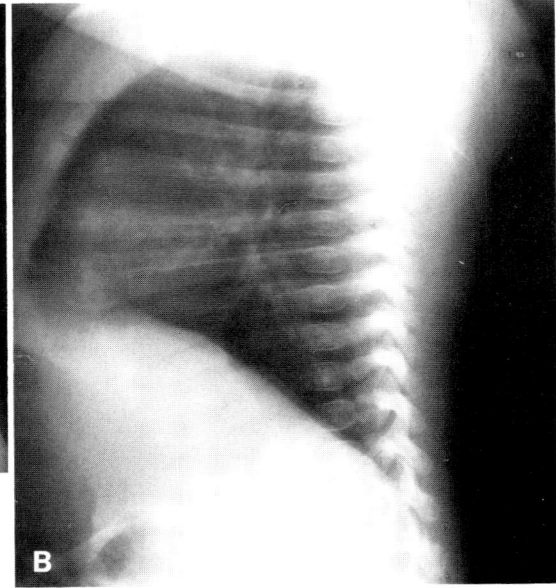

FIGURE 12. **Hyperinflation.** *A,* Frontal film shows the horizontal ribs with lung bulging between. The diaphragms are flattened from medial to lateral attachments. The pulmonary markings are increased throughout both lungs. *B,* Lateral film shows that the diaphragms are flattened from anterior to posterior attachments. The sternum is elevated away from the anterior ribs. The hila are prominent, indicating increased interstitium.

portion of the rib is inferior to the posterior rib. Hyperinflation of the chest may make the anterior rib overlap the posterior rib and even appear superior to the posterior rib. Occasionally lung may bulge outward between the ribs.

The second most popular way to evaluate inflation is to look at the configuration of the diaphragm. Everyone knows to look for "flattened diaphragms" as a sign of overinflation. The flattening is seen from anterior attachment to posterior attachment or medial attachment to lateral attachment (see Fig. 12). A small, fat child can flatten the diaphragms horizontally, but if a line is drawn from attachment to attachment, it is clear that the diaphragms are not truly flat. A radiograph depicts the dome of the diaphragm, where the beam is tangential to the superior edge. In a child whose diaphragms are truly flattened, no dome is visible and the superior margin often cannot be recognized.

An increased AP diameter on a lateral radiograph is also an indication of hyperinflation. Because the sternum usually projects close to the anterior ribs in a child who is normally inflated (see Fig. 4), space between the anterior ribs and the sternum suggests hyperinflation (see Fig. 12).

Once the degree of inflation has been determined, evaluation of the markings may begin. In normally inflated lungs, normal markings branch and taper from the hilum and do not usually extend into the outer third of the lung (see Fig. 4). Moreover, on the lateral film, the hilum is not clearly outlined. Markings that look too prominent and a visible hilum indicate the presence of interstitial fluid or inflammation. Of the many possible causes of prominent interstitial densities, the most common is viral inflammatory disease. This pattern in pulmonary disease is much more common in children than in adults.

Consolidated infiltrates are usually easier to identify unless they are small and behind the heart. **The heart is a uniform gray density. One should be able to account for every density one sees through and behind the heart.** An unexplained density overlying the cardiac silhouette on the AP film indicates an infiltrate or atelectasis in the left lower lobe (Fig. 13), whereas an unexplained density overlying the heart on the lateral film indicates an infiltrate in the right middle lobe or the left lingula. The anterior film helps to localize the infiltrate in such situations.

The density of the spine on the lateral film is also helpful in identifying the presence of an infiltrate. In a normal patient the upper thoracic spine looks whiter than the lower thoracic

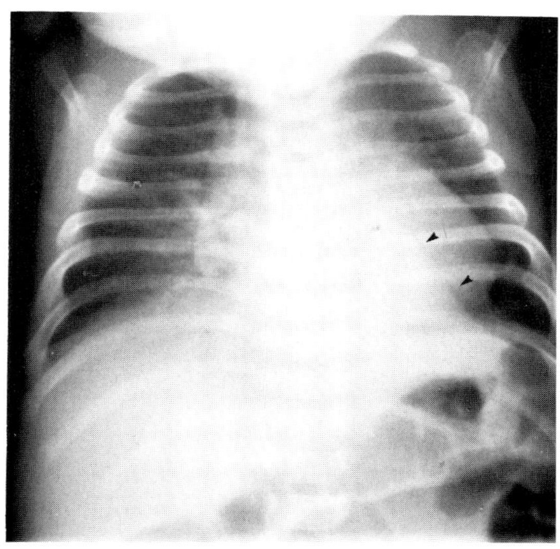

FIGURE 13. **Atelectasis of the left lower lobe.** Frontal radiograph shows a triangular density behind the heart, which represents the collapsed left lower lobe (*arrowheads*). An air bronchogram in the density shows that the airways are crowded. The remainder of the lungs are hyperinflated with interstitial densities. The child has cystic fibrosis.

spine. The upper arm overlies the upper thoracic spine and absorbs some of the x-ray beam so that the vertebral bodies look whiter. Very little soft tissue overlies the lower thoracic vertebral bodies, which thus generally look darker. Therefore, if the lower thoracic vertebral bodies appear white or if an area overlying the lower thoracic spine looks whiter than the vertebrae above, a lower lobe infiltrate must be suspected. Again, the anterior projection helps to localize the infiltrate.

By now the reader should be convinced of the necessity of obtaining both the frontal and lateral projections. Much information is lost if the clinician orders only a frontal projection.

Radiologists frequently refer to parenchymal densities on radiographs as either "interstitial" or "alveolar." These terms do not refer to histology but rather to the radiographic pattern, which is helpful in determining a differential diagnosis. The term interstitial was used earlier in this section to describe the pattern of increased markings. Another term used to describe the same pattern is "peribronchial thickening or cuffing." In children this pattern most commonly indicates viral infection or allergy. On a single examination it is almost impossible to determine whether such changes are acute or chronic; thus sequential studies are essential.

Alveolar density describes a pattern that obscures the normal vascular markings in a localized area and frequently contains air bronchograms. An air bronchogram is an air-filled airway surrounded by airless alveoli. Air bronchograms are nonspecific and may be seen in pneumonia, pulmonary edema, or atelectasis. Consolidation often can be distinguished from atelectasis because of the spacing or crowding of the air bronchogram (Fig. 13). Often both conditions occur together. The term alveolar is also used to describe the perihilar pattern in a patient with congestive heart failure or shock lung.

No discussion of radiographic patterns is complete without mention of the "miliary" pattern. A miliary pattern is an interstitial pattern with nodules distributed throughout the chest. The nodules are uniform in size, measuring approximately 2 mm in diameter, and resemble millet grain seeds (Fig. 14). This pattern is nonspecific and may be seen in several infections, but the first item on the differential diagnostic list should be miliary tuberculosis, a disease whose incidence is on the rise. Only after this diagnosis has been

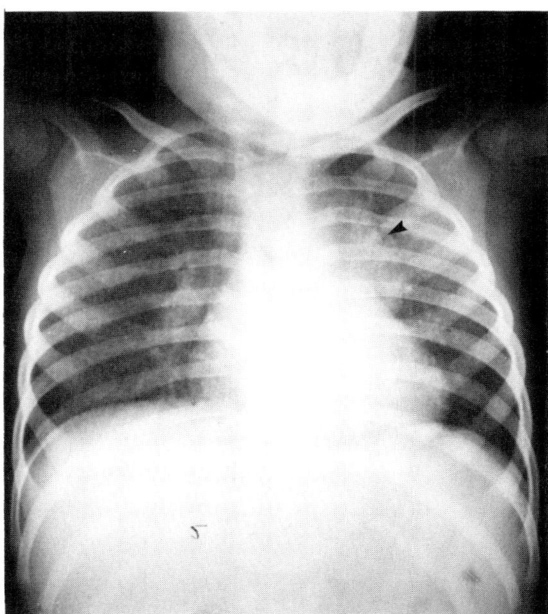

FIGURE 14. **Miliary tuberculosis.** Frontal radiograph of a 1-year-old child shows a find nodular pattern throughout the lungs. The density along the left side of the mediastinum probably represents mediastinal adenopathy (*arrowhead*).

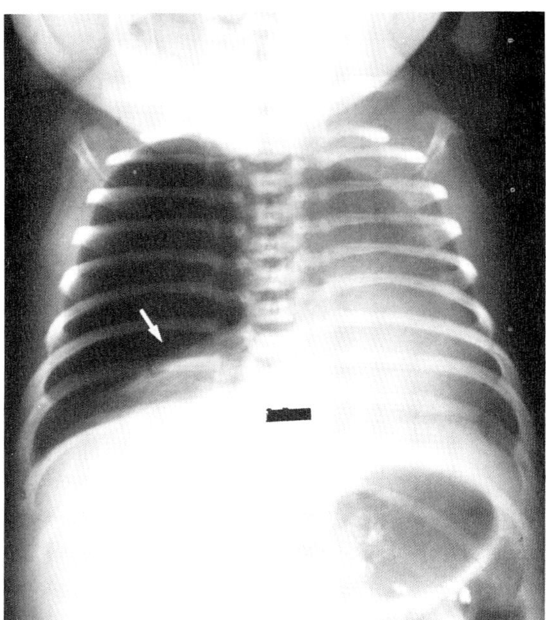

FIGURE 15. **Congenital lobar emphysema.** Frontal radiograph of a 6-day-old infant shows the marked hyperexpansion and hyperlucency of the right upper lobe. The mediastinum is shifted to the left, and the right lower and middle lobes are compressed (*white arrow*).

excluded should others be considered. A miliary pattern may also occur with chronic granulomatous disease (CGD) and other granulomatous diseases, and acquired immune deficiency syndrome (AIDS).

Examination of the chest radiograph of a child must take into account the symmetry of lung volume. It is possible for the hemithoraces to appear asymmetric because of asymmetry of the chest wall or overlying musculature. If the lungs are of different size and the mediastinum is shifted, it may be difficult to determine which lung is abnormal. Is the smaller lung too small, or is the larger lung too large? If one lung is too small, the child may have an abnormality of the pulmonary vasculature, such as a hypoplastic artery or abnormal venous drainage. If one lung or a lobe is too large, the age of the patient influences the differential diagnosis. In a young infant a large lung may be caused by vascular compression of a bronchus, such as by a pulmonary sling. An overly large lobe in an infant is probably due to congenital lobar emphysema (Fig. 15). In an older child an enlarged lobe or lung may be secondary to an aspirated foreign body. A small foreign body (such as a peanut) may lodge in a large bronchus and cause localized air-trapping by a ball-valve mechanism (Fig. 16). During inspiration the intrathoracic pressure falls and the airway opens, allowing air to enter the lung, but during expiration the intrathoracic pressure increases and the airway collapses, causing the lung to remain expanded. An expiratory film should be part of the ideal radiographic evaluation if a foreign body is suspected, but it is difficult to obtain in an uncooperative child (all children under the age of 3 years fit this description). The radiologist can fluoroscope the child during respiration to see if the lung remains inflated on expiration. An easier approach is to obtain lateral decubitus films and to compare the dependent sides. When a patient is placed in the decubitus position, the dependent lung is forced to expire. Therefore, a dependent lung that does not empty is strongly suggestive of an airway obstruction. A foreign body may be ruled in by radiographic evidence, but it is never ruled out by a normal study.

One more word of advice: when in doubt, consult the radiologist.

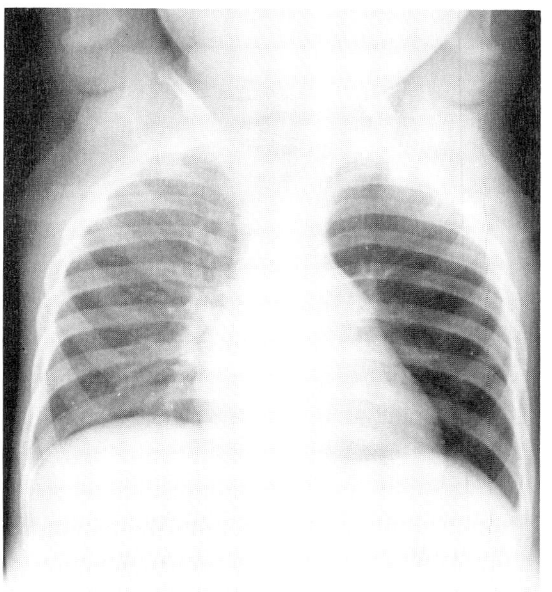

FIGURE 16. **Unilateral hyperinflation.** Frontal radiograph of a 16-month-old child shows marked asymmetry of density, with the left lung being more lucent than the right. Bronchoscopy revealed a peanut in the left main bronchus.

THE UPPER AIRWAY

Upper airway abnormalities are a common cause of respiratory distress in children. Lateral neck radiographs using a soft-tissue technique may be very helpful in making the specific diagnosis. The study is best performed during phonation with the neck extended. During phonation the vocal cords are closed, thus allowing evaluation of the larynx and the thickness of the vocal cords. Young infants may be placed supine on a sponge so that the head drops off the edge of the sponge with the help of gravity. In older children the examination may be performed in the upright position. Some authors advocate an AP radiograph of the neck, but in our experience this view has proved to be unnecessary and frequently misleading. Others advocate a technique called high kilovoltage magnification (high KV mag), which highlights the airway and filters out the bones. This technique requires a special filter that is difficult to obtain. There are few institutions where the study can be performed and even fewer where it can be interpreted correctly.

In the systematic review of the lateral neck radiograph, the first area to assess is the retropharyngeal space. In a well-positioned, properly exposed examination, the retropharyngeal soft tissues are thin (Fig. 17). In children no absolute measurement determines the normal thickness of the retropharyngeal soft tissues, which are highly compliant. Small changes in position or respiratory effort may cause dramatic change in the retropharyngeal soft tissues. When the thickness of the tissues is uncertain, fluoroscopic observation of respiration is helpful.

The next area to be examined is the nasopharynx. By 6 months of age lymphoid tissue should be present in the nasopharynx, but it should not obstruct the lumen. If the patient was phonating during the study, the palate will be "knuckled" to close off the nasopharynx. During quiet respiration the palate is relaxed, and the nasopharynx should be open. The nasopharynx should be inspected for obstruction by a foreign body.

Examination of the oropharynx should reveal a distended vallecula; frequently small nodules representing the lingual tonsils can be identified. Just beneath the vallecula is the hyoid bone, which ossifies during prenatal life but does not fuse until later in adolescence. The epiglottis, which protrudes upward through the hyoid bone and is usually thin, is connected to the arytenoid cartilages by the aryepiglottic folds, which should be paper-thin. The glottis (larynx) is found just below the arytenoid masses. The larynx is recognized by the laryngeal ventricle, which is a cigar-shaped lucency bordered on

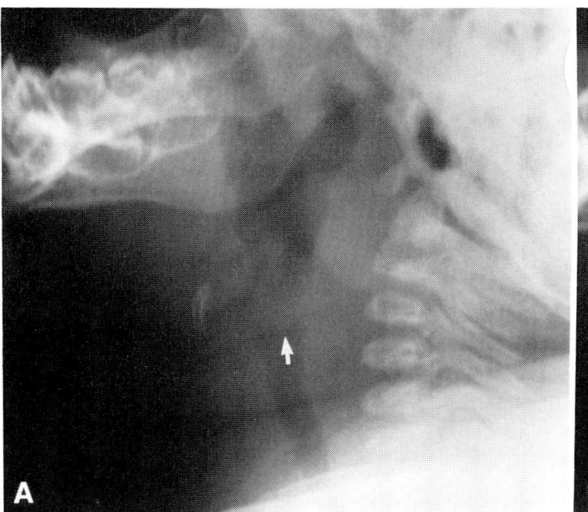

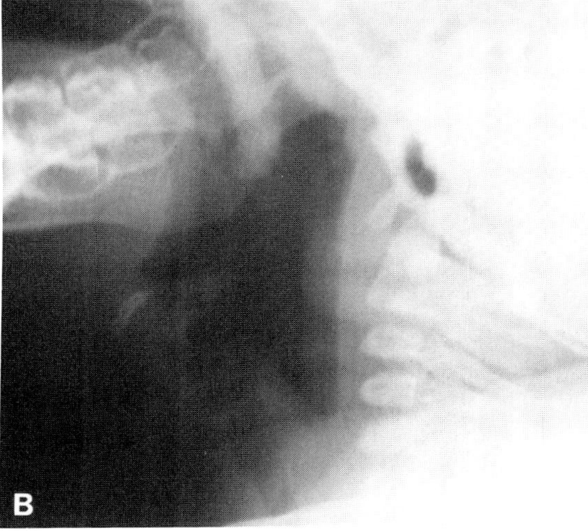

FIGURE 17. **Normal lateral neck.** Fluoroscopic images of the lateral neck during expiration (*A*) and inspiration (*B*). Note the variability in thickness of the retropharyngeal soft tissues. On the inspiratory image, note the distention of the vallecula, the shape of the epiglottis, and the thinness of the aryepiglottic folds. The undersurface of the vocal cords is sharp (*white arrow*), as are the walls of the trachea.

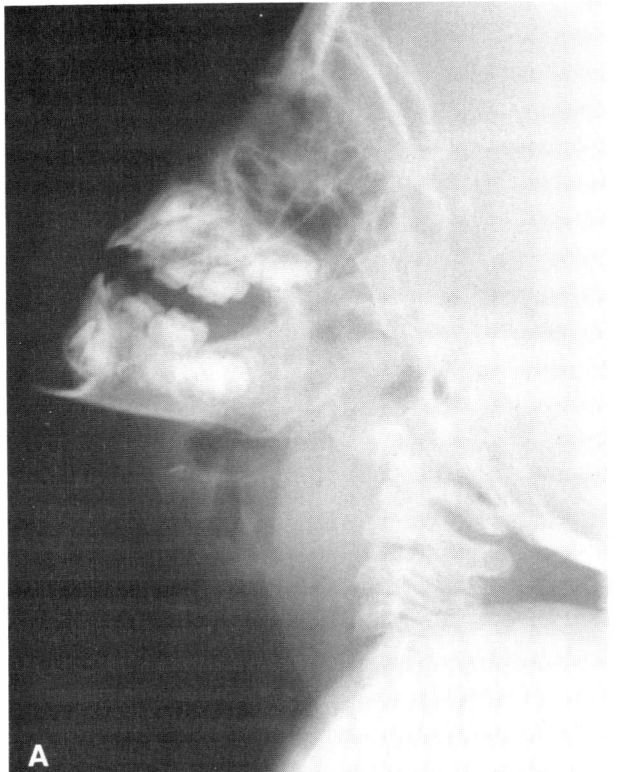

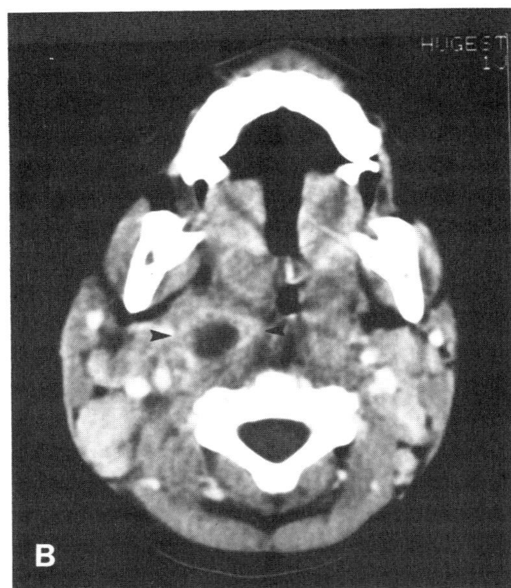

FIGURE 18. **Retropharyngeal abscess.** *A,* Radiograph of the soft tissues of the neck shows marked thickening of the retropharyngeal tissues. The neck is well extended and the hypopharynx is well distended, indicating that the swelling is real. *B,* CT scan with contrast through the neck shows the mass in the retropharynx, which is lucent at its center but shows enhancement of the wall with contrast (*arrowheads*).

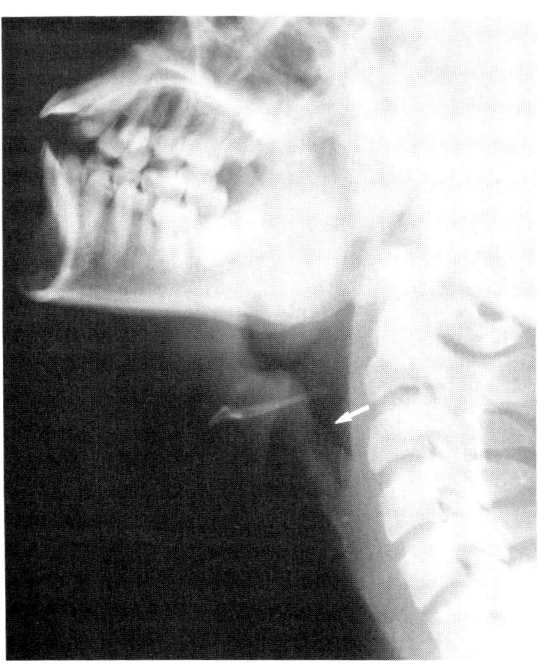

FIGURE 19. **Epiglottitis.** Lateral radiograph of the soft tissues of the neck shows enlargement of the epiglottis and thickening of the aryepiglottic folds (*white arrow*). Note that the vallecula is filled in as well.

the top by the false cords and on the bottom by the true vocal cords. These soft-tissue structures, however, are difficult to define. The undersurface of the vocal cords should be sharp, and the vocal cords should be only a few millimeters thick during phonation. The walls of the trachea below the vocal cords should be sharp, and the caliber of the trachea should be appropriate for the size of the hypopharynx (see Fig. 17). The width of the trachea varies with age, phase of respiration, and even film technique; thus, it is not possible to provide dimensions.

Retropharyngeal Abscess

Retropharyngeal abscess occurs most commonly in children between the ages of 6 months and 3 years. Patients present with high fever, drooling, and chin thrust. A lateral radiograph of the soft tissues of the neck may be helpful if the findings are dramatic (Fig. 18). The findings are often equivocal, however, because the hypopharynx is not adequately distended or the neck is not adequately extended. A repeat film or fluoroscopy may be helpful in determining the presence of soft-tissue swelling that does not change with respiration or neck position. Plain film and fluoroscopy, however, cannot help to determine whether the swelling is due to inflammation or whether an abscess is present. In this situation a CT scan of the neck may be helpful.

Epiglottitis

In a child with suspected epiglottitis, the radiograph may be helpful in confirming the diagnosis. An upright lateral film should be performed as quickly as possible. The radiographic findings, which are striking and characteristic (Fig. 19), include edema of the epiglottis and aryepiglottic folds with obliteration of the vallecula. The disease properly should be called supraglottitis, because all tissues are involved, not merely the epiglottis. In fact, it is the edema of the aryepiglottic folds rather than the epiglottis that causes compromise of the airway.

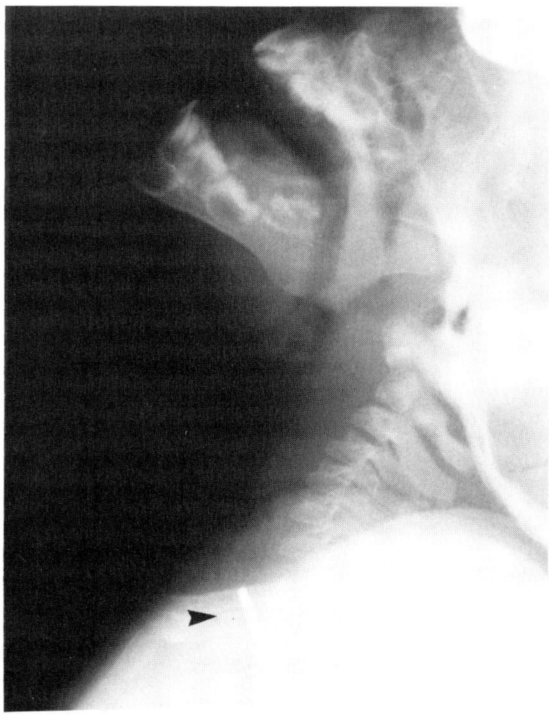

FIGURE 20. **Foreign body in esophagus.** An 8-month-old child presented with stridor. Lateral radiograph of the soft tissues of the neck shows the metallic foreign body at the thoracic inlet, causing compression of the airway at that level (*arrowhead*). The ingested coin was unsuspected before the radiograph was taken.

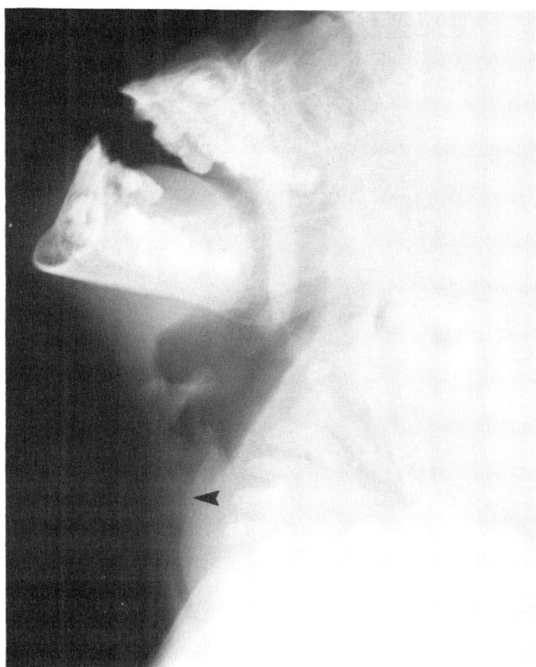

FIGURE 21. **Croup.** Lateral radiograph of the soft tissues of the neck shows marked hyperinflation of the hypopharynx and collapse of the trachea. Note the soft-tissue haziness below the laryngeal ventricle (*arrowhead*). The undersurface of the vocal cords cannot be identified, and the walls of the trachea are obscured by edema.

Croup

The role of radiology in a patient with croup is to help to identify the possible causes. The initial radiograph may exclude the presence of a radiopaque foreign body in either the trachea or the esophagus (Fig. 20). Because of the small size of the mediastinum and the compliance of the airway, foreign bodies in the esophagus as well as the trachea may cause compromise of the airway. Extrinsic impressions on the airway, such as a vascular ring (see Fig. 11), may also be excluded.

The radiographic findings of viral croup range from mild subglottic haziness to evidence of upper airway obstruction marked by distention of the hypopharynx with collapse of the trachea accompanying the subglottic haziness (Fig. 21). Such findings, however, are nonspecific. The same changes may be seen in a patient with a subglottic mass, such as a subglottic hemangioma, or a radiolucent foreign body.

SUGGESTED READING

1. Capitanio MA: From the guest editor. J Thorac Imaging 1(4):ix, 1986.
2. Felman A: Radiology of the Pediatric Chest. New York, McGraw-Hill, 1987.
3. Felson B: Chest Roentgenology. Philadelphia, W.B. Saunders, 1973.
4. Silverman F: Caffey's Pediatric X-Ray Diagnosis: An Integrated Imaging Approach, 9th ed. St. Louis, Mosby, 1992.
5. Squire LF, Novelline RA: Fundamentals of Radiology, 4th ed. Cambridge, MA, Harvard University Press, 1988.

38

WHEN THE PLAIN CHEST RADIOGRAPH IS NOT ENOUGH

Eric N. Faerber, M.D.

The plain chest radiograph is the best initial imaging technique for detecting cardiopulmonary, mediastinal, and musculoskeletal disorders of the thorax. In many instances no further investigations are necessary. Meticulous examination of the chest radiograph, however, often discloses intrathoracic masses and vascular disorders as well as abnormalities below the hemidiaphragms and in the bones and soft tissues of the thorax. These findings may necessitate further studies to arrive at a definitive diagnosis.

A wide array of imaging modalities is available, and the appropriate use of each is essential to arrive at an early diagnosis, to limit the amount of radiation exposure to the infant or child, and to be cost-effective. The choice of each study varies in different hospitals because of availability of equipment and expertise. Brief discussion of the various modalities currently available for thoracic imaging is followed by more detailed description of common thoracic disorders.

IMAGING MODALITIES

Fluoroscopy. Fluoroscopy is readily available at all hospitals. The fluoroscopic screen displays a constant image of the region under examination. The heart, lungs, tracheobronchial tree, thymus, and hemidiaphragms can be evaluated. Fluoroscopy is useful for assessment of diaphragmatic movement, air trapping, and the presence or absence of pulsation within intrathoracic masses.

Barium Swallow (Esophagogram). Barium swallow consists of the fluoroscopic visualization and roentgenographic recording of the passage of barium from the oral cavity through the esophagus to the stomach. Major indications for the use of this procedure include stridor, dysphagia, persistent vomiting, tracheoesophageal fistula, esophageal motility disorders, gastroesophageal reflux, and further evaluation of certain thoracic masses.

Bronchography. Bronchography permits direct visualization of the tracheobronchial tree under fluoroscopy. Selective sequential filling of bronchi with radiopaque contrast medium provides information about the most peripheral bronchi. We use bronchography to delineate congenital and acquired abnormalities of the trachea and bronchi and for postoperative planning.

Angiography. Angiography of the thorax includes all the procedures in which radiopaque contrast media are injected into vascular structures to characterize the vascular nature and supply of lesions, such as aortography, pulmonary angiography, bronchial arteriography, and venacavography.

The main indications for pulmonary angiography are thromboembolic disease of the lungs and acquired disease of the pulmonary arterial and venous circulation. Magnetic resonance imaging (MRI) is largely replacing angiography for the evaluation of congenital abnormalities of the pulmonary vascular tree. Previously aortography was used widely for the identification of aortic anomalies, differentiation of mediastinal masses that may have a vascular

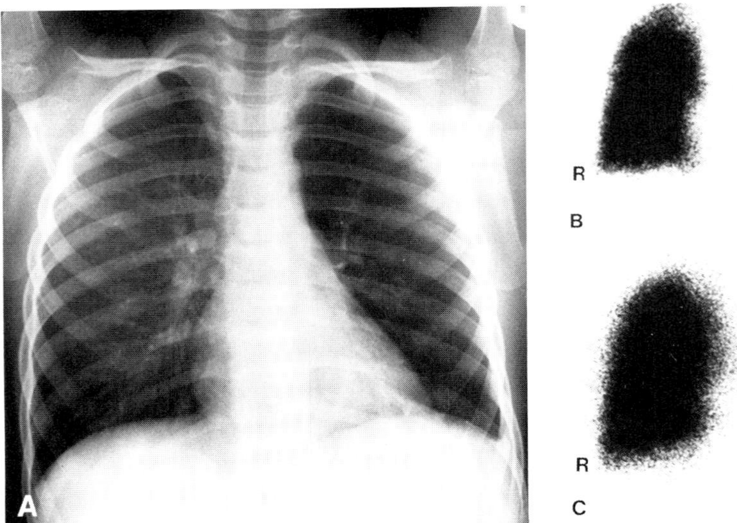

FIGURE 1. **Bronchiolitis obliterans.** *A,* Frontal chest radiograph demonstrates left upper lobe overaeration with left lower lobe volume loss. *B,* Radionuclide V-Q scan demonstrates nonperfusion of the left upper lobe and lower lobes. *C,* V-Q scan demonstrates nonventilation of the entire left upper lobe and nearly all of the left lower lobe.

cause, and identification of anomalous intrathoracic vessels. For these indications also, angiography has been replaced mainly by MRI.

Nuclear Medicine. Radionuclide scintigraphy of the lung is extremely useful in clinical situations in which regional ventilation and perfusion (V-Q) must be assessed after identification of abnormalities on the plain radiograph. When the plain radiograph demonstrates unequal inflation of the lungs, a V-Q scan may be performed to assess pulmonary function (Fig. 1). Scintigraphy is also used to assess inflammatory foci, tumor uptake, and gastroesophageal reflux.

Ultrasound. Ultrasound evaluation of the chest is limited because of the surrounding bony thorax. Ultrasound is excellent for the detection of pleural effusions and loculation (see chapter 19) and for assessment of diaphragmatic movement. Spectral and color flow Doppler are used for anatomic differentiation of pulmonary from pleural, mediastinal, and chest wall lesions. Fluid aspiration and biopsies may be performed under ultrasound guidance.

Computed Tomography. Computed tomography (CT) has rapidly emerged as a major imaging modality in the evaluation of thoracic disease, because it allows excellent soft-tissue resolution, superior density discrimination, and cross-sectional imaging of the thorax.[2] CT helps to define the origin and extent of mediastinal masses, tracheobronchial abnormalities, and chest wall masses. High-resolution CT yields information about the airway, pulmonary parenchyma, and vasculature not available from plain chest radiographs.

Magnetic Resonance Imaging. MRI is the most recent diagnostic technique available. It is especially appealing in infants and children because of the lack of ionizing radiation. The inherent contrast between blood and vascular walls or cardiac chamber walls is excellent, thus obviating the need for intravenous contrast medium. MRI has the added advantage of being able to image in three planes: transaxial, coronal, and sagittal. The role of MRI in evaluating thoracic disorders in infants and children is evolving; already, however, it is widely used in the evaluation of cardiac, vascular mediastinal, hilar, and chest wall abnormalities. MRI is an important tool in the evaluation of congenital heart disease as well as the procedure of choice for evaluation of vascular rings.[3,4]

Mediastinal masses are visualized optimally by CT or MRI.[6] MRI, however, is the modality of choice for demonstrating the extradural extension and spinal cord displacement of neurogenic tumors in the posterior mediastinum. The chest wall is effectively evaluated by MRI because of the very high soft-tissue contrast. Lipoma, lymphangioma, hemangioma, and malignant tumors are easily detected. MRI is relatively nonspecific for pulmonary parenchymal disease.

TABLE 1. Summary of Important Mediastinal Masses

Anterior: the four Ts
- Thymus, normal and abnormal
- "Terrible" leukemia and lymphoma
- Teratoma
- Thyroid-retrosternal

Middle: ABV
- Adenopathy
- Bronchopulmonary foregut malformations
- Vascular anomalies

Posterior
- Neurogenic tumors

IMAGING OF THORACIC DISORDERS

Mediastinal Masses

Mediastinal masses detected on plain chest radiography may be located within the anterior, middle, or posterior compartments (Table 1). Because the appearance of a mass on plain chest radiography is often nonspecific, further studies are necessary to define the exact location of the mass and to characterize its nature. **CT is particularly helpful in the work-up of anterior and middle mediastinal masses, whereas MRI**

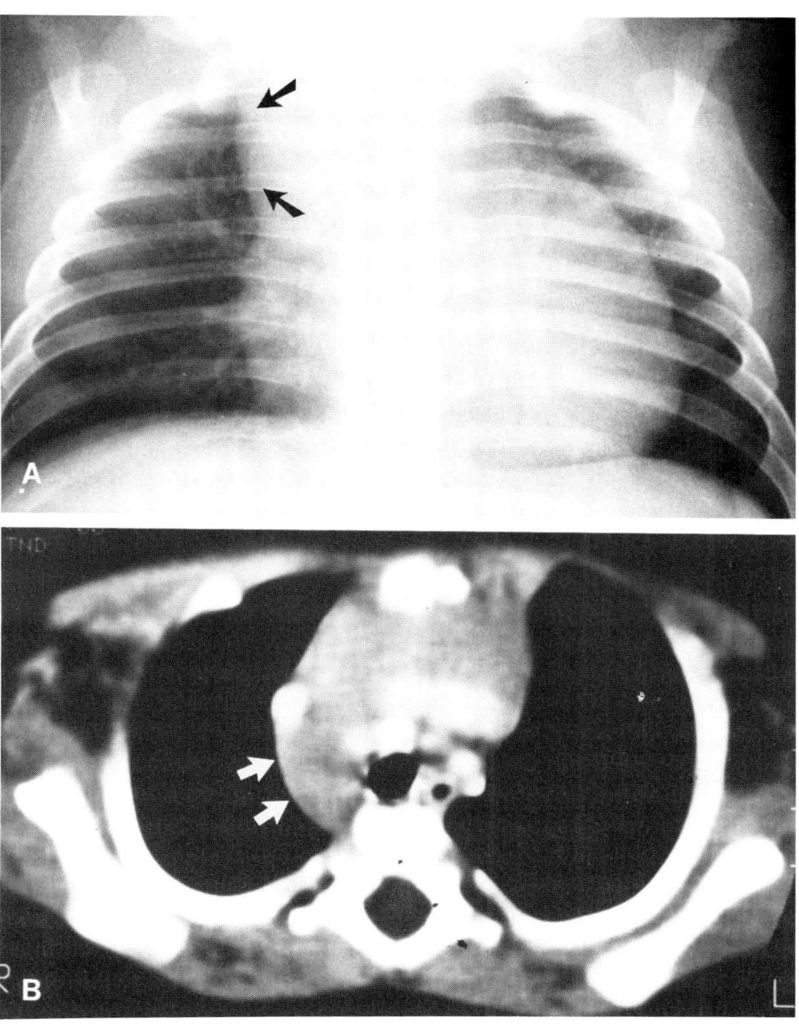

FIGURE 2. **Normal thymus with posterior extension.** *A*, Frontal chest radiograph demonstrates a right-sided mediastinal mass (*arrows*). *B*, Contrast-enhanced CT of the chest shows a uniform soft-tissue mass with a smooth lateral margin extending from the anterior to the posterior mediastinum (*arrows*). (From Faerber EN: The role of computed tomography in pediatric chest disease. J Thorac Imaging 1:70–77, 1986; with permission).

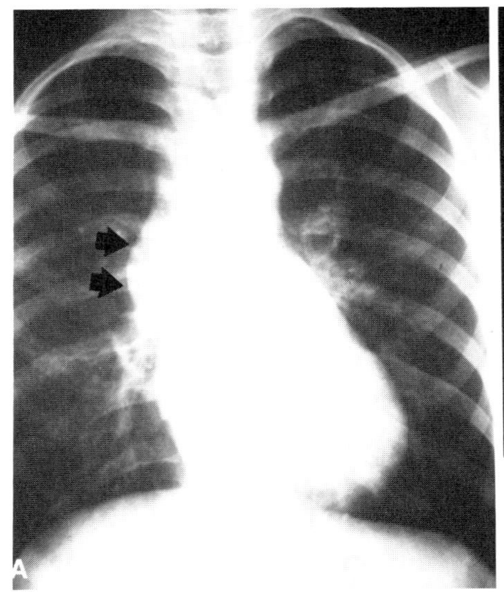

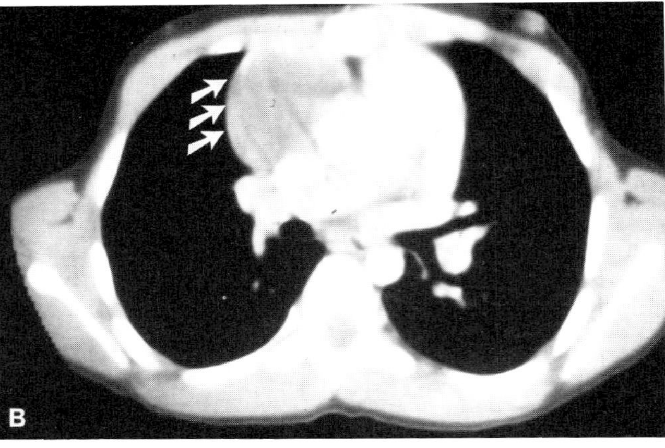

FIGURE 3. **Thymic cyst.** *A*, Frontal chest radiograph demonstrates a mass in the region of the right lobe of the thymus (*arrows*). *B*, Contrast-enhanced CT shows a large cystic mass of low density in the right thymic lobe (*arrows*).

is mandatory for posterior mediastinal masses in order to demonstrate intraspinal extension.

Anterior Mediastinal Masses

The anterior mediastinum is bounded superiorly by the clavicles, inferiorly by the diaphragm, anteriorly by the sternum, and posteriorly by the anterior surface of the heart and great vessels. The contents include the thymus, lymph nodes, nerves, muscles, and sternum.

The normal thymus may have numerous configurations, often simulating mass lesions (see chapter 37). Occasionally the normal thymus may extend from the anterior mediastinum to the posterior mediastinum. This normal variant is best demonstrated by CT (Fig. 2) or MRI. Thymic cysts are rare in childhood. They are most commonly developmental in origin, representing tubular remnants of the third pharyngeal pouch. The plain chest radiograph may demonstrate mild mediastinal widening due to the anterior mediastinal location of the mass. CT demonstrates a well-defined mass of low density characteristic of a cyst (Fig. 3). A large anterior mediastinal mass that is found to be mainly of fat origin on CT is usually a thymolipoma (Fig. 4), whereas the presence of mixed elements such as calcium, soft tissue and fat are more characteristic of a teratoma (Fig. 5).

The most common abnormal anterior mass is lymphoma (Hodgkin's or non-Hodgkin's) or leukemia. These lesions cannot be differentiated radiographically. The thymus may be infiltrated by tumor and enlarged (Fig. 6). There is, however, a wide spectrum of anterior mediastinal masses, including cystic hygroma, retrosternal thyroid, histiocytosis (Fig. 7), hemangioma, germ-cell tumors, and hematoma.

Middle Mediastinum

The middle mediastinum extends from the posterior surface of the heart and great vessels to the anterior surface of the thoracic vertebrae. The contents of this compartment are the posterior heart and pericardium, the aorta and its thoracic branches, major systemic thoracic veins, pulmonary arteries and veins, trachea and mainstem bronchi, phrenic and vagus nerves, and lymph nodes. Two major disease entities are encountered in the middle mediastinum: lymphadenopathy and the spectrum of bronchopulmonary foregut malformations.

Lymphadenopathy. Lymphadenopathy accounts for the majority of middle mediastinal masses. Node involvement is usually due to malignancy or inflammation.

Lymphomas. Approximately one-third of children with Hodgkin's lymphoma have mediastinal adenopathy at the time of diagnosis. All mediastinal nodes, with the exception of paracardiac and posterior mediastinal nodes, are involved more commonly by Hodgkin's than by non-Hodgkin's lymphoma.

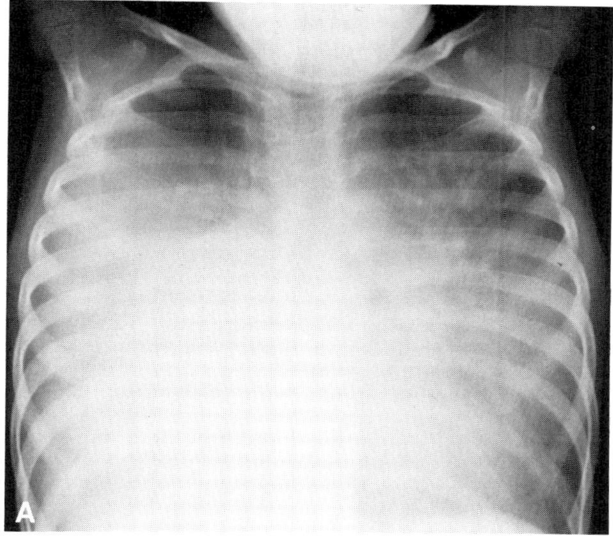

FIGURE 4. **Thymolipoma.** *A*, Frontal chest radiograph shows apparent cardiomegaly with bilateral pulmonary opacification. *(Cont., below.)*

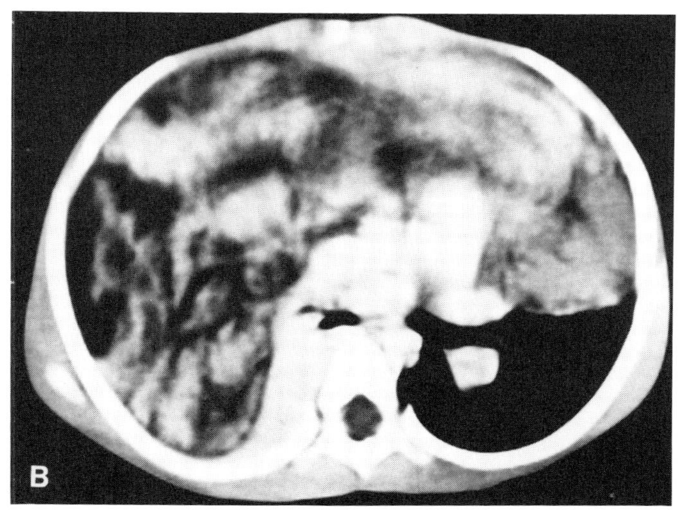

FIGURE 4 *(Cont.).* *B*, Contrast-enhanced CT demonstrates a large mass of varying densities. Islands of thymic tissue are located between low-density areas representing adipose tissue. (From Faerber EN: Pediatr Radiol 20:196, 1990; with permission.)

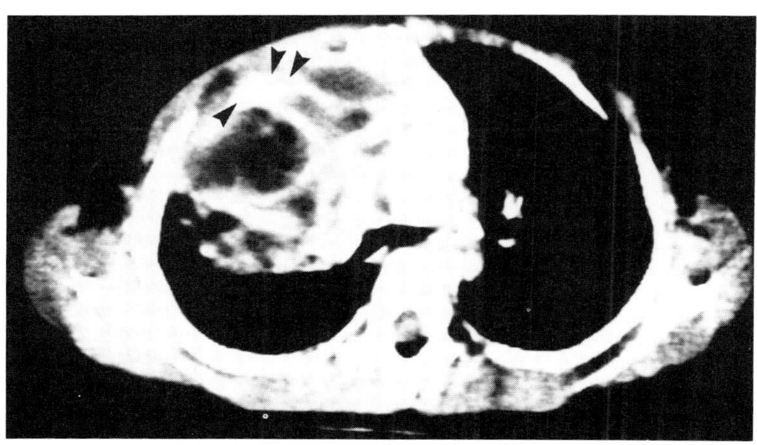

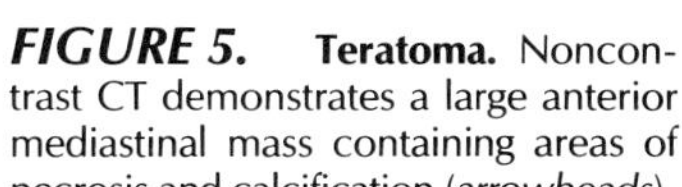

FIGURE 5. **Teratoma.** Noncontrast CT demonstrates a large anterior mediastinal mass containing areas of necrosis and calcification (*arrowheads*).

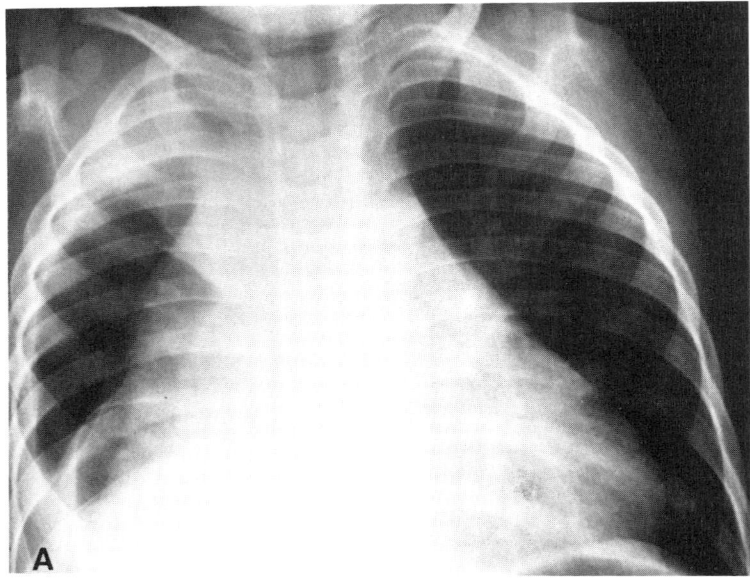

FIGURE 6. **Leukemic infiltration of the thymus.** *A*, Frontal chest radiograph demonstrates a right upper lobe atelectasis, right pleural effusion, and right-sided mass. *(Cont., below.)*

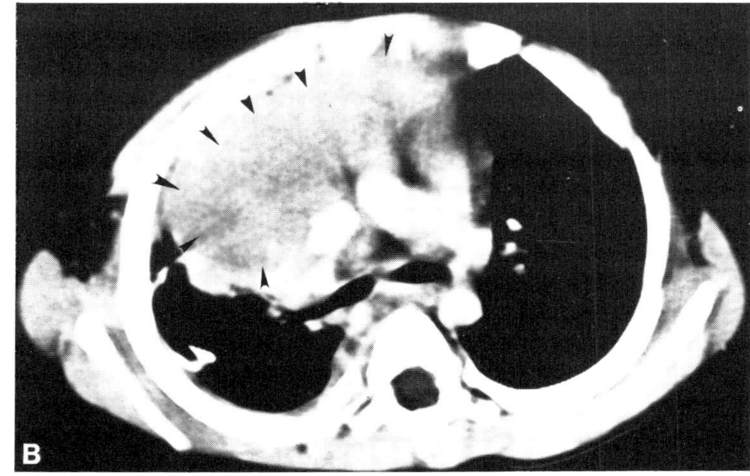

FIGURE 6 *(Cont.).* *B*, Contrast-enhanced CT (after thoracentesis) demonstrates enlargement of the thymus, which is of uniform low density (*arrowheads*).

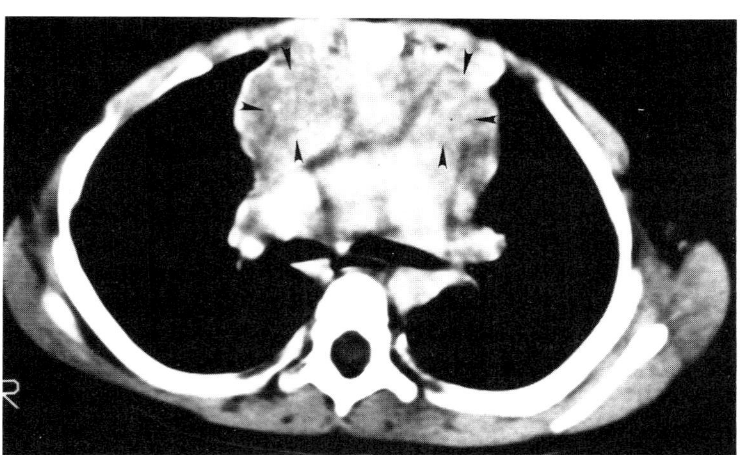

FIGURE 7. **Histiocytosis-X.** Contrast-enhanced CT demonstrates an anterior mediastinal mass of low density (*arrowheads*). The plain chest radiograph is demonstrated in Fig. 2, chapter 19).

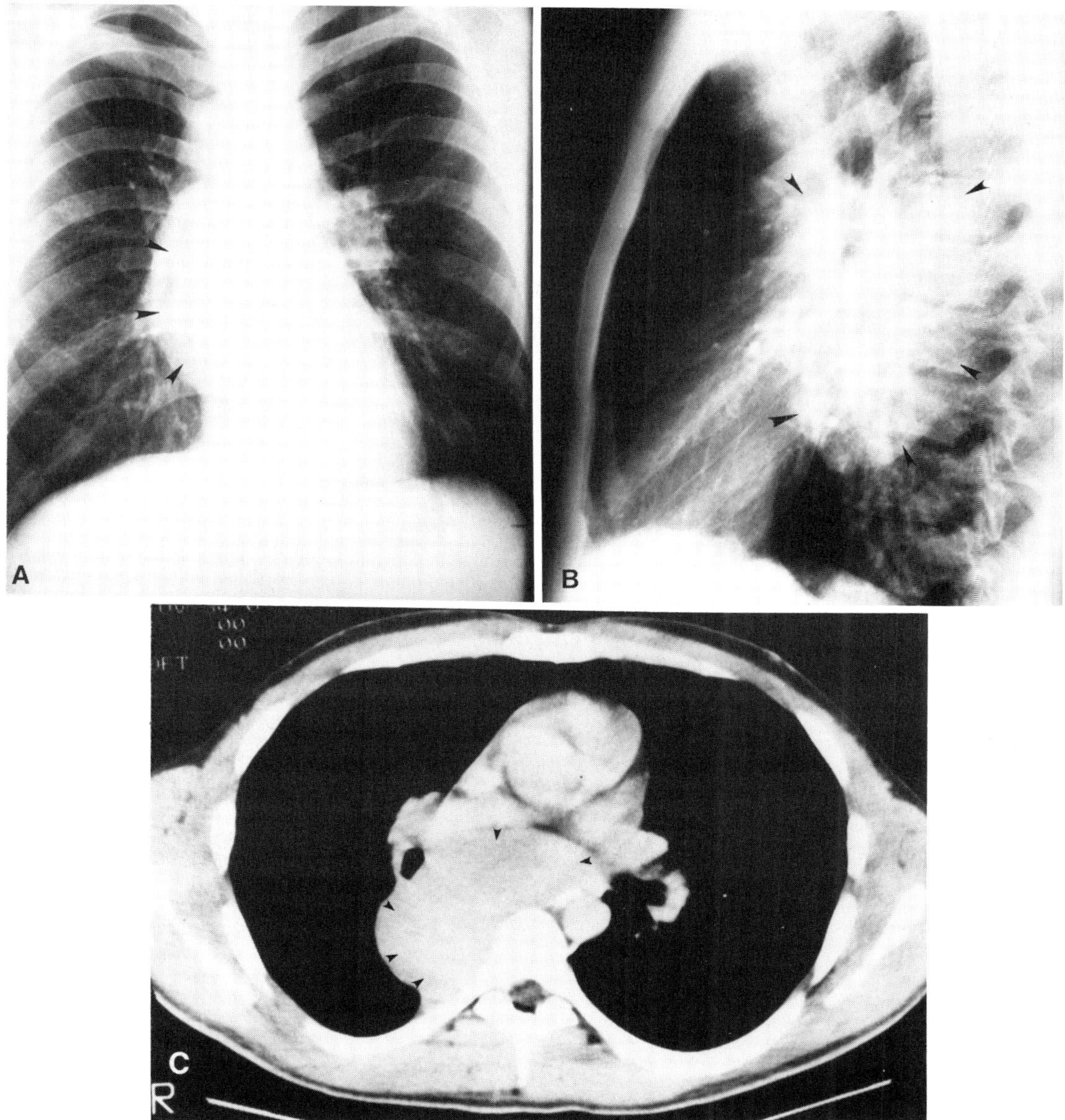

FIGURE 8. **Lymphoma.** Frontal (*A*) and lateral (*B*) chest radiographs demonstrate middle mediastinal adenopathy (*arrowheads*). *C*, Contrast-enhanced CT demonstrates middle and posterior mediastinal adenopathy.

Lymph nodes on CT are masses of soft-tissue density (Fig. 8). They are readily distinguished from vascular structures, which are enhanced by intravenous administration of contrast medium. On MRI lymph nodes are similar to muscle in signal intensity on T1-weighted images but become brighter than muscle and similar to fat in signal intensity on T2-weighted images. The absence of signal in pulmonary vessels is a further distinguishing feature.

Non-Hodgkin's lymphoma, a heterogeneous group of malignancies with worse prognosis, cannot be differentiated from Hodgkin's disease by CT or MRI.

Metastatic Lymphadenopathy. Metastatic lymphadenopathy results mostly from neuroblastoma, Ewing's sarcoma, osteogenic sarcoma, and Wilms' tumor.

Inflammatory Lymphadenopathy. Inflammatory lymphadenopathy is usually associated

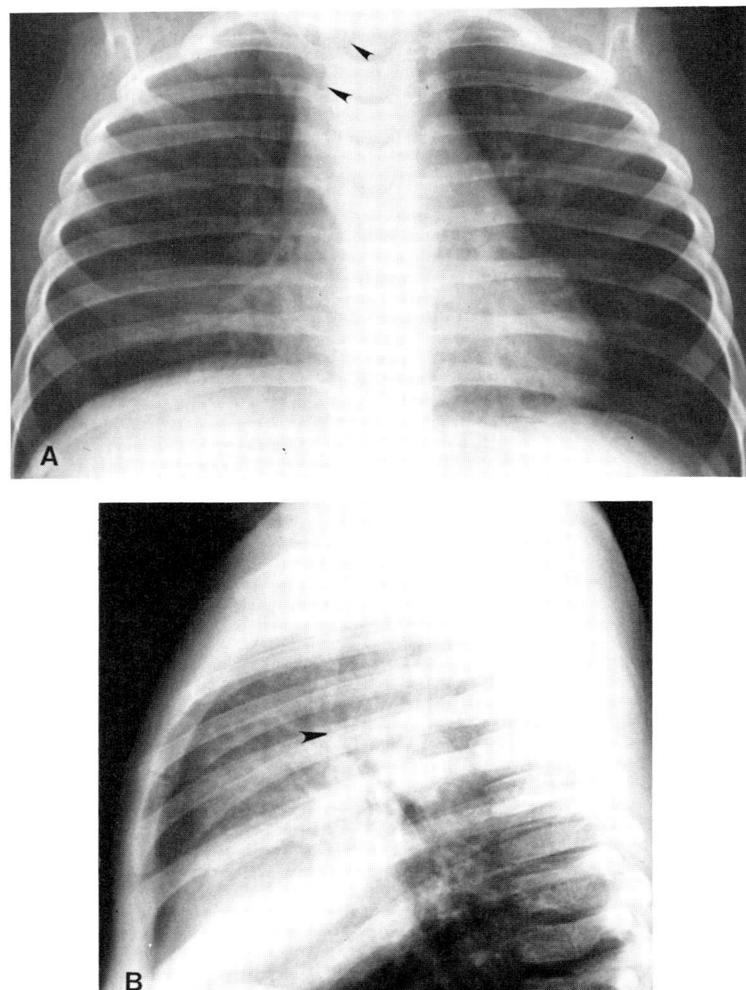

FIGURE 9. **Bronchogenic cyst.** *A,* Frontal chest radiograph demonstrates lateral deviation of the trachea by a soft tissue mass (*arrowheads*) *B,* Lateral radiograph demonstrates anterior displacement and bowing of the trachea by the mass (*arrowhead*). (*Continued on facing page.*)

with focal pulmonary disease, usually granulomas such as tuberculosis, sarcoidosis, and histoplasmosis.

Bronchopulmonary Foregut Malformations. Bronchopulmonary foregut malformations are a spectrum of varied disorders with a common embryology. The foregut is the origin of both the tracheobronchial tree and esophagus. The lung bud develops as a ventral outpouching of the foregut. Later in development a lateral fold separates the ventral trachea from the dorsal esophagus. Abnormal budding of the foregut leads to the formation of bronchogenic cysts. Esophageal duplication cysts result from the endodermal outpouching of the developing esophagus. Failure of separation of the primitive foregut from the notochord with which it was closely associated may result in sequestered portions of the foregut within the spinal canal, which lead to formation of neurenteric cysts.

The spectrum of bronchopulmonary foregut malformations[4] includes:

1. Pulmonary sequestration, both intralobar and extralobar
2. Pulmonary sequestration with partial or complete enteric communication
3. Intestinal duplications (esophageal and other gastrointestinal types)

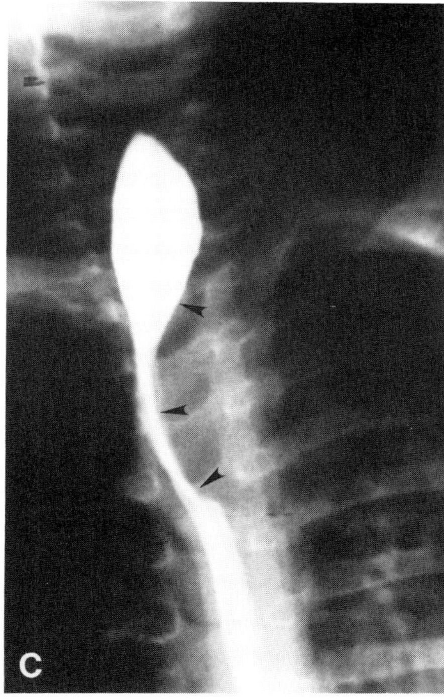

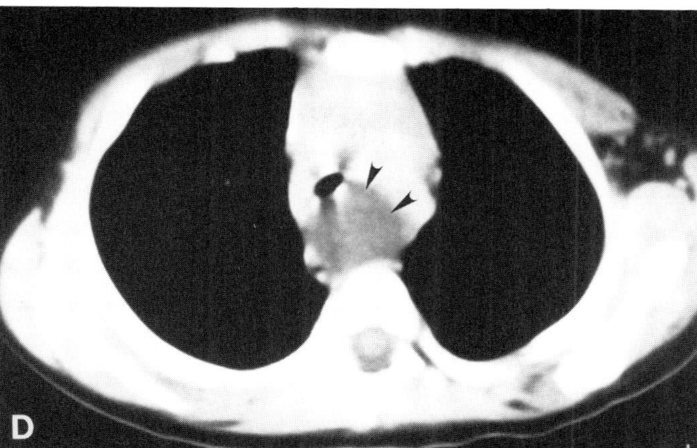

FIGURE 9 *(Cont).* *C*, Barium swallow demonstrates extrinsic compression of the esophagus by the mass. *D*, Contrast-enhanced CT demonstrates a low-density mass posterior to the displaced trachea (*arrowheads*).

4. Bronchogenic cyst
5. Tracheoesophageal fistula with or without fistula
6. Neurenteric cyst

Bronchogenic Cyst. The bronchogenic cyst is the most common foregut duplication cyst (Fig. 9). The chest radiograph usually demonstrates a well-defined soft-tissue mass, round or oval in shape, near the carina. Barium swallow demonstrates displacement or compression by the cyst. CT, however, is more helpful in assessment of the nature and extent of the cyst and demonstrates a well-defined avascular mass. Many cysts are of water density, but the cyst content may have increased density due to mucoid material or milk with calcium content. Curvilinear calcification may occur within the cyst wall but is rare. A cystic lesion has a similar appearance on MRI, with low-to-intermediate signal intensity on T-1 weighted images and high signal intensity on T-2 weighted images.

Esophageal Duplication Cyst. Esophageal duplication cysts result from abnormal vacuolization of the esophageal lumen. They usually occur in the middle mediastinum but also may occur in the posterior mediastinum.

Chest radiograph demonstrates a sharply marginated mass of water density. CT demonstates a low-density mass with smooth borders located close to the esophagus. MRI shows the visual signal characteristics of a cyst, much like those of the bronchogenic cyst described above.

Neurenteric Cyst. Neurenteric cysts represent a residual connection between the foregut and the spinal canal. The cysts are located in the middle or posterior mediastinum and are often right-sided. Numerous vertebral anomalies may be present, including butterfly vertebrae, hemivertebrae, or scoliosis, and are visible on the plain chest radiograph. **CT and MRI are the modalities of choice for assessment of the cyst, intraspinal involvement, and vertebral abnormalities.**

Posterior Mediastinum

The posterior mediastinum extends from the anterior surface of the thoracic vertebrae to the posterior chest wall. This compartment contains the thoracic duct, descending thoracic aorta, hemiazygous veins, sympathetic chain, spinal column, and nerve roots.

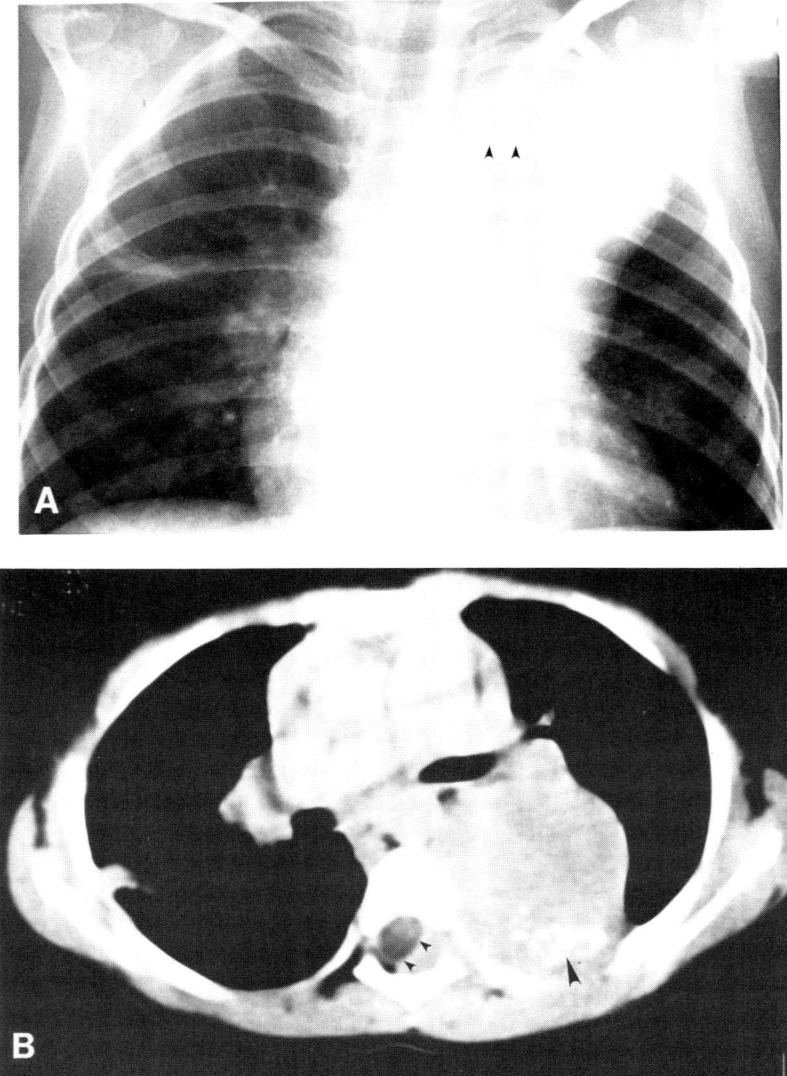

FIGURE 10. *A*, Frontal chest radiograph demonstrates a large posterior mediastinal mass. Note rib space widening and rib erosion (*arrowheads*). *B*, Contrast-enhanced CT demonstrates a large posterior mediastinal mass containing calcification (*large arrowhead*). Extradural extension of the mass displaces the spinal canal (*small arrowheads*). (*Continued on facing page.*)

Neurogenic Tumors. The vast majority of posterior mediastinal masses are neurogenic in origin and may be divided into three groups:

1. Sympathetic ganglia derivatives, including neuroblastoma, ganglioneuroblastoma, and ganglioneuroma;
2. Peripheral nerve derivatives, including neurofibroma and neurilemmoma; and
3. Paraganglion cell derivatives, which are rare in children.

Neurogenic Tumors Arising from the Sympathetic Nervous System. Sympathetic ganglia derivatives include neuroblastoma (Fig. 10), ganglioneuroblastoma, and ganglioneuroma. Neuroblastoma is the most common of the three, with 10–15% occurring within the thorax. It is a highly malignant tumor, although prognosis is more favorable if the tumor is diagnosed before the child is 1 year of age. The age range for neuroblastoma extends from under 2 years (40% of patients) to the preschool children, whereas ganglioneuroblastoma and ganglioneuroma occur in older children. Neuroblastoma usually presents late, when it produces

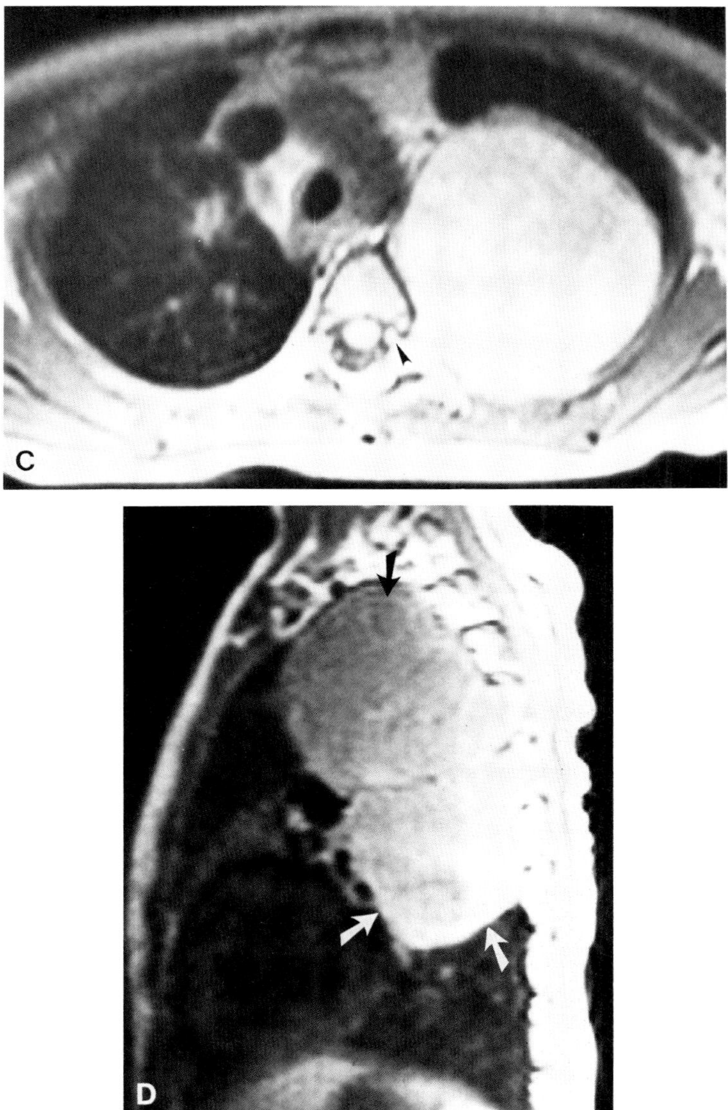

FIGURE 10 *(Cont.).* *C,* Transaxial intermediate-weighted MRI demonstrates the posterior mediastinal mass with intraspinal extension (*arrowhead*). *D,* Coronal T1-weighted MRI demonstrates the superoinferior extent of the mass (*arrows*).

signs and symptoms due to local invasion or compression, metastases to other sites, or paraneoplastic syndromes.

The imaging appearances of all three tumors of neurogenic origin is similar. The plain chest radiograph usually demonstrates a posterior mediastinal mass that is paravertebral in location. Focal calcification is seen in about one-third of cases. Spreading and thinning of adjacent posterior ribs may be seen (see Fig. 10).

CT is the modality of choice for initial evaluation of thoracic neuroblastoma. A soft-tissue paravertebral mass is seen. CT readily demonstrates calcification that may not be evident on plain radiographs as well as adenopathy, spinal canal involvement, and chest wall invasion. **MRI is superior to CT in the demonstration of intraspinal extension and chest wall invasion** (see Fig. 10).

Peripheral Nerve Tumors. Neurofibromas tend to occur in patients with the systemic form of the disease rather than as isolated lesions. They are more often bilateral. The chest radiograph may demonstrate the neurofibroma in addition to other associated abnormalities, such as scoliosis or the slender "ribbon" ribs. CT and MRI also demonstrate presence of the soft-tissue masses but are superior to chest radiographs in demonstrating paravertebral masses with intraspinal extension.

Vascular Rings and Anomalies of the Great Vessels

Vascular rings and anomalies of the great vessels should be suspected when abnormal configurations of the trachea and esophagus are noted on the initial chest radiographs.[1]

Aberrant Left Pulmonary Artery (Pulmonary Sling)

The aberrant left pulmonary artery results from obliteration or failure of normal development of the left sixth aortic arch. Because the left pulmonary artery fails to develop, the arterial supply of the left lung is derived from an anomalous vessel that originates from the right pulmonary artery. The aberrant artery passes between the trachea and esophagus. Hypoplasia or dysplasia of the trachea and main bronchi is frequently present.

The varied appearances of a pulmonary sling on plain chest radiograph (Fig. 11) include:

1. Anterior bowing of the trachea at the level of the carina
2. Indentation on the anterior portion of the esophagus
3. Low left hilum with mainstem bronchi showing a horizontal "inverted" T-shaped pattern
4. Hyperlucent right lung in neonates and infants

The indentation on the esophagus is usually shown by esophagogram (Fig. 11). This study, however, may be normal if the indentation is transient. The diagnosis may be confirmed by CT or pulmonary arteriography. **MRI is now becoming the modality of choice**, because it demonstrates the origin and cause of the left pulmonary artery and the associated airway anomalies.

Double Aortic Arch

A double aortic arch is the most common cause of a symptomatic vascular ring in infants and young children. There are two types of double aortic arch: (1) complete functioning double aortic arch and (2) double aortic arch with interruption of the left arch at the varying positions and fibrous continuity of the interrupted segment.

Complete Functioning Double Aortic Arch. With persistence of both the right and left

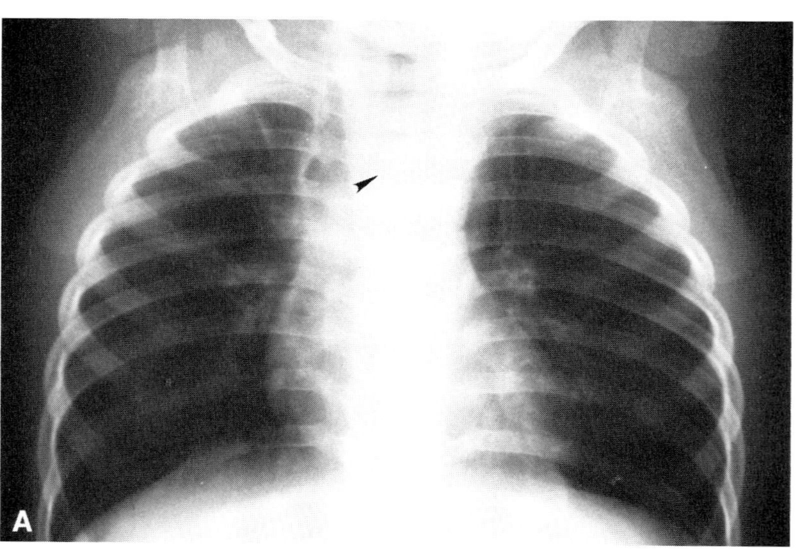

FIGURE 11. **Pulmonary sling.** *A*, Frontal chest radiograph demonstrates a midline trachea with right-sided deviation (*arrowhead*) before return to the midline.
(Continued on facing page.)

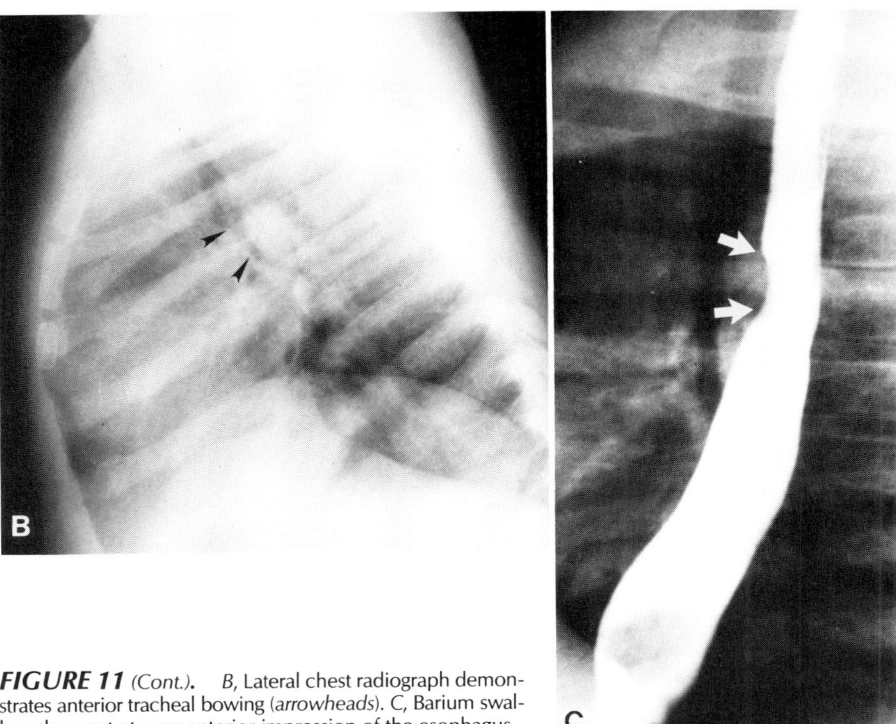

FIGURE 11 *(Cont.).* *B,* Lateral chest radiograph demonstrates anterior tracheal bowing (*arrowheads*). *C,* Barium swallow demonstrates an anterior impression of the esophagus.

aortic arches, the two vessels arise from the ascending aorta and course distally on each side of the trachea and esophagus to join posteriorly, usually into a left descending aorta. The plain chest radiograph may appear normal in infants. In older children the appearance of a double aortic arch may simulate a right aortic arch, although narrowing of the trachea may be observed in a lateral chest radiograph. Displacement of the trachea to the left and narrowing of the distal trachea may be seen on a chest radiograph using high kilovoltage and added filtration techniques. Barium swallow demonstrates lateral and posterior indentations on the esophagus. The right and posterior indentations are more prominent because of the larger right arch.

Abnormalities found on chest radiograph and esophagogram may provide sufficient information for some clinicians, without recourse to further imaging studies. Aortography and MRI further confirm the diagnosis. MRI in axial and coronal planes provides valuable preoperative information about vascular abnormality and is noninvasive (Fig. 12).

Double Aortic Arch with Partial Atresia of the Left Arch. Regression of varying segments of the left aortic arch is accompanied by fibrous continuity of the segments to complete the vascular ring. Atresia between the left common and subclavian arteries or atresia distal to the left subclavian artery is a common variation. Chest radiograph shows a prominent right aortic arch in frontal projection. Barium swallow also shows lateral impressions on the esophagus, more prominent on the right side, and a prominent posterior indentation. Both angiography and MRI demonstrate the lack of patency of the left arch with a left innominate artery. An aortic diverticulum may be seen at the junction of the right aortic arch and upper descending aorta in one of the subtypes of this anomaly.

Aberrant Right Subclavian Artery

Aberrant origin of the right subclavian artery is a common malformation of the aortic arch. The artery arises from the left descending thoracic aorta and courses behind the esophagus superiorly to the right side. Congenital heart disease of varying types may frequently coexist. Barium swallow demonstrates an

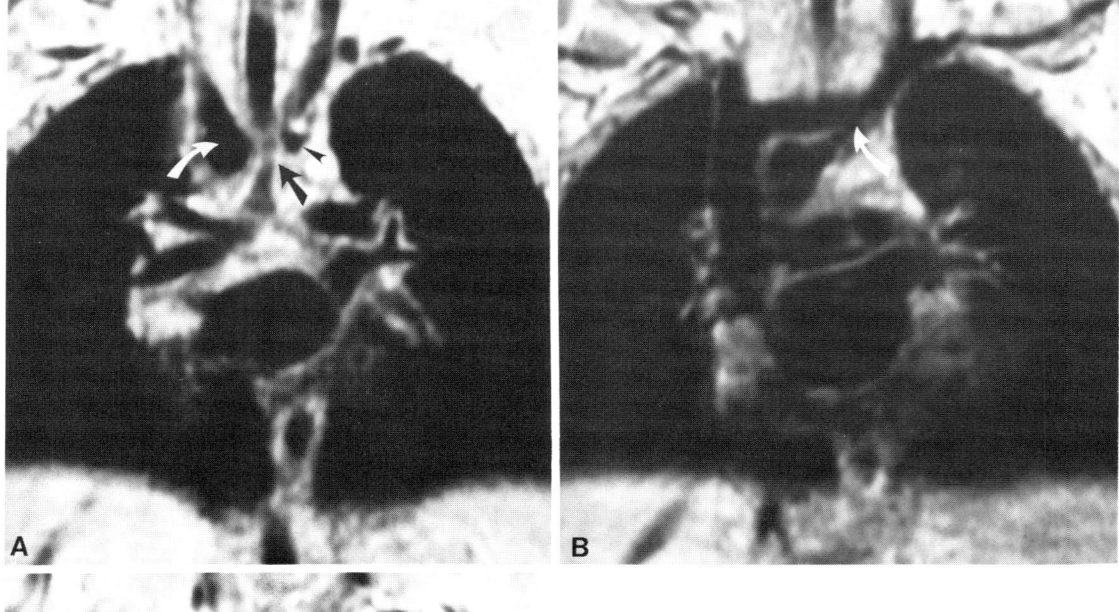

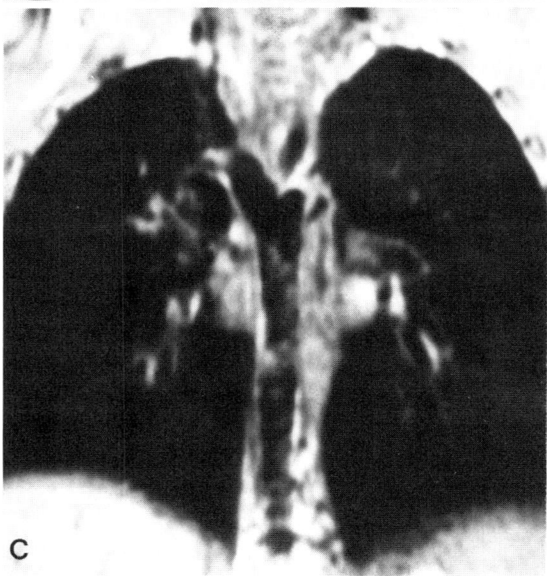

FIGURE 12. **Double aortic arch.** *A*, Coronal T1-weighted MRI demonstrates a dominant right aortic arch (*white arrow*) and smaller left aortic arch (*black arrow*). Note tracheal compression (*arrowhead*). *B*, Coronal T1-weighted MRI demonstrates small left aortic arch (*arrow*). *C*, Coronal T1-weighted MRI demonstrates fusion of the two arches above the descending aorta.

oblique defect on the esophagus on frontal projection and a smooth posterior impression of the esophagus on lateral projection (Fig. 13). The appearance of this vascular abnormality is well demonstrated on MRI (Fig. 13).

Recurrent Infection

The presence of recurrent or persistent pulmonary consolidation in the same anatomic site, especially the lung base, should alert the clinician and radiologist to the diagnosis of **pulmonary sequestration**, a congenital abnormality that is considered part of the spectrum of bronchopulmonary foregut malformations. The underlying abnormality is a mass of nonfunctioning pulmonary tissue without connection to either the bronchial tree or the pulmonary arteries. The arterial supply usually arises from a branch of the abdominal aorta. The venous drainage is variable and may be through the pulmonary veins, inferior vena cava, or azygos system. There are two types of sequestration: intralobar and extralobar. Each has a distinct clinical presentation.

Intralobar Sequestration

Intralobar sequestration is contiguous to normal lung parenchyma. The sequestered lung tissue lies within the pleural covering of the normal lungs, with which it communicates because of infection. **The most common location is the paravertebral gutter, with two-thirds of cases on the left side and most of the remainder on the right side.** The upper lobes are rarely involved. Bilateral involvement is infrequent.

The disorder is discovered usually because of repeated or persistent pulmonary infection or less frequently as an incidental finding on chest radiograph. Other presentations include congestive heart failure due to a right-to-left shunt or hemoptysis, if there is a connection with the bronchial tree.

The plain chest radiograph demonstrates a soft-tissue mass of varying size and configuration. The mass may be cystic, simulating a congenital cystic adenomatoid malformation of the lung. An upper GI series should be performed to exclude communication with the gastrointestinal tract.

Demonstration of the arterial supply to the sequestered segment is important for diagnostic and surgical purposes. Angiography, traditionally the modality of choice (Fig. 14), is now being replaced by MRI.

Extralobar Sequestration

Extralobar sequestration is separate from normal lung parenchyma and invested with a separate pleural covering. In the vast majority of cases it is contiguous with the left hemidiaphragm; it is usually unilateral. Patients with extralobar sequestration are usually asymptomatic. The diagnosis is made after the observation

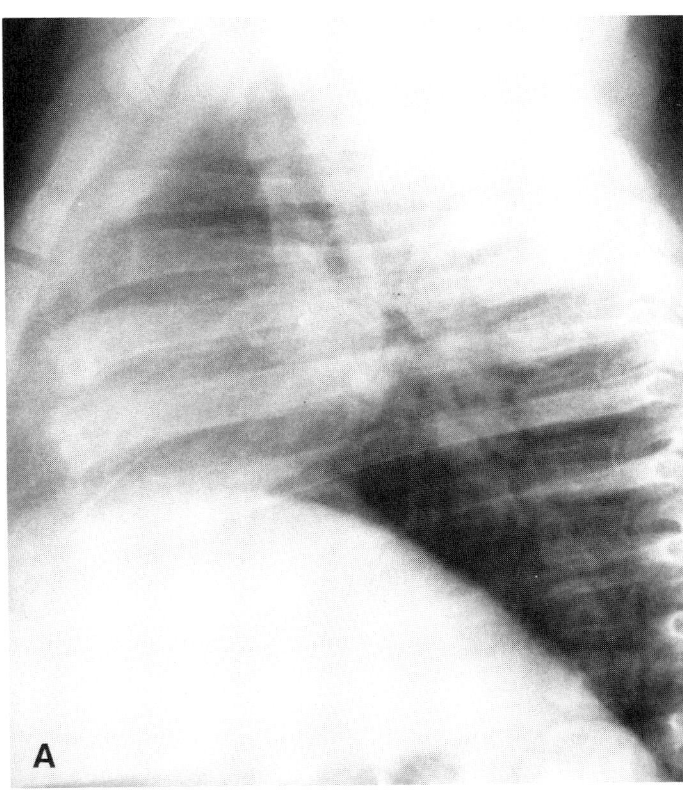

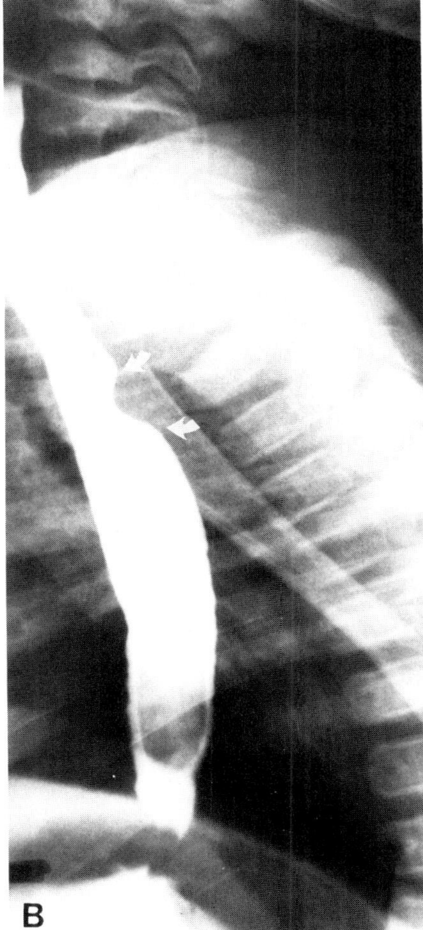

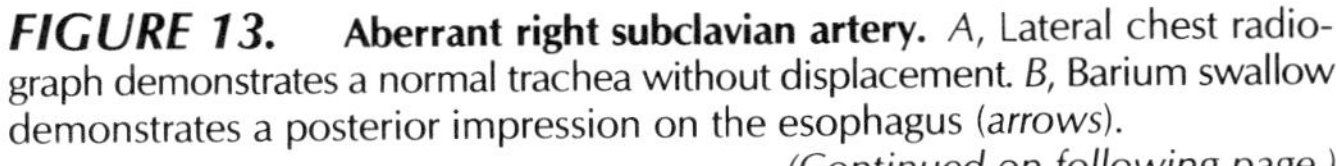
FIGURE 13. **Aberrant right subclavian artery.** *A*, Lateral chest radiograph demonstrates a normal trachea without displacement. *B*, Barium swallow demonstrates a posterior impression on the esophagus (*arrows*).

(Continued on following page.)

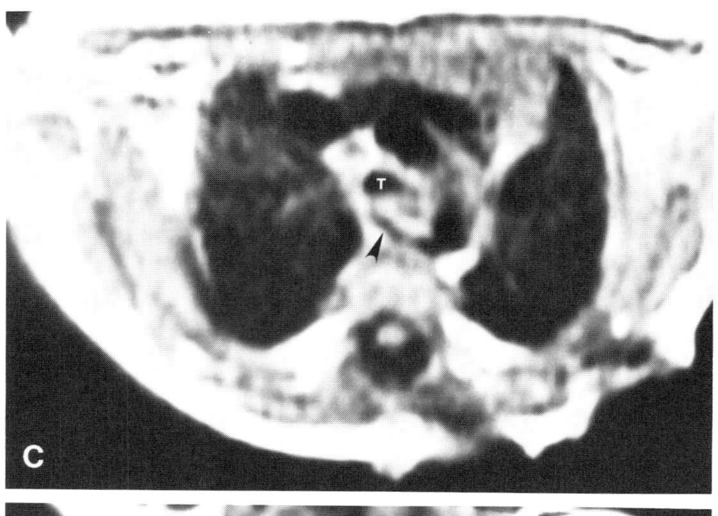

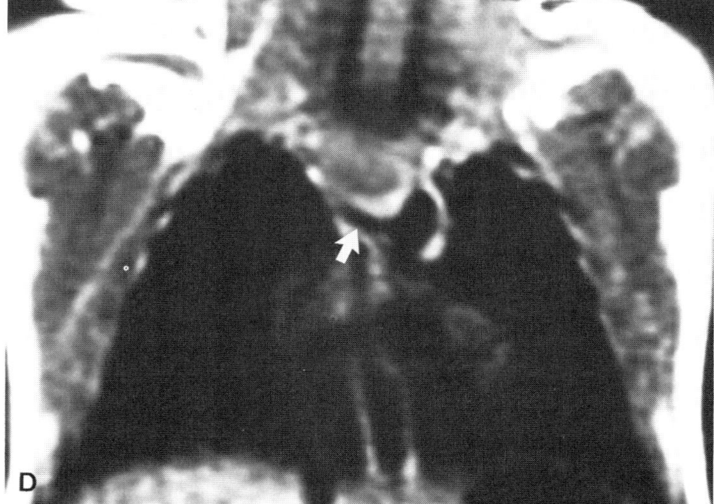

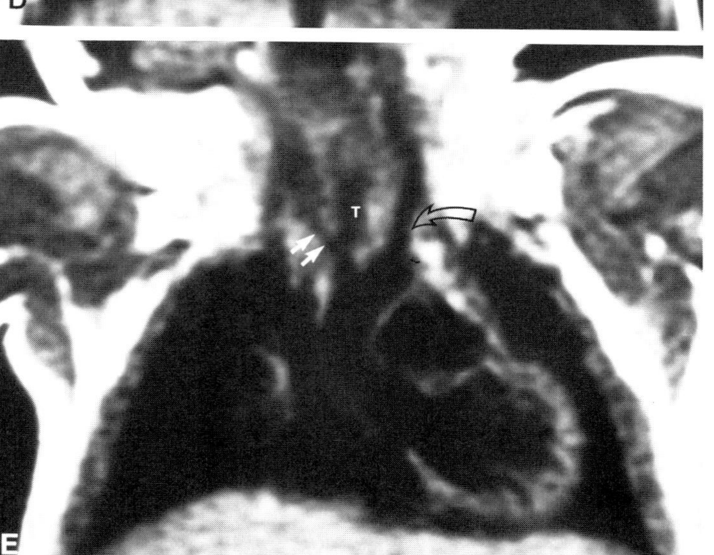

FIGURE 13 *(Cont.).* *C*, Transaxial T1-weighted MRI demonstrates the aberrant right subclavian artery (*arrowhead*) behind the trachea (T). *D*, Coronal T1-weighted MRI demonstrates the aberrant right subclavian artery (*arrow*) posterior to the trachea. *E*, Coronal T1-weighted MRI demonstrates the left common carotid artery (*curved white arrow*) and right subclavian artery (*white arrows*) anterior to the trachea (T).

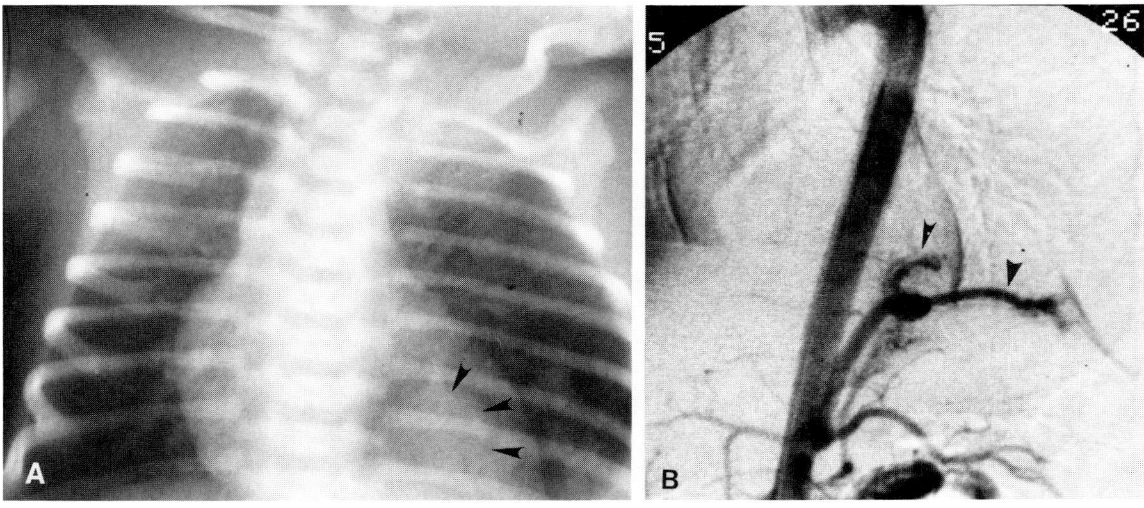

FIGURE 14. **Pulmonary sequestration.** *A,* Frontal chest radiograph demonstrates a soft-tissue mass over the left lower lobe (*arrowheads*). *B,* Digital subtraction angiography demonstrates vascular supply from the descending aorta (*arrowheads*). A combination of both intra- and extralobar sequestration was found at surgery.

of a mass at or below the hemidiaphragm. Diaphragmatic hernia is an abnormality in almost one-third of cases, and association with tension hydrothorax has been demonstrated.

Bronchiectasis

Bronchiectasis is an irreversible disorder characterized by local dilatation of the bronchial tree, usually due to infection. A reversible form may occur with acute pneumonia. Reid[7] identified three types: (1) cylindrical (the least severe form), (2) varicose, and (3) cystic or saccular (the most severe form).

The chest radiograph is usually abnormal in most cases of bronchiectasis and indicates the need for further radiologic investigation. In a small percentage of cases the chest radiograph is normal, but a high index of suspicion of underlying bronchiectasis prompts further studies. The chest radiographic findings vary with the severity of the disease. Thickening of the bronchial wall is noted as ring and tramline shadows. If mucoid impaction is also present, the dilated airways appear as round or oval opacities when they are viewed end on. The cystic changes may have a honeycomb appearance. Air-fluid levels are seen in advanced cases of cystic bronchiectasis.

Radionuclide perfusion scans with technetium 99m have been used to complement chest radiographs. A normal chest film together with a normal perfusion scan excludes the diagnosis of bronchiectasis.

CT of the chest is now the modality of choice for demonstrating bronchiectasis (Fig. 15). High-resolution CT (HRCT) has proved to be a sensitive and specific technique for establishing the diagnosis of bronchiectasis and, because it is noninvasive, has largely replaced bronchography.[5]

Significant bronchial dilatation is easily recognized on CT by comparing bronchial size with the size of an accompanying pulmonary vessel, provided the lung is aerated and the bronchi are patent. If the lung is consolidated and the bronchi are filled with fluid, the CT appearance may not be as obvious. The bronchi appear dilated with administration of contrast medium.

Cystic bronchiectasis is characterized on CT by bronchial dilatation with strings or clusters of cysts, which may be fluid-filled. In cylindric bronchiectasis, dilated thick-walled bronchi extend toward the periphery. On axial projection the combination of dilated bronchus and pulmonary arterial branch produces a signet ring appearance. Varicose bronchiectasis appears as beaded bronchial walls when the bronchi are parallel to the sectional plane.

Although now bronchography is usually replaced by CT, it is often useful for surgical

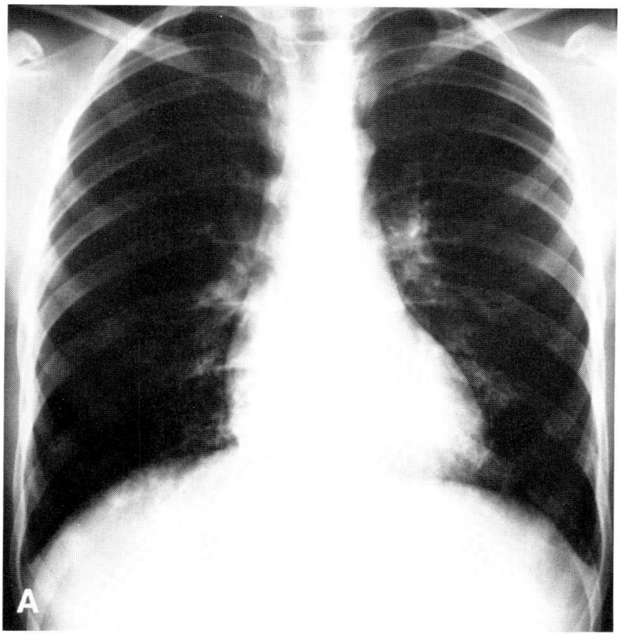

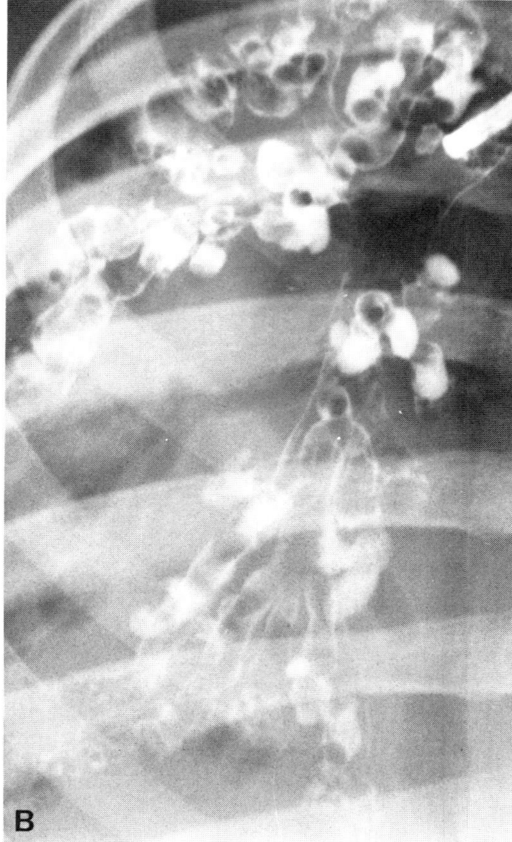

FIGURE 15. **Cystic fibrosis with bronchiectasis.** *A*, Frontal chest radiograph demonstrates bibasilar interstitial densities, thickened bronchial walls, and cystic changes. *B*, Bronchogram demonstrates multiple ectatic bronchi. *(Cont., below.)*

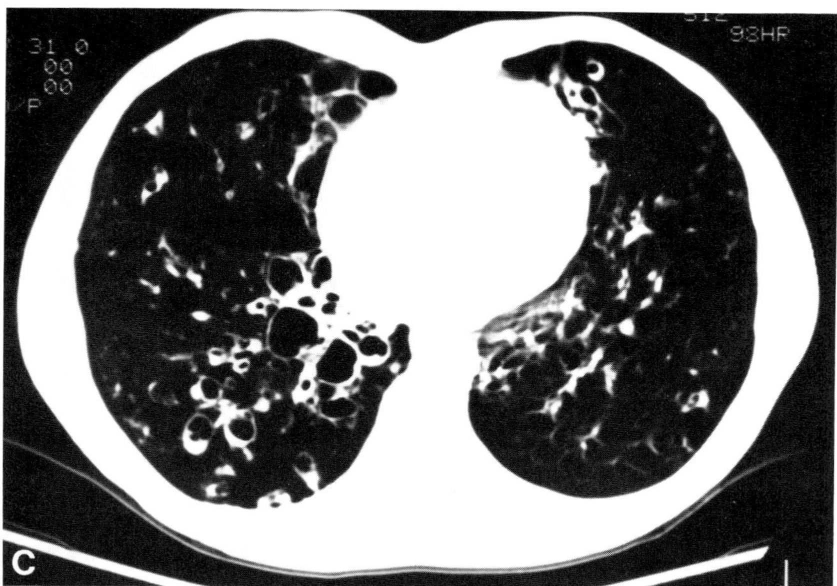

FIGURE 15 *(Cont.).* *C*, High-resolution CT demonstrates diffuse bronchiectasis. The signet ring appearance is found in cylindrical bronchiectasis.

planning. The two main contrast agents are oily dionsil (which is now less readily available) and nonionic water-soluble contrast media. The varicose and cystic (saccular) types conform to their pathologic descriptions (see Fig. 15). The cylindrical type shows tubular dilatation with a smooth outline.

SUGGESTED READING

1. Berdon WE, Baker DH: Vascular anomalies of the infant lung: Rings, slings and other things. Semin Roentgenol 7:39–64, 1972.
2. Faerber EN: The role of computed tomography in pediatric chest disease. J Thorac Imaging 1:70–77, 1986.
3. Jaffe RB: Magnetic resonance imaging of vascular rings. Sem Ultrasound CT MR 11:206–220, 1990.
4. Kuhn JP, Slovis TL, Silverman FN, Kuhns LR: Diseases of the airways and abnormalities of pulmonary aeration. In Silverman FN, Kuhn JP (eds): Caffey's Pediatric X-ray Diagnosis. St. Louis, Mosby, 1993, pp 490–492.
5. Kuhn JP: High resolution computed tomography of pediatric pulmonary parenchymal disorders. Radiol Clin North Am 31:533–551, 1993.
6. Meza MP, Benson M, Slovis TL: Imaging of mediastinal masses in children. Radiol Clin North Am 31:583–604, 1993.
7. Reid LM: Reduction in bronchial subdivision in bronchiectasis. Thorax 5:233–247, 1950.

39

ALLERGY EVALUATION: WHO, WHAT AND HOW

Robert K. Bush, M.D., and James E. Gern, M.D.

More than 50 million Americans suffer from allergic rhinitis, the single most common chronic disease of adults and children. Allergic factors frequently contribute to the pathogenesis of asthma, which affects 20–30 million Americans. Recognition of allergic factors may lead to a reduction in morbidity and mortality as well as in cost of treatment.

Allergic children typically start to become sensitized to respiratory allergens and to develop allergen-specific IgE antibodies around the age of 2 years. Children younger than 2 years may become sensitized to food allergens; however, **it is rare for food allergy to present solely with respiratory symptoms.** Skin test reactivity is progressively acquired in childhood and is common from the ages of 2–8 years, with peak prevalence between 15 and 25 years.

Studies have shown a strong correlation between skin reactivity to inhaled allergens and allergic rhinitis. Asymptomatic children with positive skin tests have a 50% risk of developing rhinitis and a 5% chance of developing asthma in the next 5 years. Thus, sensitization to inhalant allergens is highly correlated with the presence of allergic rhinitis.

THE LINK BETWEEN ASTHMA AND ALLERGY

The precise role of allergen exposure in asthma is not known, but a mounting body of evidence suggests that it is an extremely important factor, particularly in childhood. In children younger than 2 years who have not yet become sensitized to aeroallergens, viral respiratory infections are more likely to trigger episodes of wheezing. In children older than 2 years, allergy assumes an increasing importance, not only in the persistence and severity of asthma, but possibly in its development as well.

Studies have shown that children born to at least one parent with allergic rhinitis or asthma or exposed to high levels of dust mite allergens are at high risk for developing asthma. Moreover, a striking correlation has been demonstrated between serum IgE levels standardized for age and sex and the presence of asthma in all age groups. In addition, airway hyperresponsiveness, defined as sensitivity of the airways to nonspecific irritants, has been linked to serum IgE levels even in asymptomatic individuals. The likelihood of developing IgE-mediated hypersensitivity appears to have a genetic basis, but persistent exposure to allergens such as dust mite, animal dander, or fungi may be necessary for the development of asthma. Sensitivity to dust mite and cat dander in particular are risk factors for the development of asthma in children up to the age of 13 years. A recent report also has demonstrated that in some patients sensitivity to the fungus *Alternaria alternata* may be associated with particularly severe episodes of asthma, leading to respiratory arrest and death. Such individuals have skin test reactivity and elevated specific IgE antibodies to *A. alternata*. Thus, allergen exposure in sensitized asthmatic patients can trigger acute and severe episodes of asthma.

An estimated 50–85% of asthmatic patients have specific IgE antibodies to one or more inhalant allergens. The prevalence of specific IgE antibody to dust mites, cockroach, grass, pollen, ragweed pollen, and cat dander, as well as positive skin reactions to dust mite antigens, has been found to be several times more common in individuals with asthma than in healthy individuals. Furthermore, the severity of childhood asthma also correlates with the number of positive skin tests. For example, children with positive skin tests to multiple antigens are more likely to have daily rather than intermittent symptoms of asthma. In sensitized individuals, allergen exposure enhances the inflammatory changes in the airways, leading to increased asthma symptoms. Chronic, low-intensity allergen exposure typical of indoor allergens, such as house dust mites and animal danders, may lead to chronic asthma that is refractory to treatment unless the exposure is reduced or eliminated. In contrast, intense allergen exposure may precipitate sudden and severe life-threatening episodes of asthma. During seasons of high pollen counts sensitized asthmatic patients have an increased risk of developing acute episodes.

ROLE OF ALLERGY TESTING AND TREATMENT OF ACUTE DISEASES

Allergen avoidance is one of the mainstays of therapy for allergic diseases. Identification and removal of the offending allergens may improve symptoms and reduce the need for medication. In adults and children sensitive to dust mites, allergen avoidance decreases the incidence of symptoms and the need for medication. Avoidance also improves pulmonary function and reduces bronchial hyperresponsiveness.

Immunotherapy, although controversial, may be an important adjunct to the management of allergic rhinitis and possibly asthma in selected patients. Numerous studies have demonstrated a beneficial effect of immunotherapy, particularly in the treatment of seasonal allergic rhinitis. Patients with sensitivity to pollen, grasses, trees, and weeds are most likely to benefit from immunotherapy. Data supporting its use in the treatment of asthma are not as convincing. **For patients who continue to have symptoms in spite of avoidance measures and medical therapy, immunotherapy may be considered.** Several studies have shown beneficial effects of immunotherapy in children with sensitivity to house dust mites and pollen-induced asthma. Evidence for improvement after treatment with animal danders and fungi is less convincing.

Mechanisms of Allergy

A brief review of the mechanism of IgE-mediated sensitivity helps to appreciate the methods of allergy testing. The development of IgE antibody to specific antigens, termed allergens, is not completely understood. The allergens, which are usually proteins or glycoproteins, are first recognized and processed by cells such as macrophages or B-lymphocytes (antigen-presenting cells) and then presented to CD4-positive lymphocytes (T-helper cells) in the context of the major histocompatibility (MHC) class II molecules. Through generation of interleukin-4 (IL-4), these lymphocytes activate B-lymphocytes that mature into plasma cells that produce IgE antibody specific for the antigen.

Circulating specific IgE antibodies can then bind to the Fc receptor for IgE (FcEI) found on mast cells and basophils. The mast cells are abundant in the conjunctiva and gastrointestinal tract, as well as throughout the respiratory tree. This process is known as sensitization and requires exposure to the antigen on more than one occasion. Both genetics and the frequency and intensity of allergen exposure contribute to the likelihood of developing an allergic response to a particular antigen.

When the sensitized individual is reexposed, the allergen bridges the IgE molecules on the surface of the mast cell and triggers the release of histamine as well as the generation of other biochemical inflammatory mediators of the allergic reaction, such as leukotrienes and prostaglandins. These biologically active compounds induce the typical symptoms of allergic disease through their effects on sensory nerves (sneezing and itching); on the vascular system (tissue edema, which produces nasal congestion and airway narrowing); on airway smooth muscle (bronchoconstriction); and on mucous glands (increased secretion).

In addition to vasoactive compounds, the allergic reaction produces chemotactic factors that attract inflammatory cells, such as eosinophils, into the site of the reaction. Exposure to allergens in sensitized individuals may result in both immediate onset of symptoms (within minutes to 1 hour) and a late-phase response that occurs 4–6 hours after allergen exposure and generates an inflammatory reaction. The late-phase response has been linked to the symptoms of chronic disease.

Most clinically useful tests for the presence of allergen-mediated disease use methods for detecting allergen-specific IgE antibody, such as allergen skin testing or the radioallergosorbent test (RAST or RAST analogs). Other tests, such as basophil histamine release assays, are used primarily for research purposes.

DIAGNOSIS OF ALLERGIC RESPIRATORY DISEASES

As with all diseases, the diagnosis of allergic respiratory diseases is based on a carefully performed history and physical examination and is then confirmed by appropriate testing procedures.

History

The history is the fundamental part of the evaluation of the patient. Symptoms such as cough, sneezing, ocular pruritus, nasal congestion, and clear rhinorrhea occurring either chronically or in a seasonal pattern are suggestive of respiratory allergy. Children with respiratory allergies tend to have more frequent episodes of upper respiratory infections, otitis media, and sinusitis. Children with asthma frequently have a history of recurrent "pneumonia" or "bronchiolitis" before their asthma is recognized.

Certain aeroallergens are prevalent during different parts of the year and may precipitate seasonal respiratory symptoms. In the northern and eastern parts of the country, tree pollen is common in the early spring from March through May, grass pollens occur from late April into July, and ragweed is prevalent from mid-August to frost. In other geographic areas, such as California, the grass pollen season lasts for many months. Symptoms during the winter months suggest a possible sensitivity to house dust mites or animal dander. Precipitating factors such as lawn mowing may suggest sensitivity to either mold or grass pollen. Symptoms associated with farming-related activities may suggest fungal allergy.

The family history is important because allergic diseases seem to have an inherited pattern.

The environmental history for children should always include the school, day-care or caretaker's environment. Day-care attendance predisposes children to frequent upper respiratory infections that may be misconstrued as allergy. Areas of high humidity (>50% relative humidity) are good habitats for fungi and house dust mites. Carpets placed on cement floors, as in basement rooms, are prime habitats for the dust mite. Information regarding heating and air conditioning of the home are also relevant. Tobacco smoking by either parents or caretakers may cause or worsen allergic rhinitis and asthma.

Physical Examination

Conjunctival vascular dilatation, erythema, and chemosis are suggestive of allergic conjunctivitis. Some children have "allergic shiners," which are dark circles under the eyes due to venous engorgement and poor drainage of the suborbital vasculature. Examination of the tympanic membranes may reveal serous effusions of the middle ear. The nasal mucosa may have a pale or blue tinge due to edema of the tissues. Nasal polyps suggest the possibility of underlying cystic fibrosis. A transverse crease across the bridge of the nose is caused by rubbing the nose repeatedly to relieve nasal itching.

Mouth breathing suggests nasal obstruction. In patients with asthma, the anteroposterior diameter of the chest may be increased as a result of pulmonary hyperinflation. The presence of eczema is also suggestive of an allergic diathesis.

Laboratory Tests

Elevation of the blood eosinophil count is suggestive but not diagnostic of allergic disease. Elevation of the total eosinophil count may be seen in patients with allergic rhinitis and in some patients with asthma, even without evidence of an allergic component to the disease. A nasal smear for eosinophils is sometimes useful. During active allergic rhinitis, the eosinophil count may exceed 25% of the total cell count. Some patients with the nonallergic rhinitis with eosinophilia syndrome (NARES), an entity of unknown etiology, also have eosinophilia in nasal secretions.

Elevation of the total serum IgE level may be suggestive of but is not specific for allergic disease. Overlap in the total serum IgE levels among patients with asthma or allergic rhinitis and healthy individuals is considerable. Thus, in general, total serum IgE levels are of little diagnostic value. A more effective diagnostic test is the detection of specific IgE antibodies with an appropriate panel of allergen skin tests or in vitro methods.

METHODS OF ALLERGY TESTING

Two methods are used for the detection of IgE-mediated sensitivity: in vitro tests, such as the RAST or RAST analogs, and in vivo tests, such as the prick/puncture or intradermal skin test.

In vitro Testing

The RAST or RAST analogs are in vitro tests designed to detect the presence of allergen-specific IgE antibodies. The test involves the coupling or absorption of an allergenic protein onto a solid-phase support, such as microcrystalline cellulose, paper disks, sepharose beads, or nitrocellulose. Human serum is then incubated with the solid-phase antigen. The allergen-specific IgE antibodies are detected by the addition of anti-human IgE antibodies labeled with radioactive iodine or an enzyme. If radiolabeled materials are used, the amount of radioactivity bound to the solid phase is usually compared with a control serum. With the enzyme-linked assays, a colorimetric method such as spectrophotometry is used to detect the amount of IgE binding to the solid phase.

The RAST and RAST analogs are useful in patients who cannot undergo skin testing because of extensive skin disease, such as atopic dermatitis; in patients with marked dermatographism that inhibits interpretation of skin test; or in patients unable to discontinue mediation, such as antihistamine therapy, that may interfere with interpretation of the skin test.

The sensitivity of the RAST or RAST analogs is comparable to skin testing (in the range of 70–90%) if they are performed by an experienced laboratory with good quality control. Quality control may be a problem, especially with regard to the extent of binding of the antigen to the solid-phase support system. The test is also somewhat limited by the relatively small number of allergens available for testing. Other disadvantages of RAST testing include relatively high cost compared with skin testing and a turn-around time of several days.

TABLE 1. Indications and Contraindications for Allergen Skin Testing

Indications	Contraindications
Inhalant sensitivity	**Absolute**
Allergic rhinitis	Beta-adrenergic receptor blocking agent therapy
Asthma	Pregnancy
Food sensitivity	Inability to discontinue antihistamine
Atopic dermatitis	Generalized skin disease
Urticaria	**Relative**
Anaphylaxis	History of anaphylaxis
Drug reactions	Dermatographism
Penicillin sensitivity	
Local anesthetic reactions	
Stinging insect anaphylaxis	

Skin Testing

Indications

Indications for skin testing include the detection of sensitivity to inhalant allergens in the case of allergic rhinitis and asthma (Table 1). Skin testing for food antigens may be considered in cases of atopic dermatitis, urticaria, and anaphylaxis and possibly for diagnosing suspected food reactions that produce respiratory symptoms in infants. Other well-established indications for skin testing include adverse drug reactions to penicillin and local anesthetics and anaphylaxis to stinging insects.

Contraindications

Skin testing is absolutely contraindicated in patients receiving beta-blocker therapy (e.g., propranolol, metoprolol) (Table 1). A systemic reaction to skin testing in such a patient would prove fatal if resuscitative efforts with epinephrine were unsuccessful.

Pregnancy is also a contraindication to skin testing. Although the risk for anaphylaxis is small, such an event may harm the fetus. Occasionally patients may be unable to discontinue antihistamine therapy, which increases the likelihood of false-negative results. Finally, relative contraindications include generalized skin diseases, such as extensive atopic dermatitis, that make interpretation difficult; a history of allergen-induced anaphylaxis; and dermatographism.

Selection of Skin-Testing Methods (Table 2)

Skin testing can be divided into two major techniques: prick-puncture and intradermal testing. Prick skin tests are simple, rapid, relatively painless, and less expensive compared with other methods. Prick skin tests are more specific than intradermal tests because of the fewer false-positive reactions. Intradermal tests are more sensitive than the prick method because of the fewer false-negative results. Therefore, intradermal tests are preferred when maximal sensitivity is desired. Adverse reactions are more common with intradermal testing because of the larger dose of antigen administered; prick skin testing, therefore, should be done first to minimize the risk of systemic allergic reactions.

Skin testing should follow several principles:

1. The patient's symptoms and signs should be consistent with an IgE-mediated disease (e.g., allergic rhinitis, asthma).

2. Allergic extracts should be safe and reliable.

3. Extracts should be at a concentration that does not produce nonspecific irritant reactions.

4. Testing techniques should be reproducible and associated with minimal trauma.

5. Skin test responses must be interpreted in conjunction with clinical history.

6. Positive (histamine or codeine) and negative controls should be included.

Many factors affect skin test response (Table 3). **Usually, skin tests to inhalant allergens are negative in children under the age of 2 years; thus routine testing in this age group is not indicated.** The patient's specific IgE antibody titer to the particular allergen may also affect the response, although the skin test is contingent on a number of factors, including total IgE concentration, the ability of the mast cells to degranulate and release their histamine content, and the effect of chemical mediators, such as histamine, on the target tissue, namely the blood vessels in the skin. Skin testing provides a more comprehensive evaluation of the effect of the allergic reaction than simply measuring specific IgE antibodies in the sera.

The site of the skin test also may influence the results. The skin of the upper back tends to be more reactive than the skin of the forearms. The quality of the extracts currently available for allergen skin testing presents some problems. Currently there are no standardized reagents for evaluating tree pollens, fungi, or animal danders other than cat. Reasonably good quality extracts are available for ragweed, grass pollen, dust mites, and cat dander, although additional testing reagents are being standardized.

TABLE 2. Selection of Skin Test Method

1. Prick skin tests are more specific than intradermal testing (i.e., fewer false positives).
2. Intradermal tests are more sensitive than prick method (i.e., fewer false negatives).
3. Prick skin testing should precede intradermal testing to decrease risk of anaphylactic reactions.
4. Prick skin tests are simple, rapid, and inexpensive.
5. Prick skin tests usually produce little discomfort.
6. Intradermal tests may be more reproducible.

TABLE 3. Factors Affecting Skin Test Response

- Age of patient
- Specific IgE titer
- Test site—upper back more reactive than forearm
- Quality of extracts—no standardized reagents for many allergens
- Presence of dermatographism
- Use of medications
  - Antihistamines inhibit skin test response for variable periods
    - Astemizole—6 weeks
    - Hydroxyzine, terfenadine—5 days
    - Other antihistamines—1-3 days
    - Tricyclic antidepressants—5 days
  - Prolonged use of topical corticosteroids may blunt response
- Test technique
  - Prick more specific
  - Intradermal more sensitive

Use of medications also may affect the skin test results. Antihistamines may suppress skin test responses for variable periods. Certain antihistamines, such as astemizole, may inhibit the skin test for up to 6 weeks. Hydroxyzine and terfenadine may suppress skin test reactivity for 5 days, and other antihistamines may have effects lasting from 1–3 days. Tricyclic antidepressants, although not commonly used in the treatment of children, may affect the skin test response for up to 5 days. Prolonged use of topical corticosteroids also may have suppressing effects.

CONSIDERATION OF SPECIFIC ALLERGENS FOR TESTING

In selecting allergens for testing, either by in vivo or in vitro methods, several factors should be considered. The first consideration is the likelihood that identification of allergens will improve the quality of the patient's care, either by avoidance measures or by immunotherapy. Second, skin testing or in vitro testing also may be used as a predictor for when the patient's symptoms may worsen so that medical therapy can be escalated at appropriate times. Third, the specific allergens used in the testing depend on the nature of the allergens found in the area where the patient resides. Pollens from trees, grasses, and weeds vary in different portions of the United States. Thus a knowledge of the botany of the area in which the patient lives is useful in determining which materials to select for testing and possibly for treatment with immunotherapy. Finally, the availability of suitable extracts for testing should be considered. Currently in the United States, only a limited number of allergens have been standardized for allergenic composition and concentration.

House Dust Mites

Because sensitivity to house dust mites is a major cause of allergic respiratory disease, testing for this allergen is extremely important. The two major species of house dust mites that are available in the United States are *Dermatophagoides pteronyssinus* and *D. farinae*. Standardized materials for these extracts are available for testing.

Clinical data clearly indicate that control measures to diminish environmental exposure to house dust mites decrease symptoms and the need for medication in sensitized patients (see chapter 13). Furthermore, placebo-controlled, double-blind immunotherapy trials have shown a decrease in rhinitis and asthma symptoms in children with sensitivity to house dust mites. Thus, dust mite testing should be performed in any patient suspected of allergic respiratory disease.

Animal Danders

Cat Dander

Large numbers of children are exposed to domestic cats. Sensitivity to cat dander has been linked to the development of asthma in children. Because avoidance of exposure is a major form of therapy, testing for cat dander sensitivity is very important.

The major allergen responsible for cat dander sensitivity is the protein *Fel d I*. Currently available extracts in the United States are standardized for concentration of *Fel d I*. A small percentage of patients with cat dander sensitivity develop IgE antibody to cat serum albumin. Two principal forms of cat dander allergy extracts are available: an epithelial-derived preparation that contains mainly *Fel d I* and cat pelt extracts that contain larger quantities of albumin. Both preparations contain adequate amounts of *Fel d I* to detect most sensitive individuals.

Immunotherapy trials with cat dander extracts have shown some benefit in selected individuals, although the preferred method of treatment is avoidance of exposure.

Dog Dander

Sensitivity to dogs is less common than sensitivity to cats. A link between sensitivity to dog dander and asthma has not yet been demonstrated. The major allergens responsible for dog allergy are less well characterized than cat antigens, although the protein *Can f I* has now been identified as an important allergen. Currently available extracts in the United States are not standardized for allergenic composition or concentration; therefore, they are subject to variability.

No studies show significant improvement of patients treated with immunotherapy for sensitivity to dog dander. Therefore, avoidance of exposure to the animal is the best treatment.

Other Animal Danders

Other domestic pets, such as rabbits, hamsters, and gerbils, also may cause allergic symptoms in children. Extracts available for testing are not standardized. Avoidance of exposure appears to be the best treatment at the present time, because no data are available to support the use of immunotherapy.

Pollens

Grass

Grass pollens are among the most common causes of allergy worldwide, affecting an estimated 10–30% of allergic patients. Numerous species have been implicated in allergic disease, including June or Kentucky bluegrass, rye, timothy, red top, and sweet vernal grass, among others. In certain portions of the United States, particularly in the South and Southwest, other species of grasses, such as Bermuda and Johnson grass, may be important. The allergenic components of most species of grass pollen have extensive cross-reactivity. However, Johnson and Bermuda grass, which cross-react with other species, also possess unique allegenic components. In general, mixtures of grass pollen extracts will identify patients with sensitivity to grass pollen. Testing for individual grass pollens is seldom needed because of the high degree of cross-reactivity.

Avoidance measures for grass pollen are not entirely successful because they are wind-borne and travel large distances. Closing windows and running an air conditioner may be beneficial during the grass pollen season. In the Pacific Northwest and along the western U.S. coast the grass pollen season lasts for several months, whereas in the Midwest and Northeast the season lasts for about 2 months.

Double-blind, placebo-controlled trials of immunotherapy with grass pollen extracts have shown beneficial effects. Although not currently standardized, most grass pollen extracts are potent materials that detect the presence of allergen-specific IgE antibodies in most sensitive individuals.

Trees

Tree species responsible for allergic disease vary according to geographic location. The most important tree pollens in North America are from deciduous trees, including birch, beech, oak, maple, elm, willow, poplar, aspen, olive, and ash trees. The mountain cedar, a coniferous tree, found in abundance in Texas and parts of the southwestern United States, also accounts for seasonal allergic rhinitis and asthma. Tree pollen seasons typically occur in the early spring and usually are of relatively brief duration (4–6 weeks).

Extracts of standardized allergens for tree pollens are not available in the United States. Thus selection of appropriate testing materials depends on the experience of the physician.

Avoidance of exposure is predicated on keeping the pollen outdoors by closing the house and using air conditioning.

Immunotherapy trials have demonstrated some benefit in a few patients with rhinitis and asthma induced by mountain cedar, and other studies from Europe indicate that rhinitis and asthma due to birch pollen are amenable to immunotherapy.

Weeds

The major weed pollen in the United States is ragweed. The two major forms are short ragweed (*Ambrosia artemisiaefolia*) and giant ragweed (*A. trifida*), although other species are found in different locales throughout the United States. Other weeds that cause difficulty include the amaranths and chenopods. The cross-reactivity of weed pollens appears to be extensive, although some possess unique allergens.

Avoidance techniques again include keeping the pollens outdoors during the season and using air conditioning. The use of air cleaners apparently has little benefit in the treatment of allergic rhinitis and asthma. Immunotherapy trials conducted with ragweed extracts demonstrate clinical improvement in the majority of treated patients. Standardized extracts of ragweed have been available for a number of years; other weed pollens, however, have not been standardized.

Fungi

An extensive number of fungi are allergenic. Unfortunately, the complexity of these allergens has prevented the availability of standardized extracts. Most of the extracts are of poor quality; except in a few instances, their use as either testing or treatment reagents is somewhat questionable. The most important species appear to belong to the families *Cladosporium, Alternaria, Aspergillus,* and *Penicillium.* Many other fungi, including species of *Basidiomycetes,* may be important in certain locations. Unfortunately, no extracts for testing *Basidiomycetes* are commercially available.

Immunotherapy trials with *Cladosporium* and *Alternaria* have shown some benefit. These fungi are found primarily in outdoor environments, where they live on decayed plant vegetation. *Aspergillus* and *Penicillium,* on the other hand, are classified as indoor allergens. They grow best in moist areas, such as bathroom tiles and window sills. Therefore, reduction in indoor humidity, treatment of infected areas with dilute solutions of chlorine bleach, and removal of contaminated materials such as carpeting or wood may be useful in reducing the exposure levels.

Insects

A growing body of evidence suggests that in economically deprived populations, especially in inner-city areas, cockroach allergen may be an important precipitant of asthma. Positive skin test responses and specific IgE antibodies to whole body extracts of cockroaches have been found in several studies of asthmatic children.

No standardized extracts of cockroach allergens are available, but the allergenic components derived from these insects are under investigation.

The limited data from immunotherapy trials preclude a definitive statement regarding the efficacy of this treatment. Measures to control cockroach populations in the home are somewhat difficult but may be useful in decreasing symptoms in sensitized individuals.

Foods

Food allergy is seldom the cause of isolated respiratory symptoms, but the possibility may be considered in young infants who seem to have respiratory difficulties after ingestion of milk or other foods. Because many food extracts are nonstandardized, their potency and quality are questionable. In some instances, a prick skin test after direct application to the skin of fresh foods, such as fruit or vegetable, may be useful. Once the allergen is identified, avoidance is the appropriate course of action, because immunotherapy has not been demonstrated to be efficacious and may be extremely hazardous.

TABLE 4. Approaches and Precautions for Skin Testing

Approaches
- Select high quality extracts of appropriate concentrations.
- Include positive and negative controls.
- Perform tests on normal skin; evaluate for dermatographism.
- Record results at proper time (10–15 min).

Precautions
- Skin tests should never be performed unless a physician is immediately available to treat untoward reactions.
- Emergency equipment and medications should be available.
- Do not conduct testing if patient is experiencing marked symptoms.
- Be aware of patient's current medications, i.e., beta-blockers (increase risk of fatal anaphylaxis), antihistamines (blunt skin test response).

RISKS OF SKIN TESTS

In general the risks of skin tests are minimal. However, fatal cases of anaphylaxis have occurred in some individuals undergoing skin testing to inhalant allergens. Local infections are extremely rare.

Because of the risk of serious systemic reactions to skin tests, certain approaches and precautions need to be considered (Table 4). **Skin tests should never be performed unless a physician is immediately available to treat untoward reactions**; emergency equipment and medications should be readily at hand. The patient experiencing marked symptoms should not be tested.

PRICK SKIN TEST PROCEDURE

Various devices have been used to perform prick skin testing (Table 5). The most commonly

TABLE 5. Prick Skin Test Procedure

Devices
25–27 gauge needles, blood lancets, multitest devices, bifurcated needles
Extracts
1:10 to 1:20 W/V in 50% glycerine
Control
Histamine base 1 mg/ml diluent
Number of Tests
For inhalants—up to 70
For foods—up to 50

W/V = weight per volume.

TABLE 6. Intradermal Skin Test Technique

Devices
Unitized 0.5 ml hubless syringes with 26–30 gauge needles, disposable after one-time use
Extracts
Stabilized with 0.3% human serum albumin at 1:100–1:1000 W/V (1000 protein nitrogen units)
Volume injected
0.01–0.05 ml
Controls
Histamine base at 0.1 mg/ml or codeine phosphate
Diluent
Number of Tests
For inhalants—up to 30 tests
Not appropriate for food allergens

W/V = weight per volume.

used methods employ bifurcated needles, blood lancets, commercially available multitest devices, and hollow 25-27 gauge needles. Needles cannot be used repetitively, because the antigens will be contaminated if used for more than one test. If solid tip needles are used, they should either be used only once or thoroughly wiped between each prick test. The extracts used in prick skin testing are usually 1:10 to 1:20 weight per volume extracts in 50% glycerine. Control solutions include histamine base at a concentration of 1 mg/ml and the diluent used to prepare the extract. The number of skin tests applied usually should not exceed 50-70 pricks for inhalant allergens. Due to the higher frequency of false-positive tests, skin tests with food extracts should be limited to those implicated by history or food diary.

INTRADERMAL SKIN TESTING

The devices used for intradermal skin testing are unitized, 0.5-ml hubless, disposable syringes with 26-30 gauge needles (Table 6). Needles should be discarded after use because of possible contamination by infectious agents. Extracts used in intradermal skin testing are usually stabilized with 0.3% human serum albumin at concentrations ranging from 1:100-1:1000 weight per volume (1,000 protein nitrogen units [PNU]). The volume injected is usually 0.1-0.05 ml. Positive controls include histamine base at 0.1 mg/ml or codeine phosphate; the human serum albumin diluent is used as a negative control. The appropriate number of tests for inhalant allergens should not exceed 25-30. Intradermal testing is not appropriate for food allergens because of the large percentage of false-positive test results.

INTERPRETATION

Various methods have been used to interpret skin test results (Table 7). Most methods

TABLE 7. Interpretation of Skin Test Results

Prick		Intradermal		
Grade	Wheal	Grade	Wheal	Erythema (mm)
0	≤ Negative control	0	< 5 mm	< 5
1	1 mm > control	±	5–10 mm	5–10
2	2–4 mm > control	1	5–10 mm	11–20
3	5 mm > control	2	5–10 mm	21–30
4	Wheal with pseudopods	3	5–10 mm or with pseudopods	31–40
		4	> 15 mm or with many pseudopods	> 40

TABLE 8. Common Errors in Skin Testing

1. Tests are placed too closely together.
2. Amount of pressure applied for puncture tests is not uniform.
3. Too much allergen extract is applied.
4. Too many sites are done at one time.
5. Highly sensitive patients are not checked frequently for possible systemic reactions.
6. Poor quality reagents are used.
7. Inappropriate allergens are used for testing (e.g., tobacco smoke extracts, facial tissue extracts)

compare the response with the positive histamine control. In the prick method wheals that are bigger than the control response by 2 mm or more are clinically significant. With intradermal testing a wheal size from 5-10 mm with a flare of 21 mm or greater is usually considered clinically significant.

COMMON ERRORS IN SKIN TESTING

Common errors in skin testing include placing the tests too closely together; applying too much allergenic extract, which may create large reactions that spill over to the adjacent test site; and testing too many sites done at one time (Table 8). In addition, if pressure applied for puncture tests is not uniform, variations may result. Occasionally poor quality reagents are used as well as inappropriate allergens, such as tobacco smoke extracts or facial tissue extracts. Highly sensitive patients who are not closely monitored for possible systemic reactions may be potential victims of fatal complications.

SUGGESTED READING

1. Bernstein IL: Proceedings of the task force on guidelines for standardizing old and new technologies used for the diagnosis and treatment of allergic diseases. J Allergy Clin Immunol 82:487-526, 1988.
2. Burrows B, Martinez FD, Halonen M, et al: Association of asthma with serum IgE levels and skin test reactivity to allergens. N Engl J Med 320:271-277, 1989.
3. Bush RK, Huftel MA, Busse WW: Patient selection. In Lockey RF, Bukantz SC (eds): Allergen Immunotherapy. New York, Marcel Dekker, 1991, pp 25-49.
4. Bush RK: The role of allergens in asthma. Chest 101:378S-380S, 1992.
5. Bush RK, Ritter MW: Allergen immunotherapy for the patient with allergic rhinitis. Immunol Allergy Clin North Am 12:107-124, 1992.
6. Council on Scientific Affairs: In vivo diagnostic testing and immunotherapy for allergy. Report 1, Part I. JAMA 258:1363-1367, 1987; Report 1, Part II. JAMA 258:1505-1508, 1987.
7. Duff AL, Platts-Mills TAE: Allergens and asthma. Pediatr Clin North Am 39:1277-1291, 1992.
8. Morgan WJ, Martinez FD: Risk factors for developing wheezing and asthma in childhood. Pediatr Clin North Am 39:1185-1203, 1992.
9. Nelson HS: Diagnostic procedures in allergy: Allergy skin testing. Ann Allergy 51:411-418, 1983.
10. Position Paper: Allergy testing. Ann Intern Med 110:317-320, 1989.
11. Sears MR, Burrows B, Flannery EM, et al: Relationship between airway responsiveness and serum IgE in children with asthma and in apparently normal children. N Engl J Med 325: 1067-1071, 1991.
12. Settipane RJ, Hagy GW, Settipane GA: Long-term risk factors for developing asthma and allergic rhinitis: A 23-year follow-up study of college students. Allergy Proc 15:21-25, 1994.
13. Smith TF: Allergy testing in clinical practice. Ann Allergy 68:293-301, 1992.
14. Sporik R, Holgate ST, Platts-Mills TAE, Cogswell JJ: Exposure to house-dust mite allergen (*Der pI*) and the development of asthma in childhood. N Engl J Med 323:502-507, 1990.
15. VanArsdel PP Jr, Larson EB: Diagnostic tests for patients with suspected allergic disease. Ann Intern Med 110:304-312, 1989.

40

RAPID LABORATORY DIAGNOSIS OF VIRAL AND BACTERIAL RESPIRATORY INFECTIONS

Adamadia Deforest, Ph.D., and Joel E. Mortensen, Ph.D.

More than 200 different viruses have been shown to infect the human respiratory tract. Viral infections account for more illnesses in the respiratory tract than in any other organ system. **Viruses are responsible for approximately 75% of all cases of acute respiratory illness and over 50% of physician office visits each year.** Although they vary in size, symmetry, nucleic acid type, lability, and method of replication, each virus can cause a spectrum of clinical syndromes, ranging from a minor upper respiratory infection (the common cold) to pharyngitis, laryngitis, laryngotracheobronchitis (croup), severe bronchiolitis, and pneumonia.

Each of the above clinical syndromes can be caused by several different viral agents; therefore, identification of the specific virus causing illness in an individual patient is seldom possible on clinical grounds alone.

Viruses have a typical seasonal distribution. For example, the incidence of influenza virus infection peaks each year in the United States from mid to late December. Infection with parainfluenza virus type 3 (P3) occurs throughout the year but peaks in the winter months. Parainfluenza virus types 1 and 2 (P1 and P2) appear most frequently in the fall months; usually one of the two serotypes predominates each year. Respiratory syncytial virus (RSV) appears every winter in epidemics, starting in December, peaking in January and February, and tapering off in March.

Fortunately, of the 200 viruses capable of infecting the human respiratory tract, only seven (the adenoviruses, influenza A and B, P1, P2, P3, and RSV) are responsible for most of the severe diseases seen in infants and young children. Early identification of a respiratory virus in the course of an infection is essential for the prompt institution of available antiviral therapy (such as ribavirin for RSV). Early identification also helps to avoid unnecessary antimicrobial therapy and reduces medical costs by avoiding unnecessary tests and reducing the length of hospitalization. Precise viral diagnoses also alert the community at large to the presence of influenza viruses and the need for immunization and prophylaxis, especially in high-risk populations.

A number of bacterial agents are also important pathogens of the respiratory tract and are discussed below. One of the most important causes of acute infection of the upper respiratory tract is group A, beta-hemolytic *Streptococcus pyogenes.* Statistically, it is the most common cause of acute bacterial pharyngitis. Prompt and precise detection of this organism is important because of the risk of rheumatic fever and its complications after infection.

COLLECTION OF CLINICAL SPECIMENS

The single most important factor in obtaining a precise laboratory diagnosis is the collection

and transport of an adequate specimen to the laboratory in a timely manner.

Because viruses are cell-associated, specimens containing large numbers of ciliated epithelial cells are essential for optimal recovery of the virus and detection of the antigen. **The preferred specimen for the identification of respiratory viruses in infants and children is a nasopharyngeal aspirate or nasopharyngeal washing (NPW).** Detailed instructions for obtaining such specimens are given in Figure 1. Alternatively, a nasopharyngeal swab or a throat swab may be collected. A throat swab, which is appropriate if pharyngitis is present, is adequate for recovering enteroviruses, adenoviruses, and herpes simplex virus. Throat washings are useful for the diagnosis of influenza infections, but difficult to collect from infants and young children. Other specimens that are appropriate in special clinical circumstances include tracheal and bronchial aspirates or washings and lung biopsy or autopsy materials. It is important that specimens collected by swab be submerged into a sterile tube containing viral transport medium (VTM) immediately after collection. Specimens should be kept cold in a refrigerator or on wet ice at 4°C and transported to the laboratory as quickly as possible. **Specimens should not be frozen.** Several respiratory viruses lose infectivity on repeated cycles of freezing and thawing.

The timing of specimen collection is critical. Most viruses are shed in respiratory secretions for only 3–7 days after the onset of clinical symptoms; thus specimens must be collected **as early as possible in the course of the illness.**

Nasal Wash: Syringe Method

Materials: Saline
3-5 ml syringe*
2" 18-20 gauge tubing*
Viral Transport Medium (VTM)
Specimen container

1. Fill syringe with saline; attach tubing to syringe tip.
2. Quickly instill saline into nostril.
3a. Aspirate the recoverable nasal specimen. Recovery must occur immediately, as the instilled fluid will rapidly drain.
3b. (alternate) In appropriate cases, patients may tilt head forward to allow specimen to drain into suitable sterile container.
4. (if aspirated) Inject aspirated specimen from syringe into suitable dry, sterile specimen container or one containing VTM, according to virology laboratory requirements.

A

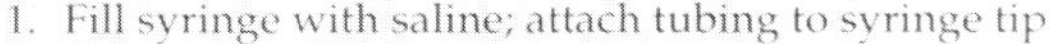
*Length and diameter of syringe, tube or bulb as appropriate for infant, child or adult

Nasal Wash: Bulb Method

Materials: Saline
1-2 oz. tapered rubber bulb*
Viral Transport Medium (VTM)
Specimen container

1. Suction 3-5 ml saline into a new sterile bulb.
2. Insert bulb into one nostril until nostril is occluded.
3. Instill saline into nostril with one squeeze of the bulb and immediately release bulb to collect recoverable nasal specimen.
4. Empty bulb into suitable dry, sterile specimen container or one containing VTM, according to virology laboratory requirements.

B

FIGURE 1. For all four procedures illustrated below, patient's head should be inclined 70 degrees backward from the vertical for proper specimen recovery. *A,* Nasal wash: syringe method. *B,* Nasal wash: bulb method. *(Continued on facing page.)*

Vacuum-assisted Nasal Aspirate Method

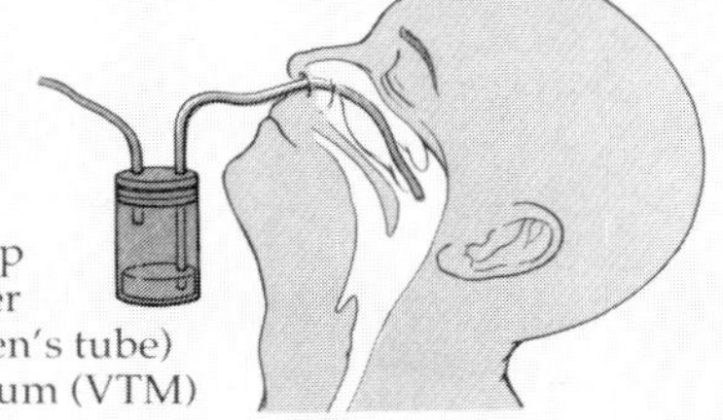

Materials: Portable suction pump
Sterile suction catheter
Mucus trap (i.e., Luken's tube)
Viral Transport Medium (VTM)

1. Attach mucus trap to suction pump and catheter, leaving wrapper on suction catheter; turn on suction and adjust to suggested pressure.
2. Without applying suction, insert catheter into the nose, directed posteriorly and toward the opening of the external ear. **NOTE**: depth of insertion necessary to reach posterior pharynx is equivalent to distance between anterior naris and external opening of the ear.
3. Apply suction. Using a rotating movement, slowly withdraw catheter. **NOTE**: catheter should remain in nasopharynx no longer than 10 seconds.
4. Hold trap upright to prevent secretions from going into pump.
5. Rinse catheter (if necessary) with approximately 2.0 ml VTM; disconnect suction; connect tubing to arm of mucus trap to seal.

Patient Age	Catheter Size (French)**	Suction Pressure
Premature infant	6	80-100 mmHg
Infant	8	80-100 mmHg
Toddler/Preschooler	10	100-120 mmHg
School Age	12	100-120 mmHg
Adolescent/Adult	14	120-150 mmHg

**To determine length of catheter tubing, measure distance from tip of nose to external opening of ear.

C

Nasopharyngeal Swab Method

Materials: Mini-Tip **Culturette**® Brand Collection and Transport System *or*
Nasopharyngeal swab with synthetic fiber tip
1-2 ml Viral Transport Medium (VTM)
Specimen container

1. Insert swab into one nostril.
2. Press swab tip on the mucosal surface of the mid-inferior portion of the inferior turbinate (see sketch), and rub the swab tip several times across the mucosal surface to loosen and collect cellular material.
3. Withdraw swab; insert into **Culturette**® or container with VTM.

D

FIGURE 1 *(Cont.).* *C,* Vacuum-assisted nasal aspirate method. *D,* Nasopharyngeal swab method. (From Becton Dickinson Microbiology Systems, Cockeysville, MD, with permission.).

The sensitivity of culture for *S. pyogenes* depends on collection of an adequate throat swab. **The swab should be vigorous and must include the posterior pharynx and each tonsillar area.** Swabs should be placed into a transport medium and transported to the laboratory within a few hours of collection.

Specimens aspirated from closed spaces such as sinuses and the middle ear should be quickly placed into a transport system that protects anaerobic bacteria from the deleterious effects of oxygen. These specimens should be transported to the laboratory and inoculated on appropriate media as quickly as possible. Other specimens appropriate for specific bacterial pathogens are discussed below.

IDENTIFICATION OF VIRAL PATHOGENS

Serologic Diagnosis

The serologic approach to viral diagnosis is rarely used today. The major drawback to this diagnostic approach is the requirement for (1) an acute specimen collected early in the course of the disease and (2) a convalescent specimen collected 2–3 weeks later. Furthermore, in young infants, passively acquired maternal antibody may complicate the interpretation of serologic data. Serologic diagnosis is not clinically useful in the management of viruses with short incubation periods, including most respiratory viruses.

Serologic diagnosis is the method of choice, however, for the diagnosis of infection with Epstein-Barr virus (EBV). A specific diagnosis can be made with one serum specimen, collected as early as possible in the acute stage of infection. Presence of IgM antibody to the viral capsid antigen (VCA) and absence of IgG antibody to the Epstein-Barr nuclear antigen (EBNA) are indicative of a current or very recent infection. Presence of IgG antibodies to both VCA and EBNA indicates past infection with this virus.

Cytopathology

Cytopathology, the oldest method used for rapid viral diagnosis, depends on the formation of inclusion bodies in the infected host cell during viral replication. The best examples of this technique are the demonstration of herpes simplex inclusions in cells collected from the base of a skin vesicle (Tzanck preparation) and of cytomegalovirus (CMV) inclusions in lung biopsy or autopsy materials. Cytopathology is not generally useful for the major respiratory viruses.

Electron Microscopy

Electron microscopy has been widely used in Canada, England, and Australia for the rapid diagnosis of many viral infections. The technique also has played an important role in the recognition of several important human pathogens that grow poorly or not at all in conventional cell-culture systems (e.g., hepatitis viruses, rotaviruses, coronaviruses). **A major limitation of electron microscopy is the absolute requirement that virus be present in the clinical specimen in high titer. Electron microscopy is rarely used today to diagnose respiratory infections; it has been replaced by newer, less costly, more rapid, and more sensitive techniques described below.**

Isolation of Viruses in Cell Culture

The traditional method for the laboratory diagnosis of viral infections is isolation and identification of the pathogen after inoculation of the clinical specimen into various cell cultures, such as primary monkey kidney cells and human fetal lung fibroblasts. The inoculated cultures are observed daily under low-power magnification for evidence of cytopathic effect (CPE) or the ability of the infected cells to adsorb erythrocytes (hemadsorption). The time required to detect CPE varies as follows: herpes simplex, 1–7 days; RSV, 2–14 days; parainfluenza, 5–7 days; adenovirus, 7–21 days; CMV, 10–42 days. The time required to detect hemadsorption with influenza and parainfluenza virus infections is 5–9 days.

Cell culture has been replaced in recent years with more rapid assays that produce results within 90 minutes to 2 days after receipt of the clinical specimen. These newer, more rapid methods have greatly expanded the ability to diagnose respiratory infections. **Virus isolation in cell culture, however, remains the "gold standard" by which newly developed assays are evaluated.**

Culture Amplification

In an effort to shorten the time for detection of viruses in conventional cell-culture systems, two new approaches have evolved in recent years. **The first approach is to stain the cell cultures with fluorescein-tagged monoclonal antibodies** 24–48 hours after the inoculation of the clinical specimen, well before the appearance of a positive cytopathic effect or hemadsorption reaction. This technique has proved

especially useful for influenza and parainfluenza viruses.

The second approach is called spin amplification culture or shell vial culture. The clinical specimen is centrifuged onto monkey kidney cells or human lung fibroblasts growing on a coverslip in a small glass vial, called a shell vial, to increase the efficacy of the infection. The culture is then incubated for a short period of time, usually 16–72 hours, and stained for the presence of respiratory viruses using the fluorescein-tagged monoclonal antisera. This technique was originally developed to shorten the time required to detect CMV and has improved the average time for detection of CMV from 21 days with conventional tube culture to 16–30 hours with the spin-amplified technique. **Shell vial culture has recently been shown to be useful for influenza, parainfluenza, and RSV, but not adenovirus infections.**

Immunofluorescence

Immunofluorescence assays use highly sensitive and specific monoclonal antibodies coupled to a fluorescent dye. Direct (DFA) and indirect (IFA) immunofluorescent assays have greatly expanded the ability to detect the presence of viral antigens, both in inoculated cell cultures and directly in exfoliated ciliated epithelial cells from clinical specimens. **Results of immunofluorescent staining may be available within 2 hours of receipt of the specimen,** although many laboratories "batch" specimens for economic reasons.

A pooled monoclonal antibody reagent is commercially available and provides efficient simultaneous detection of influenza A and B, P1, P2, P3, all serotypes of adenovirus, and RSV. If a specimen stains positive with the pooled reagent, individual monoclonal reagents are used to identify the specific virus in the sample.

Immunofluorescent staining of nasal secretions is the most common technique currently in use for the detection of RSV infection. Immunofluorescence is very accurate compared with conventional culture; both sensitivity and specificity are high. Direct immunofluorescent staining for the detection of influenza viruses is also quite sensitive and specific, but not in 100% of cases. Direct detection of parainfluenza viruses in nasal secretions has yielded variable results, depending on the antisera used and the type of parainfluenza virus studied. Direct diagnosis of adenovirus in nasal secretions has very low sensitivity compared with culture.

Enzyme Immunoassay

The second type of rapid test commonly used in clinical virology laboratories is enzyme immunoassay (EIA), sometimes referred to as enzyme-linked immunosorbent assay (ELISA). The method uses multiple antigen–antibody reactions to detect low concentrations of viral antigen in clinical materials. The antibody used for the antigen detection is tagged with an enzyme (as contrasted with a fluorescein dye in the FA assay). The quantity of antigen in the clinical specimen is measured either visually or with a spectrophotometer after incubation with a substrate that changes from clear to colored in the presence of the bound detector antibody. The amount of color produced is directly proportional to the amount of microbial antigen present in the clinical specimen.

A variation of EIA, called membrane EIA, consists of the capture of viral antigen to the membrane surface of a test device as the clinical specimen filters through the membrane. Membrane EIA assays form the basis for many pregnancy tests licensed for home use. Membrane EIA kits have become available in the past several years for the rapid detection of RSV and influenza A virus. These assays require neither special laboratory equipment nor skilled technical personnel. Although the reagent cost per patient specimen is rather high, the results are available in 15–30 minutes, making the assays cost-effective in terms of management decisions. The above two assays are highly sensitive and specific for the rapid diagnosis of RSV and influenza A virus.

Latex Agglutination Assay

In latex agglutination assays, antiviral antibody is bound to latex particles. The clinical specimen is then mixed with the antibody-sensitized latex particles on a glass or cardboard slide. If viral antigen is present in the patient material, clumping of the latex particles occurs. The test requires only 15 minutes to perform, requires neither special equipment nor highly skilled laboratory personnel, and is inexpensive. Unfortunately, latex agglutination assays are much less sensitive than FA or EIA. There are currently no approved kits for the diagnosis of respiratory viruses.

Detection of Nucleic Acid

All living organisms, including viruses and bacteria, possess unique nucleotide sequences in their genome. Once the unique sequence of a given organism has been identified, it can be amplified and labeled (with a radioactive or chemiluminescent tag) and used as a probe to identify homologous sequences in clinical materials. At the present time, hybridization assays are available commercially for certain types of human papillomavirus and for *Chlamydia trachomatis* (see below). Probes for confirmation of herpes simplex, CMV, and *Mycobacterium tuberculosis* culture are also commercially available.

Polymerase Chain Reaction

Polymerase chain reaction (PCR) and gene amplification refer to the highly sensitive technique by which minute quantities of specific DNA or RNA sequences can be enzymatically amplified to the extent that a sufficient quantity of material is available to reach a threshold signal for detection. The technique thus can be used to detect trace amounts of nucleic acid material in clinical specimens in which microorganisms are believed to play a causative role. **The fundamental basis of this new technology, as in the nucleic acid probe described above, is that each infectious disease agent possesses a unique nucleotide sequence ("fingerprint") in its DNA or RNA composition, by which it can be identified.** PCR is the method by which repeated cycles of oligonucleotide-directed DNA synthesis of target sequences are carried out in vitro. **The end result is amplification of the viral nucleic acid present in the original clinical specimen from a few copies to as many as one million copies in less than 2 hours.** PCR promises specificity equal to and sensitivity greater than those of conventional culture for the detection of many microorganisms.

The potential for PCR as a diagnostic tool in virology is enormous. However, serious procedural obstacles remain. Because the technique is so sensitive, cross-contamination between clinical specimens may occur and not be recognized by the laboratory worker. Many investigators recommend a special room dedicated solely to PCR and separated geographically from the general clinical laboratory where specimens are processed.

These and other obstacles, such as licensing requirements, must be overcome before PCR can be used on a routine basis in the clinical virology or microbiology laboratory. At the present time, the only commercial PCR kit approved for diagnostic use is the AMPLICOR PCR kit for *C. trachomatis* developed by Roche Diagnostic Systems (see p. 279). PCR assays for many other viruses are being developed in research laboratories, and a few are currently under review by the Food and Drug Administration for diagnostic use.

IDENTIFICATION OF BACTERIAL AND OTHER RESPIRATORY PATHOGENS

Gram Stain

The Gram stain may be the best indication of the numbers and types of bacteria and somatic cells present in a clinical specimen. It can also be very useful in the preliminary identification of an organism, although caution needs to be exercised. A Gram stain is also the least expensive and most rapid test available for diagnosing bacterial infections. Its use has three major limitations: (1) it cannot detect certain organisms (viruses and chlamydia); (2) it is not useful for some specimens from sites at which extensive normal flora may resemble pathogens; and (3) **reading gram-stained smears correctly requires extensive experience.**

Group A Streptococci

In patients suspected of having infection with group A streptococci, the specimen of choice is a throat swab. A throat culture will differentiate bacterial from viral pharyngitis. If beta-hemolytic colonies are present on the initial sheep blood agar plate, restreaking a representative colony onto a second blood agar plate and determining whether growth is inhibited by an A disk (or Bacitracin disk) will accurately distinguish group A streptococci from other hemolytic streptococci. Less than 5% of group A streptococci do not exhibit a zone of inhibition, and probably no more than 1-2% of non-group A streptococci are inhibited.

The finding of low numbers of streptococci usually means that a patient is carrying group A streptococci in the oropharynx. Such individuals usually do not develop increases in streptococcal antibody titers indicative of streptococcal disease.

Direct detection of *S. pyogenes* from pharyngeal swabs is probably the most common bacteriologic test in use today. Latex agglutination and enzyme immunoassay test kits, available from many manufacturers, are used in hospital laboratories as well as clinic and private office settings.

The latex tests are not accurate and have been essentially replaced by EIA. Multiple variations on the basic EIA format exist. For example, antibody to group A streptococci may be attached to a membrane filter. The antigen is extracted from the swab with acid or an enzyme, the solution is filtered, and a detection reagent is added. If antigen is present in the clinical material, it binds to the membrane and is detected by a colorimetric reaction. Initial studies showed high sensitivity and specificity for the EIA assays, but recent studies have shown less accuracy (sensitivity of 60-95%; specificity of >90%). The EIA method is relatively easy and convenient and, if positive, does not require confirmation by culture. **Current outpatient practice consists of using a rapid screening test first and, if the result is positive, treating the patient with an appropriate antimicrobial agent. If the result of the EIA screening test is negative, a culture must be performed.** In general, a positive screening test reduces the cost of medical care. A negative screening test increases cost, because subsequently a throat swab must be cultured on a blood agar plate. **In most cases, submitting specimens for culture of group A streptococci to a reference laboratory is more cost-effective than attempting to perform such cultures in the private office setting.**

Bordetella pertussis

In recent years there has been a resurgence of *B. pertussis* infection, in large part due to declines in immunization rates. The standard procedure for laboratory diagnosis is culture of a nasopharyngeal swab. Laboratory diagnosis is complicated by the fact that the organism is extremely labile, grows only on specialized bacteriologic media, may no longer be present in respiratory secretions at the time the patient seeks medical attention, and requires 3-5 days for completion. A direct fluorescent antibody (DFA) test is also available. Although there is some variability in the accuracy of the DFA method, the result is available the same day the specimen is taken. The DFA test gives few false-positive reactions when it is used by trained personnel. The incidence of false-negative results ranges from 10-50%. Therefore, **both culture and DFA should be used for optimal speed and accuracy.** Two nasopharyngeal swabs should be collected. One swab is placed in transport medium for culture by a reference laboratory, and the other is used for preparing 3-5 smears on a glass microscope slide. The smears are allowed to air-dry for DFA testing. The DFA test is time-consuming, requires highly trained personnel for interpretation, and is best suited to hospital or reference laboratories. Several DNA probes for the rapid diagnosis of *B. pertussis* have been developed, but none is yet available for routine use.

Corynebacterium diphtheriae

The method used to collect a specimen for the culture of *C. diphtheriae* depends on the specific body site or sites affected. In general, an aggressively collected swab, piece of tissue, or pseudomembrane will yield the organism if it is present. It is important to notify the laboratory that infection with *C. diphtheriae* is suspected. Few laboratories have experience with this pathogen, and the specimen may need to be sent to a reference laboratory.

Mycobacterium tuberculosis

Diagnosis of tuberculosis relies on the growth of the causative organism from a patient specimen. This is a slow process, requiring 6-8 weeks. More rapid methods of growing *M. tuberculosis* and molecular probes for culture identification have become available recently. Kits for amplification and direct detection of mycobacterial DNA in patient specimens should be available in 1994, and techniques for detection of antimicrobial resistance markers should be available soon thereafter.

Whatever methods are used, collection of the specimen is still the single most important step in diagnosis. Acid-fast staining of direct smears yields a sensitivity of 50%, with results available in 24-72 hours. Traditional culture results are available in 6-8 weeks.

Mycoplasma pneumoniae

M. pneumoniae is a fastidious organism that is difficult to culture in the laboratory. It can be isolated from the throat and respiratory secretions by inoculation onto specialized media and incubated under microaerophilic conditions for 3-10 days. Colonies have a "fried-egg" appearance on agar media. **Isolation of *M. pneumoniae* is generally considered less reliable than diagnostic serology for two reasons: (1) isolation succeeds in only 40-90% of serologically proved cases, and (2) interpretation of isolation is difficult because of persistence of the organism in the throat for up to several weeks after an acute infection.**

Antibodies develop during infection and can be demonstrated by several methods, including complement fixation (CF), hemagglutination inhibition (HI), indirect immunofluorescent antibody assay (IFA), and enzyme immunoassay (EIA). A growth inhibition assay is quite specific but more costly and cumbersome than CF, HI, IFA, or EIA. With all of these serologic techniques, a rising antibody titer is required for diagnostic significance because of the high incidence of seropositivity in normal individuals, although a CF titer of 1:32 or greater during the acute phase of illness is suggestive of infection.

Cold hemagglutinins for group O human erythrocytes appear in about 50% of untreated patients (less so in very young patients). Titers reach a peak in the third or the fourth week after acute onset of disease. A titer of 1:64 or more supports the diagnosis of infection with *M. pneumoniae*. No specific rapid diagnostic test for this pathogen is available at the present time.

TABLE 1. Comparison of Standard Method to Rapid Methods for the Laboratory Diagnosis of Respiratory Pathogens

Pathogen	Standard Method	Rapid Method
Influenza A, B Parainfluenza 1,2 Adenovirus RSV	4-14 days	SV, 2-3 days DFA/EIA, 2-4 h
Herpes simplex	1-3 days	SV, 16-20 h DFA/EIA, 2-4 h
Cytomegalovirus	14-28 days	SV, 16-72 h
Epstein-Barr virus	Not generally done; cultures held for up to 8 wk	Rapid slide test for heterophile antibody—15 min IgM antibody to VCA in acute phase serum—1 h
Group A *Streptococcus*	24-48 h	EIA, 30 min
B. pertussis	5-7 days	DFA, 2-4 h
C. diphtheriae	3-5 days	No rapid method
M. tuberculosis	6-8 wk	Acid-fast smear, 2-4 h
M. pneumoniae	3-10 days	Cold hemagglutinins—30 min CF titer of 1:32 or greater in acute serum is suggestive of infection No rapid method
C. trachomatis	3-5 days	DFA/EIA, 2-4 h PCR, 5 h

SV = shell vial amplification; DFA = direct fluorescent assay for antigen detection; EIA = enzyme immunoassay; PCR = polymerase chain reaction.

Chlamydia trachomatis

Culture is considered the gold standard for detecting infection with *C. trachomatis.* The disadvantages of culture are two: (1) even under optimal conditions, the sensitivity is only 80% because of the extreme lability of the organism, and (2) growth is slow, resulting in a delay of 3–5 days before results are available.

Several technologies for the detection of *C. trachomatis* infection are commercially available, including DFA, EIA, and a nonisotopically labeled DNA probe. In June 1993, a kit for the detection of this agent by PCR (Roche Diagnostic Systems) was approved by the FDA for diagnostic testing, the first such PCR application licensed for clinical use in the U.S. Nonculture assays yield more rapid results (1 day) but, with the possible exception of PCR, are less sensitive than culture. In several studies to date, PCR showed a sensitivity greater than that of culture, while maintaining high specificity.

SUMMARY

Several technologic advances of the past decade now make it possible to detect many respiratory pathogens within 48 hours and several within 1–4 hours. Table 1 summarizes the laboratory procedures discussed above and compares turnaround times from receipt of specimen to reporting of result for the important viral and bacterial pathogens of the respiratory tract of infants and children.

SUGGESTED READING

1. Buck GE: Nonculture methods for detection and identification of microorganisms in clinical specimens. Pediatr Clin North Am 36:95–112, 1989.
2. Costello MJ, Smernoff NT, Yungbluth M: Laboratory diagnosis of viral respiratory tract infections. Lab Med 24:150–157, 1993.
3. Dennehy PH: New tests for the rapid diagnosis of infection in children. Adv Pediatr Infect Dis 8:91–129, 1993.
4. Domingues EA, Taber LH, Couch RB: Comparison of rapid diagnostic techniques for respiratory syncytial and influenza A virus infections in young children. J Clin Microbiol 31:2286–2290, 1993.
5. Michaels MG, Serdy C, Barbadora K, et al: Respiratory syncytial virus: A comparison of diagnostic modalities. Pediatr Infect Dis J 11:613–616, 1992.
6. Miller N, Hernandez SG, Cleary TJ: Evaluation of Gen-Probe amplified *Mycobacterium tuberculosis* direct test and PCR for direct detection of *Mycobacterium tuberculosis* in clinical specimens. J Clin Microbiol 32:393–397, 1994.
7. Olsen MA, Shuck KM, Sambol AR, et al: Isolation of seven respiratory viruses in shell vials: A practical and highly sensitive method. J Clin Microbiol 31:422–425, 1993.
8. Ray CG: Respiratory viruses. In Sherris JC (ed): Medical Microbiology: An Introduction to Infectious Diseases, 2nd ed. New York, Elsevier, 1990, pp 499–516.

41

OFFICE PULMONARY FUNCTION TESTING

Julian L. Allen, M.D.

Because evaluation of lung function can be performed conveniently in adults, general practitioners and internists often have some form of spirometric equipment in the office to monitor patients with chronic obstructive lung disease. Office spirometry is not commonly performed in children, but this is likely to change. With increasing frequency practitioners are called on to care for children with various chronic lung diseases, such as asthma, bronchopulmonary dysplasia, and cystic fibrosis. Thus, although pulmonary function tests in children in the past were performed primarily in pediatric pulmonology centers, lung function testing has a role in the office both as a screening procedure and as a way to follow children with chronic lung disease. This chapter discusses the uses of office pulmonary function testing, including indications, interpretation of the common tests of lung function in children, and practical considerations in the performance of such tests.

INDICATIONS FOR PULMONARY FUNCTION TESTING (Table 1)

Lung function testing is not a means of diagnosing a specific disease, but it may point the clinician in the direction of a correct diagnosis by characterizing the physiology of the disease process. Determination of whether the primary derangement is in lung volumes or flow rates distinguishes restrictive lung disease from obstructive lung disease, respectively. Furthermore, pulmonary function testing is useful in suggesting the site of airflow obstruction, i.e., the upper or lower airways, as well as in monitoring the course of the disease process in patients with chronic lung disease. Response to therapeutic interventions, such as administration of bronchodilators or diuretics, can be assessed. In addition, lung function testing can be used to monitor lung growth and the potential effects of environmental factors such as passive smoking.

The growth of a given lung volume (such as vital capacity) or flow rate (such as FEV_1) may be viewed in much the same way as the more common growth measurements, e.g., height, weight, and head circumference. Percentile charts recently have been developed for recording growth of pulmonary function measurements[7] (Fig. 1). Just as a change in growth percentiles for height and weight should be cause for concern, a change in percentiles of lung function should alert the physician to the possibility of a problem with lung and/or airway growth. For example, a flow rate that crosses percentiles downward over time may mean either that an underlying airway disease process is worsening or that airway growth is not proceeding at an appropriate rate.

MEASUREMENT OF LUNG VOLUMES AND FLOW RATES

***Spirometry* is the most commonly performed lung function test in children over the age of 4 or 5 years.** An understanding of the physiologic principles underlying spirometry is imperative for the proper performance and interpretation of flow-volume curves. The maneuver itself is a

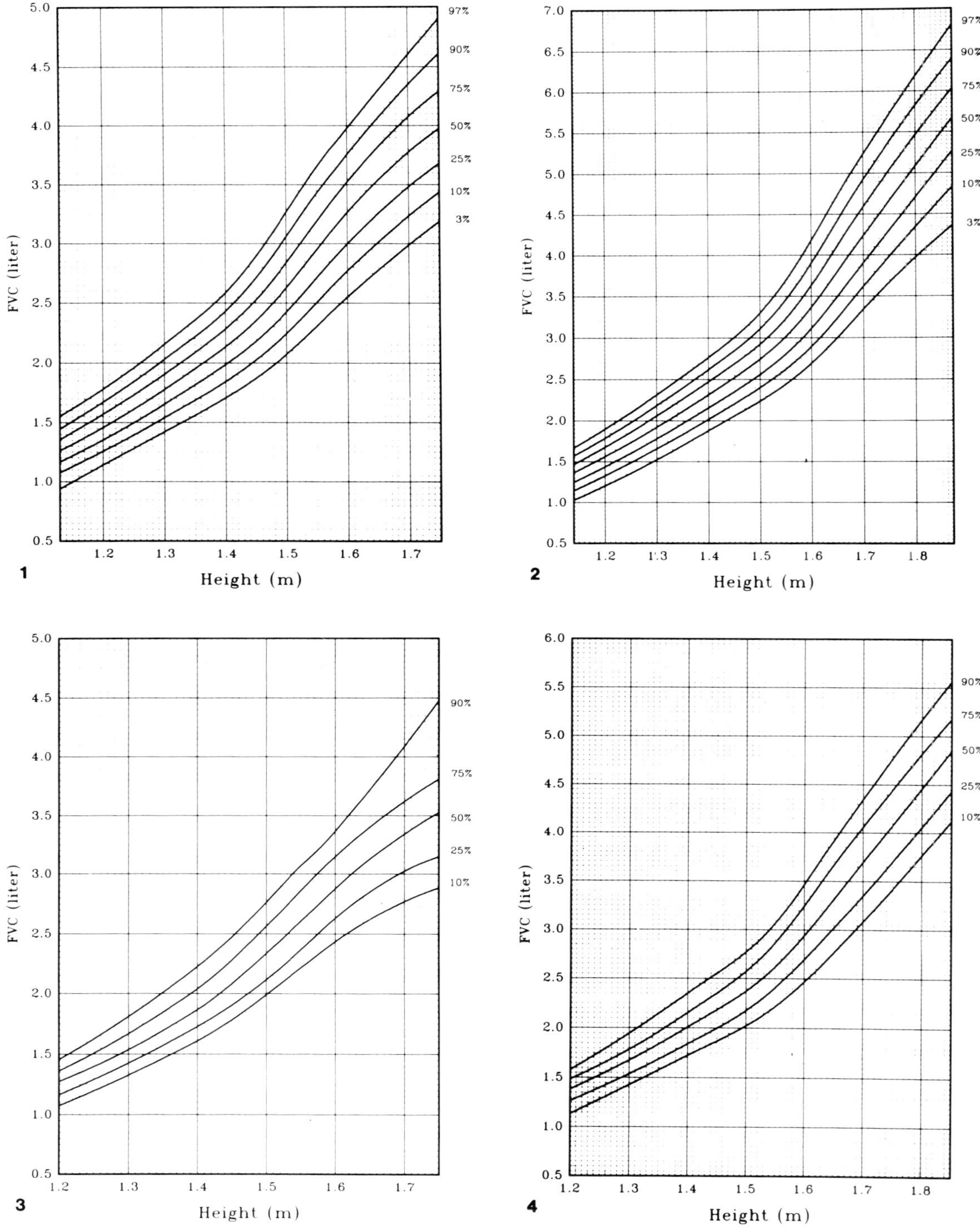

1. The smoothed percentiles of FVC by height; white girls, Six Cities, United States.
2. The smoothed percentiles of FVC by height; white boys, Six Cities, United States.
3. The smoothed percentiles of FVC by height; black girls, Six Cities, United States.
4. The smoothed percentiles of FVC by height; black boys, Six Cities, United States.

FIGURE 1. Race- and sex-specific percentile curves of forced vital capacity (FVC) and forced expiratory volume in one second (FEV_1) for children between the ages of 6 and 18 years. (From Wang X, Dockery DW, Wypij D, et al: Pulmonary function between 6 and 18 years of age. Pediatr Pulmonol 15:75–78, 1993, with permission.) *(Continued on facing page.)*

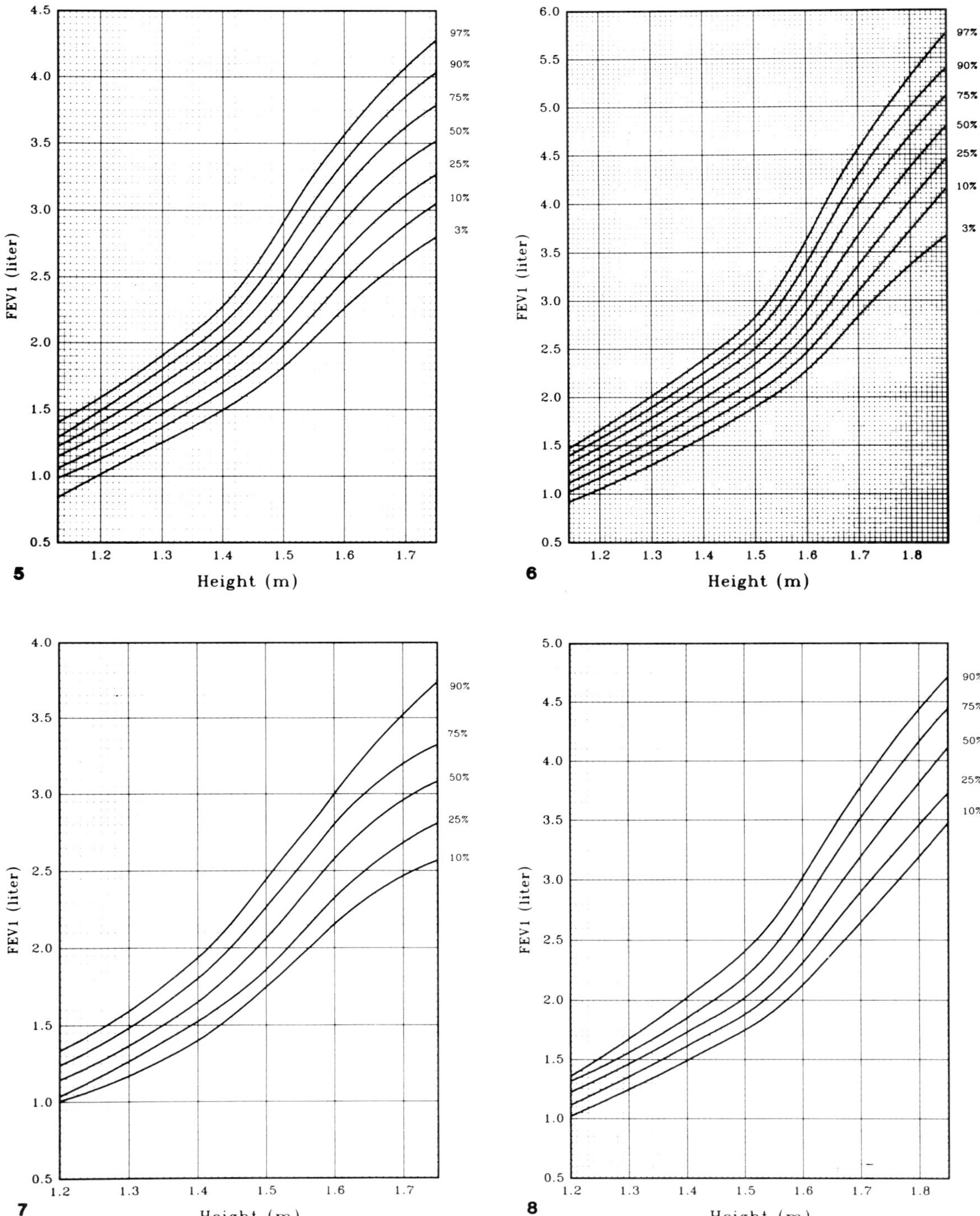

5. The smoothed percentiles of FEV_1 by height; white girls, Six Cities, United States.
6. The smoothed percentiles of FEV_1 by height; white boys, Six Cities, United States.
7. The smoothed percentiles of FEV_1 by height; black girls, Six Cities, United States.
8. The smoothed percentiles of FEV_1 by height; black boys, Six Cities, United States.

***FIGURE 1** (Cont.).*

TABLE 1. Indications for Pulmonary Function Testing in Children

1. To characterize physiology (obstructive versus restrictive disease)
2. To aid in localizing site of airflow obstruction (central versus peripheral)
3. To monitor course of chronic lung disease over time
4. To measure response to therapeutic interventions
5. To assess airway reactivity
6. To monitor lung growth and effects of environmental factors (e.g., passive smoking)
7. For preoperative assessment

simple one: the child is asked to inhale the biggest possible breath (to total lung capacity [TLC]) and to breathe out completely (to residual volume [RV]) as quickly and forcefully as possible. Expired volume is plotted in liters on the Y axis and as a function of time (in seconds) on the X axis. From the resulting curve, a number of measurements can be obtained. The forced vital capacity (FVC) is the total amount of air that can be exhaled by the patient from a maximal inhalation; it is the difference between TLC and RV (Fig. 2). Because the residual volume is the amount of air left in the lungs at the completion of such a maneuver, obviously it cannot be measured by spirometry; because total lung capacity includes the residual volume (see Fig. 2), obviously it, too, cannot be measured by simple spirometry. Residual volume, total lung capacity, and functional residual capacity (FRC, the normal resting lung volume at normal end-expiration) must be measured by other methods, such as helium dilution or body plethysmography, that generally are available only in specialized pulmonary function laboratories. However, once FRC is measured by either technique, residual volume and total lung capacity can be derived from the spirogram.

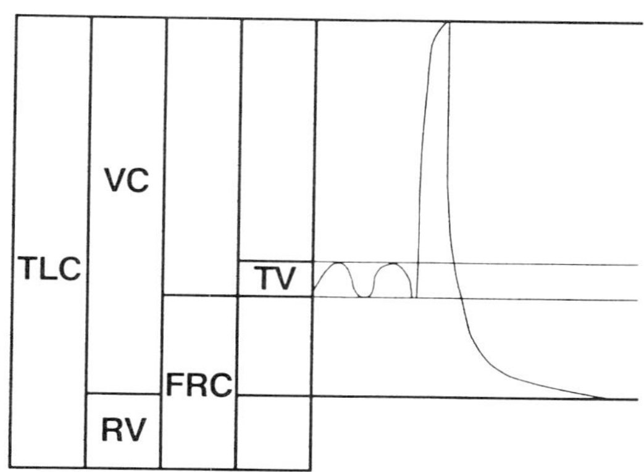

FIGURE 2. Subdivisions of lung volume. TLC = total lung capacity; VC = vital capacity; RV = residual volume; FRC = functional residual capacity; TV = tidal volume.

Because flow is volume moved per unit of time, the forced-volume time plot can be used to derive flow rates as an index of airway size. An instantaneous flow rate can be calculated from the volume-time plot by taking the slope of the line tangent to the curve at the desired lung volume. Flow rates commonly measured from the volume-time plot include the forced expiratory volume in one second (FEV_1) and the maximal mid-expiratory flow (MMEF) rate (Fig. 3, *right*). The FEV_1 sounds like a volume, but in fact it is a flow rate—the volume expired in the first second of a forced exhalation. The MMEF (also known as the forced expiratory flow from 25–75% expired volume [$FEF_{25-75\%}$]) is the slope of the line connecting the point on the volume-time plot at 25% expired volume with the point on the plot at 75% expired volume; it is therefore approximately the average flow rate over the mid portion of the vital capacity during a forced maneuver. Although these are the two most commonly measured flow rates, an infinite number of instantaneous flow rates can be derived from the volume-time plot, most conveniently by constructing a maximal expiratory flow volume (MEFV) curve (Fig. 3, *left*).

The *flow-volume curve* is derived from the volume-time plot and gives no information not already contained in the volume-time plot. The flow-volume curve is useful, however, because it allows ready recognition of various sorts of lung pathophysiology on the basis of specific alterations of curve shape (see below). The flow rates most commonly measured from the MEFV curve are peak flow and maximal flow (Vmax) at 25%, 50%, and 75% of VC (see Fig. 3).

INTERPRETATION OF LUNG FUNCTION TESTS

The two classic subdivisions of lung function test abnormalities are obstructive disease (i.e., disease primarily affecting airways) and

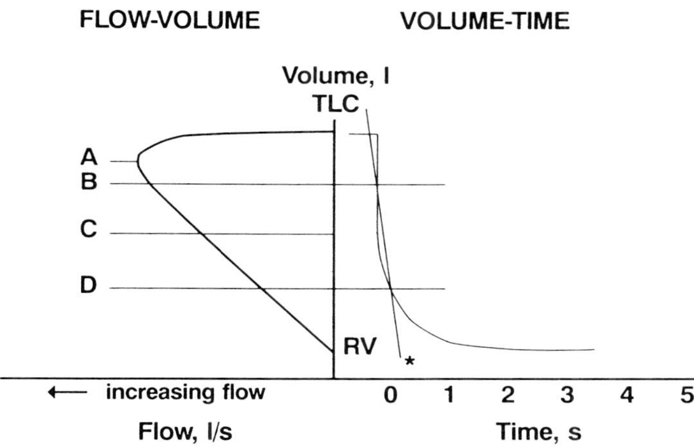

FIGURE 3. Translation of the volume-time spirogram to a flow-volume curve. *Right,* Volume–time spirogram. The FEV_1 is the volume expired in the first second of expiration. The maximal mid-expiratory flow rate (MMEF) is the slope of the straight line (asterisk) connecting the points on the volume-time curve that correspond to 25% and 75% of expired volume from total lung capacity (TLC) to residual volume (RV) (see test). *Left,* Flow-volume curve. The flow represents the instantaneous slope of the volume-time curve (*right*) at a given lung volume. Flows depicted at labeled points on the flow–volume curve are: *A,* peak expiratory flow rate; *B,* $\dot{V}max_{75}$, maximal flow at 75% of VC; *C,* $\dot{V}max_{50}$; *D,* $\dot{V}max_{25}$.

restrictive disease (i.e., diseases associated with diminished lung volumes). Table 2 shows the most common alterations in the most commonly tested lung volumes and flow rates in obstructive disease (e.g., cystic fibrosis, asthma) and in restrictive disease (e.g., neuromuscular disease, interstitial lung disease, chest wall abnormalities such as scoliosis). **The sine qua non of obstructive disease is low flow rates (FEV_1, MMEF, $\dot{V}max_{25}$), which indicate obstruction of the airways. The sine qua non of restrictive disease is diminished total lung capacity.**

In *obstructive disease,* lung volumes such as TLC and RV may be high because of excessive air trapping. VC is usually low because the RV is disproportionately increased relative to the TLC. (Air trapping at RV is usually worse than that at TLC.) FEV_1 is decreased, as are MMEF and $\dot{V}max_{25}$.

The flow-volume curve adds additional information for localizing the site of airway obstruction. In simple terms, expiratory flows at high lung volumes represent central (large) airway events, whereas flows at low lung volumes represent peripheral (small) airway events. Thus characteristic alterations in the shape of the expiratory flow-volume curve are seen in patients with central and small airways disease. The clipped peak flow of central airways disease is in fact a manifestation of low flows at high lung volumes, whereas the scooped flow-volume curve of small airways disease is a manifestation of low flows at low lung volumes (Fig. 4A and B). A scooped flow-volume curve corresponds to a low $\dot{V}max_{25}$ and a low MMEF on the volume-time plot. These two indices therefore reflect small airway function.

Central airway disease may be further characterized by comparing maximal inspiratory flow to maximal expiratory flow (Fig. 4C–E). Lesions that cause variable or dynamic obstruction of the extrathoracic airway (e.g., laryngomalacia) diminish inspiratory flow more than expiratory flow (Fig. 4C); lesions that cause variable or dynamic obstruction of the intrathoracic airway (e.g., tracheo- or bronchomalacia) diminish expiratory flow more than inspiratory

TABLE 2. Patterns of Abnormality in Pulmonary Function Tests: Restrictive Versus Obstructive Disease

Measurement	Restrictive	Obstructive
Volumes		
TLC*	↓	↑
RV*	‡	↑
VC†	↓	↓
Flows		
FEV_1†	↓	↓
MMEF†	↓	↓
$\dot{V}max_{25}$†	↓	↓
Flow/volume ratio		
FEV_1/FVC†	NL	↓

* Must be measured in a pulmonary function laboratory (by body plethysmography or helium dilution technique).

† May be measured by office spirometry.

‡ May be high in neuromuscular disease (due to expiratory muscle weakness), high or low in chest wall disease, and low in interstitial lung disease.

TLC = total lung capacity; RV = residual volume; VC = vital capacity; FEV_1 = forced expiratory volume in one second; MMEF = maximal mid-expiratory flow; $\dot{V}max_{25}$ = maximal flow at 25% of vital capacity; FVC = forced vital capacity; NL = normal limits.

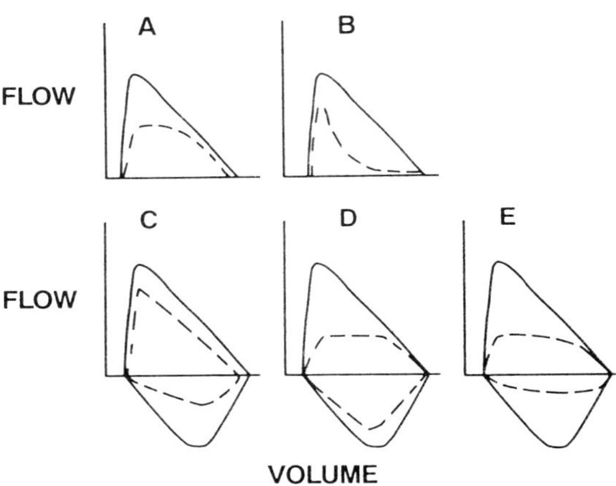

FIGURE 4. Expiratory flow volume curve alterations in (*A*) central airway disease and (*B*) peripheral airway disease. *C–E,* Inspiratory vs. expiratory flow-volume curve in various forms of central airflow obstruction. *C,* Variable extrathoracic airway obstruction, *D,* variable intrathoracic airway obstruction, and *E,* fixed central airway obstruction (extra- or intrathoracic). Solid line—normal curve. Dashed line—abnormal curve. See text.

flow (Fig. 4D). Fixed structural lesions of the central airways diminish both inspiratory and expiratory flows (Fig. 4E).

All forms of *restrictive disease* are characterized by a diminished total lung capacity and vital capacity. Because TLC cannot be measured by spirometry, at first it may appear that spirometry and the flow-volume curve would be more useful in the diagnosis of obstructive than of restrictive disease. Although this is true to a certain extent, these two simple office tests can at least suggest the presence of restrictive disease. The FEV_1 and other flows are usually diminished in restrictive lung disease.This fact does *not* indicate concomitant air flow obstruction; rather, it is a reflection of the fact that flow is a volume moved per unit of time and that if volumes decrease, so do flow rates. The crucial distinguishing spirometric measurement between restrictive and obstructive disease is the ratio of FEV_1 to FVC. In purely restrictive disease, flows are decreased in proportion to the decrease in lung volumes, and the FEV_1/VC ratio is normal (0.8) or elevated. In obstructive disease, in contrast, the FEV_1/FVC ratio is low. Thus, the combination of a low FEV_1 with a normal FEV_1/VC ratio strongly suggests restrictive disease and indicates the need for lung volume measurements in a pulmonary function laboratory.

An important part of proper interpretation of lung function testing in children is comparison with accurate normal standards. Normal standards are based on studies of normal children and usually are expressed as percent of predicted value based on the child's standing height. When standing height is not an appropriate predictor of lung function, as in patients with severe scoliosis, arm span is a better measurement. (In normal individuals, arm span is approximately equal to standing height). There are several reliable studies of normal standards in young children and adolescents.[4-8] Whatever group of normal values is used, the standards should be consistent within the laboratory. Normal standards should encompass the age range of the children being tested; predicted equations extrapolated from other height and age ranges lead to misleading results. Recent studies provide predicted values for children as young as 6 years of age; our laboratory uses these studies for predicted values.[5] In general, normal values for FEV_1, TLC, and VC should be within 80–120% of the predicted value (±2 standard deviations), whereas the MMEF should fall within 60–140%. Alternatively, recently published pulmonary growth charts for children from 6–18 years of age provide percentile values for the growth of FVC, FEV_1, FEV_1/FVC, and MMEF (see Fig. 1). A given patient should fall between the 5th and 95th percentiles to be considered normal. Furthermore, there should be no significant crossing from one percentile to another over time.

TESTS OF AIRWAY HYPERREACTIVITY

In patients with baseline obstructive disease, inhaled bronchodilator therapy should be given to see whether obstruction is reversible. The response to inhaled bronchodilators is easily assessed with office spirometry. The child can be given the usual treatment of inhaled bronchodilator after performing baseline spirometry. (This has the added advantage of enabling the practitioner to observe the child's technique of inhalation and to make any necessary modifications.) Spirometry is repeated 10–20 minutes after the inhalation treatment. An improvement in FEV_1 of >10% is generally considered evidence of airway hyperreactivity.

Conversely, in patients with normal lung function at baseline, various provocation procedures may be performed to induce bronchospasm in patients with hyperreactivity. Commonly used methods include methacholine challenge, histamine challenge, and eucapneic hyperventilation of subfreezing dry air. A decrease in FEV_1 of >10% in the third test is indicative of airway hyperreactivity.

Airway challenge testing is probably best left to specialized pediatric pulmonary centers experienced in their performance and in treatment of untoward side effects. Although rare, side effects should be promptly recognized and treated with bronchodilators. We do *not* recommend such office procedures as asking the child to run up and down the steps to elicit changes in airway function. Such nonstandardized approaches are probably not sensitive enough to diagnose or to rule out airway hyperreactivity with any degree of certainty.

Lung function testing in infants is a new and rapidly developing field. Although standardized methods and normal values are as yet hard to come by, such tests hold great promise for the evaluation of lung disorders in early infancy.[1] At present, they are best confined to specialized centers well versed in their performance and interpretation.

PRACTICAL CONSIDERATIONS

Equipment should conform to the standards recommended by the American Thoracic Society.[2] In brief, volume range for measuring vital capacity and FEV_1 should be 7 L. Accuracy should be ±3% or 0.050 liters, whichever is greater. Flow range should be 0–12 L/sec. The spirometer should be able to accumulate the FVC for at least 10 seconds. A graphic printout displaying either volume-time or flow-volume curves is necessary. Finally, there should be a minimal back pressure against which the subject must exhale.

There are various considerations in choosing among the dozens of spirometers that meet the above requirements. Nonautomated spirometers require manual calculation of flows and volumes from the raw volume-time curve. Although such instruments can be purchased for less than $2,000, we do not recommend them for the office setting because such calculations are time-consuming. Automated spirometers are preferable, because they calculate the desired lung function measurements and express them both as an absolute number in liters or liters per second and as a percent of predicted value (calculated from an internal set of reference values). These instruments usually cost between $2,000 and $5,000.

Other considerations include portability, ease of cleaning, adequate graph size (3–6 inches square for an exhalation curve), and dependable servicing by the manufacturer. A recently published monograph gives further details on comparing the various spirometers on the market.[3]

Peak flow testing should not be used as a substitute for spirometry. Peak flow is highly dependent on patient effort, and variability of the test is probably too great to allow detection of anything less than fairly dramatic changes in lung function. The initial investment in a good spirometer is certainly more costly, but the information obtained is likely to be of much more use to the practitioner.

TECHNIQUE

To be interpretable, a child's spirometry must be reproducible. The expiratory effort should last at least 3 seconds, and 3 sets of curves should be obtained with FVCs that agree to within 10% of the largest effort. Thus, the technique used to coach the subject is as important as adequacy of the instrumentation. An individual well-versed in explaining the procedure to children and enthusiastic in coaching them is an absolute necessity to obtain accurate results. The tester must walk a fine line, enthusiastically exhorting ("Blow, blow, blow, blow, blow! Harder, harder, harder! More, more, more, more, more!") without frightening a young child. Many spirometers on the market now have incentive devices to enlist the child's full cooperation, such as pictures of candles on a birthday cake that the child can blow out. Conventionally, the lower age range for children able to cooperate with spirometry is approximately 6–7 years. However, the practitioner familiar with pulmonary function testing in children can obtain interpretable results from children as young as 4 years of age.

SUGGESTED READING

1. American Thoracic Society/European Respiratory Society: Respiratory mechanics in infants: Physiologic evaluation in health and disease. A Statement of the Committee on Infant Pulmonary Function Testing. Am Rev Respir Dis 147:474–496, 1993.
2. American Thoracic Society: Standardization of spirometry—1987 update. Am Rev Respir Dis 136:1285–1293, 1987.
3. Enright PL, Hyatt RE: Office Spirometry: A Practical Guide to the Selection and Use of Spirometers. Philadelphia, Lea & Febiger, 1987.
4. Hsu HK, Jenkins DE, Hsi BP, et al: Ventilatory functions of normal children and young adults: Mexican-American, white and black. I: Spirometry. J Pediatr 95:14–23, 1979.
5. Knudson RJ, Lebowitz MD, Holberg C, Burrows K: Changes in the normal maximal expiratory flow volume curve with growth and aging. Am Rev Respir Dis 127:725–734, 1983.
6. Polgar G, Promadhat V: Pulmonary Function Testing in Children: Techniques and Standards. Philadelphia, W.B. Saunders, 1971.
7. Wang X, Dockery DW, Wypij D, et al: Pulmonary function between 6 and 18 years of age. Pediatr Pulmonol 15:75–88, 1993.
8. Weng TR, Levison H: Standards of pulmonary function in children. Am Rev Respir Dis 99:879–894, 1969.

42

PRACTICAL ASPECTS OF OXYGEN THERAPY

David Lowe, M.D.

The most common, dramatic, and life-saving intervention in critical care medicine occurs when cyanosis is overcome by oxygen therapy. Whether a patient is receiving 100% oxygen with a Mapleson D system (see p. 294) or 18% oxygen with mouth-to-mouth ventilation, oxygen is the most powerful drug provided by the clinician. This chapter reviews the causes of hypoxemia that are responsive to supplemental oxygen and the equipment that must be available, functional, and understood to provide it reliably.

OXYGEN DELIVERY TO THE TISSUES

Adequate oxygenation depends on the integrated function of the lungs, blood, and circulation to deliver as much oxygen as the tissues demand. The quantity of oxygen delivered to the tissues each minute (O_2 delivery) is equal to the oxygen content of the arterial blood (CaO_2) times the cardiac output (CO):

$$O_2 \text{ delivery (ml/min)} = CaO_2 \times CO$$

Normally, 20 ml of oxygen is contained in each 100 ml of arterial blood (CaO_2 = 20 vol%). Almost all of the oxygen is bound to hemoglobin (19.7 vol%), and a small fraction is dissolved in the plasma (0.3 vol%):

$$CaO_2 = 1.37 \times Hgb \times SaO_2 + 0.003 \times PaO_2$$

where 1.37 = volume of O_2 (ml) carried by 1 gm of fully saturated Hgb; Hgb = hemoglobin in gm/dl; SaO_2 = % oxyhemoglobin to total Hgb; 0.003 = solubility of O_2 in plasma in vol% per mmHg; and PaO_2 = arterial O_2 tension in mmHg.

Normally, only about 25% or 5 vol% of the O_2 carried by the arterial blood is extracted and consumed by the tissues. Thus the oxygen content of the venous blood (CvO_2) is about 15 vol%, with an oxygen tension (PvO_2) of 40 mmHg and an oxygen saturation (SvO_2) of 75%.

Like the base deficit that reflects the lactic acid produced by anaerobic glycolysis, the oxygen content of a mixed venous sample is a global measure of the balance between oxygen supply and demand. If oxygen delivery decreases, more O_2 is extracted from the arterial blood, lowering the CvO_2. Increased metabolic demand (fever, sepsis, trauma, exercise, hyperthyroidism, malignant hyperthermia) increases O_2 consumption and reduces the CvO_2 if there is no compensatory increase in O_2 delivery. The CvO_2 increases with systemic left-to-right shunts, cyanide toxicity (which prevents utilization of the O_2 that is delivered to the mitochondria), and decreased metabolic demand (general anesthesia, hypothermia and paralysis, brain death).

DEFINITIONS OF HYPOXEMIA AND HYPOXIA

Hypoxemia is defined as an arterial oxygen tension (PaO_2) that is below normal for age. Hypoxia exists when the oxygen tension within mitochondria is inadequate to maintain aerobic metabolism. Table 1 indicates that hypoxia may be caused by inadequate blood flow (stagnant hypoxia) and/or a low arterial oxygen content (hypoxemic hypoxia). Arterial oxygen content may be decreased as a result of a low

TABLE 1. Types of Hypoxia

Type	Effect
Stagnant hypoxia	↓ CO, normal CaO_2
Hypoxemic hypoxia	
Hypoxemic hypoxemia	↓ PaO_2, ↓ SaO_2, normal Hgb
Anemic hypoxemia	↓ Hgb, normal PaO_2, normal SaO_2
Toxic hypoxemia	↓ SaO_2, normal PaO_2, normal Hgb (↓ COHgb or metHgb)

hemoglobin (anemic hypoxemia), a low PaO_2 (hypoxemic hypoxemia), and/or a low oxyhemoglobin saturation despite a normal PaO_2 (toxic hypoxemia). Toxic hypoxemia occurs when normal hemoglobin is replaced by carboxyhemoglobin (COHgb) or methemoglobin (metHgb).

INDICATIONS FOR OXYGEN THERAPY

The most obvious indication for oxygen therapy is the presence or risk of a low PaO_2 and/or extreme anemia. Supplemental O_2 also may be indicated to improve oxygen delivery when the cardiac output is low; to lower pulmonary vascular resistance; to enhance elimination of carbon monoxide; or to accelerate the removal of nitrogen from air-containing spaces (pneumothorax, venous air embolism, bowel distention). Because compensatory increases in minute ventilation and cardiac output occur in response to hypoxemia, **oxygen therapy that improves oxygenation also is indicated to decrease the work of breathing** required to maintain a higher alveolar oxygen tension and to decrease the work of the heart required to provide an adequate delivery of oxygen.

Causes of a Low Arterial Oxygen Tension

There are six causes of a low PaO_2, most of which are responsive to supplemental oxygen:

1. Increased $PaCO_2$
2. Low ventilation-perfusion ratios
3. Low inspired oxygen concentration
4. Inadequate cardiac output
5. Profound anemia
6. Intracardiac right-to-left shunts

Increased $PaCO_2$. The oxygen tension of the inspired gas decreases in a normal stepwise fashion as it is diluted with water vapor in the upper airway and with carbon dioxide in the alveoli. With higher concentrations of carbon dioxide in the alveoli, the alveolar oxygen tension (PAO_2) decreases as predicted by the alveolar gas equation:

$$PAO_2 = (FiO_2)(P_B - 47) - PaCO_2 \div 0.8$$

Examples:

1. $100 = (0.21)(760 - 47) - 40 \div 0.8$
2. $50 = (0.21)(760 - 47) - 80 \div 0.8$
3. $613 = (1.0)(760 - 47) - 80 \div 0.8$

where PAO_2 = alveolar oxygen tension; FiO_2 = inspired oxygen fraction; P_B = barometric pressure; 47 = vapor pressure of water at 37°; $PaCO_2$ = arterial PCO_2 (an estimate of alveolar PCO_2); and 0.8 = respiratory quotient = CO_2 production/O_2 consumption (more O_2 is consumed than CO_2 is produced).

Example 1 reveals that when a child breathes room air and the PCO_2 is 40, the alveolar PO_2 is 100, and the arterial PO_2 is a little less than 100. Example 2 reveals that when a child is breathing room air and the PCO_2 rises to 80 because of airway obstruction, the alveolar PO_2 is only 50. Example 3, however, reveals that when the spontaneously breathing child is supported simply by delivering 100% oxygen, the alveolar PO_2 is extremely high and hypoxemia is corrected. By itself, the CO_2 retention is not life-threatening.

Low Ventilation-Perfusion Ratio. When airways or alveoli are totally occluded or collapsed (and no inspired gas reaches alveoli that are perfused), the ventilation-perfusion ratio (V/Q) is zero. Hypoxemia due to such true intrapulmonary shunts does not respond to supplemental oxygen. However, when atelectasis, pulmonary edema, secretions, or bronchospasm cause partial small airway obstruction and partial alveolar collapse, ventilation-perfusion ratios are below 1 but above zero. This common cause of hypoxemia responds to supplemental oxygen. The lower the V/Q ratio, the greater the venous admixture and the higher the FiO_2 required.

Low Inspired Oxygen Concentration. As indicated by the alveolar gas equation, another cause of a low PaO_2 is a low inspired oxygen concentration. An FiO_2 below 21% may occur when the barometric pressure is below 760 mmHg at high altitudes, when oxygen is consumed by a fire in a closed space, or when other gases, such as 100% nitrous oxide, are administered unintentionally.

Inadequate Cardiac Output. A low cardiac output produces a decrease in PaO_2 through a combination of two events:

1. Because a low cardiac output, by definition, means that oxygen delivery to the tissues is inadequate, the tissues extract a greater than normal amount of oxygen from the blood. As a result, the mixed venous blood is markedly desaturated.

2. To the extent that there are areas of lung with low V/Q ratios, as usually occur when the cardiac output is low, this markedly desaturated blood mixes at the level of the left atrium and contributes to arterial desaturation. Profoundly elevated oxygen consumption by the tissues (without an adequate cardiac compensation) causes hypoxemia by the same mechanism.

Profound Anemia. Profound anemia (without an adequate cardiac compensation) causes hypoxemia by a similar mechanism when markedly desaturated venous blood passes through unventilated and underventilated alveoli.

Intracardiac Right-to-Left Shunts. Increasing the alveolar oxygen tension has relatively little effect on hypoxemia that is due to cardiac defects responsible for right-to-left shunts. Increasing the FiO_2, however, may produce useful gains through the addition of appreciable amounts of dissolved oxygen.

ANTICIPATING AND DIAGNOSING HYPOXEMIA

Intervention to correct hypoxemia will be prompt and effective when it is assumed that:

1. Hypoxemia exists before cyanosis becomes obvious.

2. Anything that disturbs the child will increase the severity of any airway obstruction and the impact of the obstruction by increasing oxygen consumption and CO_2 production.

3. Until proved otherwise, agitation, anxiety, and lethargy are signs of hypoxemia, hypercarbia, or both.

4. The use of any sedative or narcotic before the patient receives adequate support (e.g., relief of airway obstruction, supplemental oxygen, positive airway pressure) not only interferes with the assessment of the child but also takes away whatever remaining ability the child has to compensate for the problem.

5. Breathing supplemental oxygen increases the amount of oxygen stored within the lungs and provides an important margin of safety by raising the PaO_2 and decreasing the rate of onset of hypoxemia.

6. Any delay in intervention is catastrophic, because respiratory insufficiency may progress rapidly to respiratory failure, respiratory arrest, and irreversible injury.

7. There is never a resuscitation situation in which the delivery of 100% oxygen is contraindicated.

Pulse Oximetry

In addition to a high level of visual surveillance with the child's shirt off and the room lights on, **any patient at risk of hypoxemia should be monitored continuously with a pulse oximeter.** This is a relatively inexpensive, safe, accurate, portable and noninvasive monitor of the hemoglobin saturation. With each beat of the heart, a visual and an auditory signal provides immediate detection of arterial hemoglobin desaturation before cyanosis is observed, allowing prompt intervention before irreversible injury occurs. An early warning of desaturation is especially important in infants and children, in whom hypoxemia develops much more rapidly than in adults.

Pulse oximetry protects patients with obvious (and not so obvious) impairment of pulmonary or cardiac function, patients with a critical airway, patients who require supplemental oxygen, and patients whose respiration may be depressed by narcotics and sedatives.

Pulse oximetry detects hypoxemia much sooner than visual observation because cyanosis is usually not detected until the PaO_2 falls to 60 mmHg, when the SaO_2 is 90% and almost no margin of safety remains. The oxyhemoglobin dissociation curve (Fig. 1) is fairly flat at a high PaO_2, and the SaO_2 does not decrease meaningfully until the PaO_2 reaches 75–80 mmHg. However, as the PaO_2 reaches 60 mmHg, the slope of the curve becomes vertical, and any further decrease in PaO_2 results in a precipitous decrease in SaO_2.

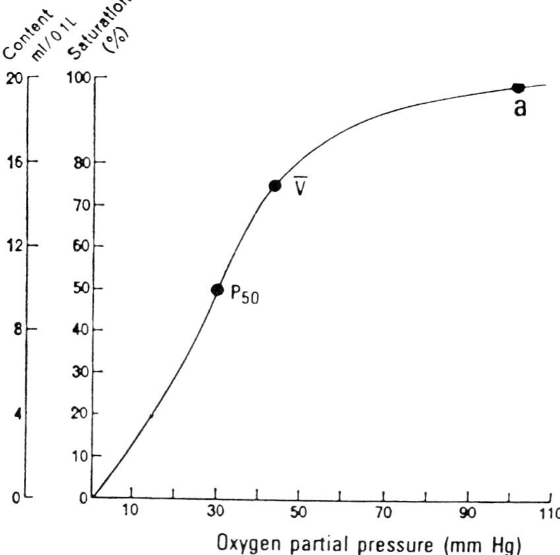

FIGURE 1. Oxyhemoglobin dissociation curve reveals the normal arterial (a) and venous ($\bar{v}$) PO_2. When the PO_2 is 40, 50, or 60 mmHg, the oxygen saturation is approximately 70, 80, or 90%, respectively.

A helpful way to estimate the relationship between the PaO_2 and the SaO_2 is to remember: 40, 50, 60—70, 80, 90. When the PaO_2 is 40, 50, or 60 mmHg, the SaO_2 is 70, 80, or 90%, respectively. Moreover, the P50 of normal hemoglobin (the PaO_2 when 50% of the hemoglobin is saturated) is 27 mmHg.

Pulse oximeters have certain limitations: (1) the signal may be lost during low perfusion conditions; (2) there may be interference with room lights and motion artifacts; (3) pulse oximetry does not differentiate between oxyhemoglobin, carboxyhemoglobin, and methemoglobin; and (4) it does not detect large changes in PaO_2 until the PaO_2 drops to 75–80 mmHg when the saturation begins to fall from 100%.

Inspired Oxygen Concentration

Patient safety demands use of an oxygen analyzer when medical gases are administered during inhalation anesthesia and mechanical ventilation. Currently available electrochemical oxygen analyzers continuously measure the concentration of oxygen in the breathing system and signal when the concentration varies from the desired level. The delivery of less than the desired FiO_2, even a hypoxic gas below 21%, is possible and likely to be catastrophic.

OXYGEN ADMINISTRATION DEVICES

The delivery of an inspired oxygen concentration above 21% requires a source of oxygen under pressure, a pressure-reducing valve, a flowmeter, tubing, and an interface with the patient (e.g., face mask with bag reservoir, nasal cannula, hood). The choice is based on the required FiO_2, the need for positive airway pressure, and the preference of the patient.

There are two sources of oxygen under pressure: central oxygen piped to a wall outlet with a float-type flowmeter in a hospital setting (Fig. 2) and a portable oxygen E cylinder mounted with a gas regulator (Fig. 3). Oxygen cylinders are painted green in the United States and white in most other countries. When completely filled to 2200 psi, an E cylinder weighs

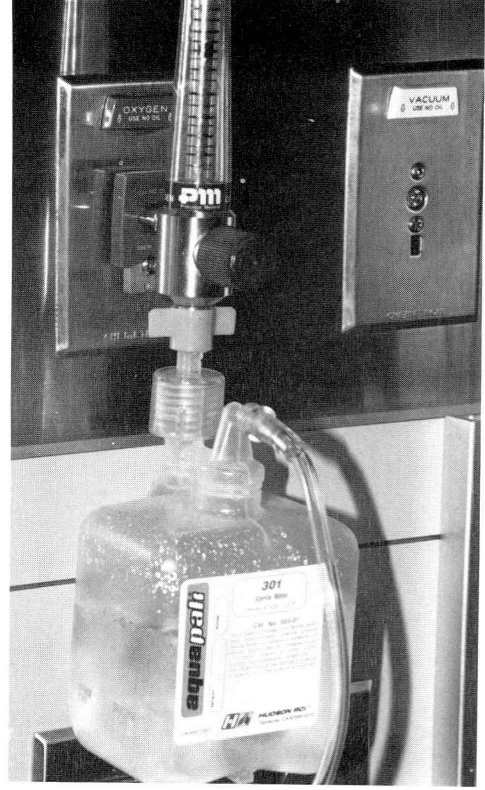

FIGURE 2. Central oxygen wall outlet with float-type flowmeter and bubble humidifier.

about 15 lbs and contains 625 liters of oxygen, which last a little more than 90 minutes at a flow of 6 L/min. The gas regulator includes a pressure gauge, a pressure-reducing valve, and a needle-valve flowmeter for controlling the flow of oxygen. The entire system is useless without a tank wrench to open (counterclockwise) the stem of the cylinder. This allows gas to exit the cylinder and to reach the gas regulator.

Being caught in a hallway, on an elevator, or in an ambulance with an empty tank of oxygen during transport of a critically ill patient from one central source of oxygen to another can be catastrophic. It is a good habit to turn on the E cylinder as the last step before departure and to turn it off as the first step on arrival. A significant delay may occur between being ready to leave and actually leaving.

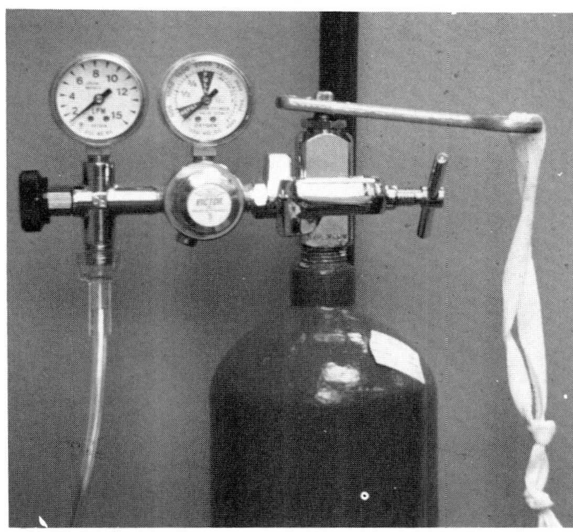

FIGURE 3. Gas regulator (pressure gauge and needle-valve flowmeter) mounted on oxygen E cylinder. A functioning system includes a tank wrench that turns the stem of the cylinder in a counterclockwise direction to allow gas to exit the cylinder and to reach the gas regulator.

HUMIDIFICATION

The upper respiratory tract normally warms and humidifies inspired air from room temperature and a relative humidity of 40% to 37°C with a humidity of 100%. If this heat and moisture exchanger is bypassed by an artificial airway, the inspired gases ultimately are heated to 37°C with 100% humidification, but at the expense of the trachea and bronchi.

Like all medical gases, 100% oxygen flows from a central source or a cylinder at room temperature with 0% humidity. The delivery of dry gas by an endotracheal or tracheotomy tube directly to the trachea leads to mucociliary dysfunction, injury of the respiratory epithelium, and thickening of secretions, perhaps requiring emergency intentional extubation for mucus plugs that cannot be adequately suctioned. Therefore, **any patient receiving medical gases through an artificial airway for more than 1–2 hours, particularly a child with a small artificial airway, should receive humidified inspired gases.**

A heat and moisture exchanger is a small, inexpensive, disposable attachment to the artificial airway that conserves some of the exhaled water and heat and returns them to the inspired gases. Although it provides limited humidification, it is especially useful during transport of an intubated patient.

Humidification approaching 100% at room temperature (<40% humidity at 37°C) can be provided by a bubble humidifier that passes a stream of gas bubbles through water. This device is often used for patients receiving oxygen via a face mask or nasal cannulas. Humidification approaching 100% at 37°C can be provided by a heated humidifier. This is the ideal device because it delivers what the patient would have received at the level of the carina if the upper respiratory tract had not been bypassed.

OXYGEN DELIVERY SYSTEMS

Self-Inflating Manual Resuscitators

A self-inflating resuscitator consists of a compressible, self-expanding bag and two valves, one that directs fresh gas from the bag to the patient and the other that prevents rebreathing of exhaled gases. The resuscitator delivers room air if no supplemental oxygen is delivered to it; 40% O_2 if 100% O_2 is delivered without a reservoir adapter; and 100% O_2 if 100% O_2 is delivered with a reservoir bag attached (Fig. 4). The reservoir collects oxygen when the bag is not filling and fills the bag with oxygen when it reexpands.

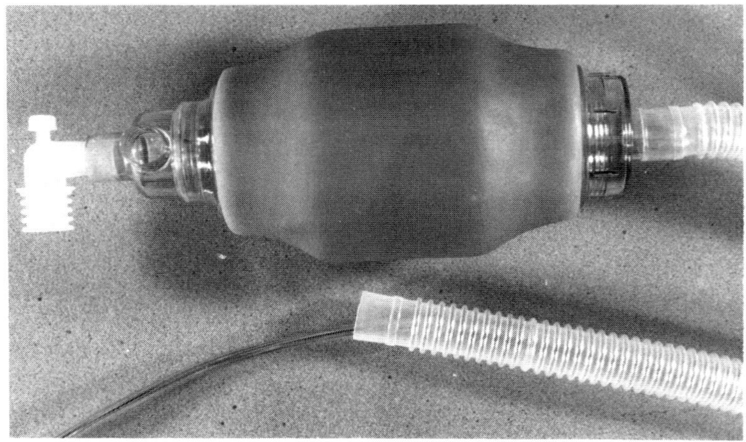

FIGURE 4. Self-inflating bag with reservoir required to deliver 100% oxygen.

The unique advantage of a self-inflating bag is that it does not require of O_2 under pressure to deliver positive-pressure ventilation. **Therefore, it is used primarily during transport and at sites of emergencies. However, it has three major disadvantages:** (1) because the bag automatically refills even if the oxygen flow has been interrupted, there is no obvious way to verify delivery of the desired FiO_2; (2) with spontaneous ventilation, the entire inspired gas may be air coming from the exhalation port rather than the bag; and (3) these bags have a preset pressure relief valve (normally set at 40 cm H_2O) that may need to be manually occluded for effective ventilation in patients with partial airway obstruction or stiff lungs who need high airway pressures for ventilation. Thus, the sicker the patient, the less useful the device becomes.

Mapleson D System

A more versatile breathing device is the Mapleson D system, which requires a source of oxygen under pressure. However, the system allows the delivery of 100% O_2 to the spontaneously breathing patient, the delivery of 100% O_2 and continuous positive airway pressure, or the delivery of 100% O_2 with positive pressure ventilation. The Mapleson D circuit consists of a fresh gas input close to the face mask or endotracheal tube, a single corrugated tube, an overflow valve, and a reservoir bag (Fig. 5).

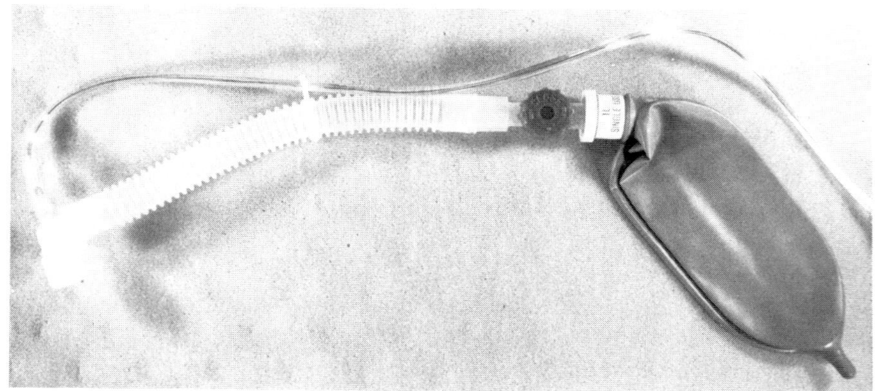

FIGURE 5. Mapleson D system consisting of a fresh gas inlet close to the face mask or endotracheal tube, a single corrugated tube, an overflow valve, and a reservoir bag.

During spontaneous ventilation, the overflow valve is open (counterclockwise), and gas is exhausted from the circuit during exhalation. Early in exhalation, dead space gas, alveolar gas, and fresh gas enter the corrugated tubing. As the reservoir bag fills, pressure within the system increases, opening the overflow valve and allowing some of this mixture to exit. On inspiration, the patient receives fresh as well as mixed gas from the corrugated tube. By turning the overflow valve in a clockwise direction, the desired continuous positive airway pressure can be established.

When used for controlled ventilation, the overflow valve is partially closed. It opens only during the higher pressures toward the end of inspiration. During exhalation, dead space gas, alveolar gas, and fresh gas enter the corrugated tubing. During the expiratory pause, fresh gas continues to enter the circuit, moving the mixed contents of the corrugated tube toward the reservoir bag. As the next breath is initiated, the patient inspires the contents of the corrugated tube: a mixture of fresh gas, dead space gas, and alveolar gas. As the pressure in the system increases, the overflow valve opens, and the contents of the reservoir bag are discharged.

The mixture of 100% O_2 and the exhaled carbon dioxide contained in the corrugated tube and the reservoir bag are determined by the fresh gas flow, the duration of inspiration and exhalation, and the tidal volume. **Rebreathing of exhaled carbon dioxide is minimal with fresh gas flows of at least 6–8 L/min,** and minute ventilation is achieved with a low respiratory rate, long expiratory pause, and large tidal volume.

When the reservoir bag is squeezed during positive-pressure ventilation, a fraction of the gas is delivered to the patient and a fraction of the gas exits the overflow valve. **It is important to ignore the sound of gas exiting the overflow valve into the room, because this sound can give a false sense of confidence. Instead, the overflow valve should be set to provide a resistance that allows the appropriate delivery of gas to the patient, as verified by observation of obvious, symmetrical chest expansion that can be viewed from across the room.**

Anesthesia Face Mask

The face mask serves as an interface between the self-inflating bag or the Mapleson D system

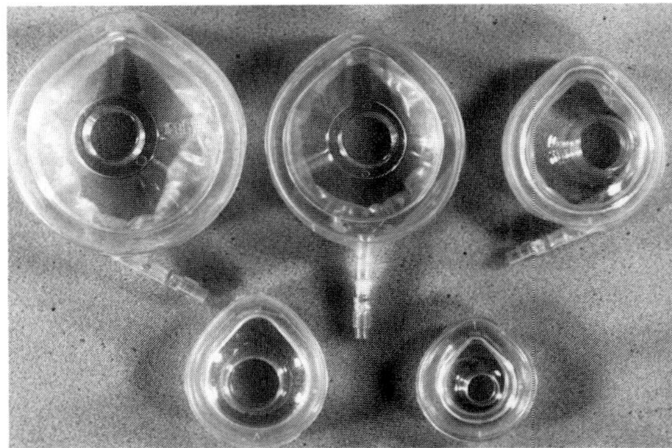

FIGURE 6. Clear, disposable anesthesia face masks conform to a child's face.

and the patient. Modern face masks have an inflatable cushion that conforms with most facial structures (Fig. 6) and provides an effective seal that prevents entrainment of ambient air and allows the administration of positive airway pressure. Clear masks allow easy recognition of vomitus. The face mask is gently applied with a downward force to acquire an adequate seal against the face as the jaw (with the head and neck in a neutral position) is lifted in the opposite direction with a greater force to eliminate soft-tissue obstruction.

Simple Face Mask

A simple face mask (Fig. 7) fits loosely and operates with O_2 flowing at 4–8 L/min. **It rarely provides over 50% O_2 at the level of the trachea in a patient who is breathing 100% O_2** from the oxygen source and room air entrained around the mask. The inspired oxygen concentration varies depending on the patient's inspiratory flow rate, the flow of oxygen into the system, the volume of the reservoir, and the fit of the mask. Simple masks are easily displaced, particularly when a patient become agitated by the effects of hypoxemia and hypercarbia.

Non-rebreathing Face Mask

Non-rebreathing face masks typically have a one-way valve between a simple face mask and a reservoir bag below the chin (Fig. 8). **Concentrations of O_2 up to 90% can be achieved** when the mask fits snugly, the flow into the system

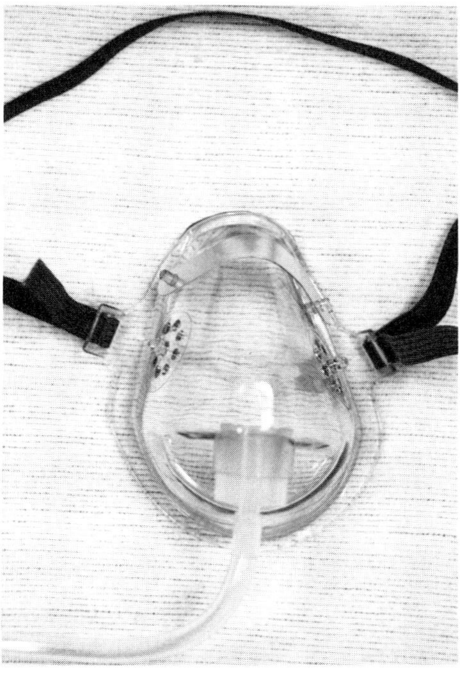

FIGURE 7. **Simple face mask** rarely provides over 50% oxygen at the level of the trachea despite 100% oxygen arriving from the oxygen source.

(6–10 L/min) exceeds the patient's minute ventilation, and the bag remains inflated, rising and falling with the respiratory cycle. Because these conditions are difficult to sustain, **endotracheal intubation may be indicated for reliable delivery of >50% oxygen for a sustained period of time.**

Venturi Mask

Based on the Bernoulli principle, Venturi masks receive oxygen at flow rates between 3 and 15 L/min through a jet orifice that can be adjusted to control the entrainment of air through port holes in the mask (Fig. 9). The size of the jet orifice and entrainment ports determines the concentration of oxygen, and the flow of oxygen determines the total flow of air and oxygen that can exceed 40 L/min. Although such high flow rates prevent rebreathing of CO_2 and **reliably deliver oxygen**

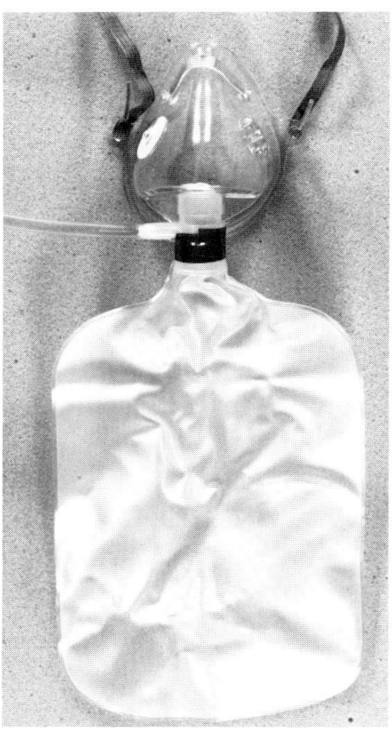

FIGURE 8. **Non-rebreathing face mask.** The patient receives supplemental oxygen from a source of oxygen under pressure and from the reservoir bag, reducing the volume of room air entrained around the tightly fitting mask.

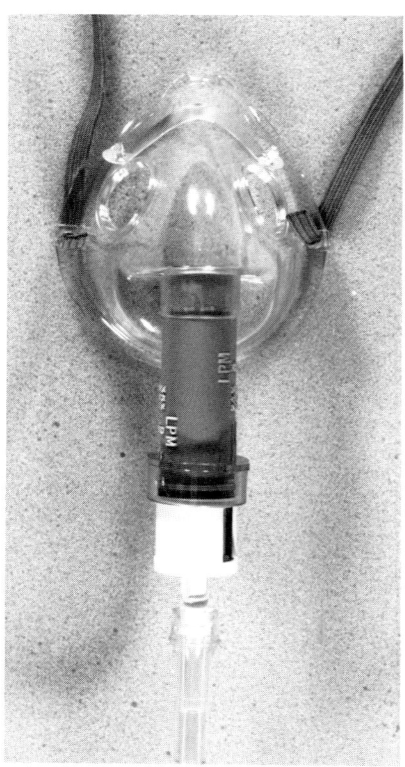

FIGURE 9. **Air entrainment (Venturi) mask** receives oxygen at high flow rates through a jet orifice that can be adjusted to control the entrainment of air through the port holes in the mask.

concentrations within a range of 24–50%, the system creates noise and a breeze that bothers many patients.

Nasal Cannula

Nasal cannulas deliver oxygen at low flow rates of 0.5–6 L/min into two prongs positioned in the anterior nares, directing oxygen flow into the nasooropharynx (Fig. 10). This anatomic dead space serves as a reservoir to maximize the FiO_2, **which reaches 22–40%** after mixing with variable amounts of room air. When the nasal airways are not completely obstructed, the tracheal FiO_2 will be the same whether the patient breathes through the nose or through the mouth.

Nasal cannulas are the least restrictive device and the easiest to secure, even in neonates. They are economic, lightweight, and usually well-tolerated. They take advantage of the humidifying properties of the nasopharynx, but external humidification is necessary when the flow rate exceeds 4 L/min. The use of nasal cannulas is limited because they deliver a relatively low, unpredictable concentration of oxygen.

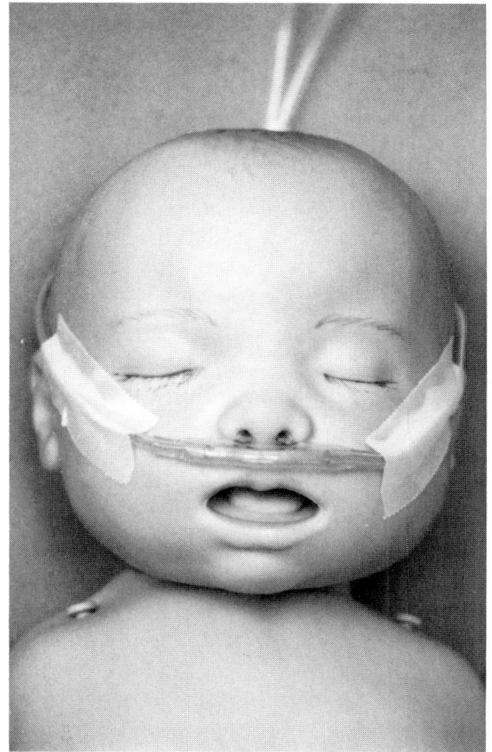

FIGURE 10. Nasal cannula with prongs properly positioned in the anterior nares. Tape secures the tubing so that it passes above the ears and behind the head.

Oxygen Hood

Oxygen hoods are small, clear plastic cylinders or boxes that enclose the head of a neonate, infant, or small child who is likely to stay relatively still (Fig. 11). Hoods allow almost full access to the child. **The volume contained within the hood is small enough to achieve precise oxygen concentrations up to 80–90%, yet large enough to provide the patient's entire tidal volume.**

The oxygen entering through a gas inlet port flushes out all of the exhaled gas through the opening for the neck if the flow rates are high (>7–10 L/min). Such high rates cause evaporative and convective heat loss, which should be minimized by heating and humidifying the inspired gases before they enter the hood. High noise levels within the hood can be minimized by the use of an air-oxygen blender and a large volume humidifier. An oxygen analyzer sensor placed within the hood near the child's mouth and nose provides a relatively accurate measure of FiO_2.

Hut Tent

Hut tents are similar to oxygen hoods, but the small tent frame has a canopy that encloses the upper half of a neonate's or infant's body. The hut tent allows hand-mouth stimulation and greater access by caretakers than the oxygen tent.

Oxygen Tent

Oxygen tents, often called croup tents or mist tents, provide an oxygen-enriched, humidified environment for older children, but their use is limited. Despite high flow rates of at least 10–15 L/min and a good seal with the large, clear plastic enclosure, **the maximal FiO_2 that can be achieved is only 40–50%**. Once the desired FiO_2 is achieved, it is difficult and cumbersome to maintain because the seal is often disrupted by a restless or uncooperative patient or by a caretaker who touches, views,

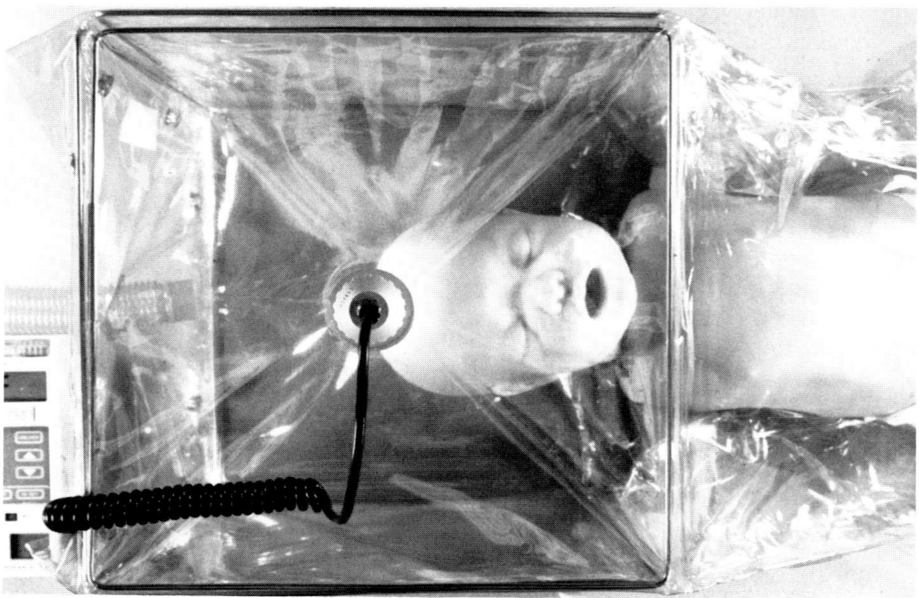

FIGURE 11. Oxygen hood with oxygen entering at high flow rates through a gas inlet port. The FiO_2 is measured by an oxygen analyzer sensor placed within the hood.

talks, or listens to the patient. Visual surveillance of the patient is particularly compromised when aerosolized gases are used. The isolation, noise, humidity, and heat loss or retention are uncomfortable for the patient.

CHRONIC OXYGEN THERAPY

There are three sources of supplemental oxygen for administration in the home: compressed gas cylinders, liquid oxygen systems, and oxygen concentrators. The selection is based on cost, convenience, and portability.

The best stationary source is the H cylinder, which weighs 130 lbs and holds 6600 liters of oxygen. The E cylinder, when filled with 625 liters and inserted within its wheeled carrier, weighs about 18 lbs; this combination is too heavy for routine ambulation but appropriate as a back-up system. Small cylinders weighing 5–10 lbs hold enough oxygen to provide 2 L/min for 1.5–3 hours.

Liquid oxygen systems in the home employ a specifically designed stationary container (like a hugh Thermos bottle) that weighs 70–160 lbs when filled with liquid oxygen stored at −297°F. Each pound of liquid oxygen becomes 342 liters of gaseous oxygen. The stationary unit is used to transfill a portable container that weighs 5–14 lbs and provides 3–13 hours of oxygen flowing at 2 L/min. These systems are the most expensive and may cause fires, freezing burns, and injury due to high pressure if the liquid evaporates in a closed space, but they are the most practical alternative for the ambulatory patient.

Oxygen concentrators remove nitrogen from room air to produce variable concentrations of oxygen up to 96% at flows as high as 6 L/min. Because most concentrators are relatively stationary, a 50-foot tubing can be used to give the child mobility within the home. Refilling is unnecessary, but routine maintenance is required.

HAZARDS AND TOXICITY OF OXYGEN THERAPY

Parenchymal Pulmonary Oxygen Toxicity. Like any drug, oxygen may cause major complications. Exposure to high inspired oxygen concentrations over long periods of time produces clinical dysfunction and pathologic changes similar to adult respiratory distress syndrome. A reasonable attitude is to assume that concentrations over 50% for more than 2 days may produce toxic changes. In practice, such concentrations are rarely maintained at the level of the trachea without an endotracheal or tracheotomy tube.

Bronchopulmonary Dysplasia. Bronchopulmonary dysplasia is a chronic lung disease that follows the respiratory distress syndrome in some premature neonates as a result of high positive airway pressures, overdistention of lung, and increased FiO_2. The FiO_2 should be restricted to minimize the severity of brochopulmonary dysplasia but always sufficient to prevent hypoxemia and to provide an appropriate margin of safety.

Absorption Atelectasis. Nitrogen helps to stent alveoli that tend to collapse. When high concentrations of inspired oxygen approaching 100% are sustained for a period of hours (only with an artificial airway), nitrogen is rinsed out of alveoli and oxygen is absorbed from underventilated and nonventilated alveoli that are more predisposed to collapse. Absorption atelectasis is negligible with the administration of 90% rather than 100% oxygen, positive airway pressure with positive end-expiratory pressure (PEEP), and effective chest physiotherapy and suctioning.

Acute Effects on the Airway and Central Nervous System. Reversible ciliary dysfunction, impaired mucus clearance, cough, dyspnea, and substernal pain develop after healthy volunteers receive 100% oxygen for several hours. Similarly, reversible neurologic problems, such as paresthesia, nausea, vertigo, muscle twitching, decreased level of consciousness, and even seizures, occur after several hours of exposure to at least 2 atmospheres of hyperbaric oxygen.

Retinopathy of Prematurity. Immature retinal vessels constrict in response to a high PaO_2 and may cause irreversible ischemic damage to the retina. The FiO_2 should be regulated carefully to maintain a normal rather than an elevated PaO_2 in neonates who have or may have immature retinal vessels (all infants less than 36 weeks postconceptual age [PCA], 20% at 40 weeks PCA, and none after 44 weeks PCA). In all cases, the appropriate margin of safety that supplemental oxygen provides to avoid hypoxemia must be considered as a higher priority.

SUGGESTED READING

1. Aloan CA: Respiratory Care of the Newborn. Philadelphia, J.B. Lippincott, 1991.
2. Dorsch JA, Dorsch SE: Understanding Anesthesia Equipment. Baltimore, Williams & Wilkins, 1994.
3. Koff PB, Eitzman D, Neu J: Neonatal and Pediatric Respiratory Care. St. Louis, C.V. Mosby, 1993.
4. Luce JM, Pierson DJ, Tyler MI: Intensive Respiratory Care. Philadelphia, W.B. Saunders, 1993.
5. Scanlon C, Spearman CB, Sheldon RL, et al: Egan's Fundamentals of Respiratory Therapy. St. Louis, Mosby-Year Book, 1990.
6. Shapiro BA: Oxygen therapy. In Clinical Application of Respiratory Care, 4th ed. St. Louis, Mosby-Year Book, 1991.
7. West JB: Pulmonary Pathophysiology—The Essentials. Baltimore, Williams & Wilkins, 1982.

COMMENTARY

by Daniel V. Schidlow, M.D.

Oxygen is one of the most effective and misunderstood therapeutic agents. Its effects can be easily measured, dosages can be rationally calculated, and its benefits are clearly perceived. Yet the use of oxygen is often plagued with irrational decisions and undue concerns.

The prescription of oxygen therapy may engender feelings of anxiety or despair. Patients with cystic fibrosis, for example, often view this type of treatment as the herald of irreversible progression toward death. Discontinuation of oxygen administration becomes a much anticipated rite of passage for children with bronchopulmonary dysplasia, and reinstitution of such treatment causes great anxiety among parents. Toxicity is a concern to health professionals that may lead to premature discontinuation of therapy. More damage is done, however, by insufficient than by excessive use, especially in the treatment of chronic lung diseases. Failure to treat appropriately chronic or recurrent hypoxemia leads to serious consequences, ranging from easy fatigability and headaches to stunted growth, cor pulmonale, and heart failure.

Growing numbers of children supported by some type of technology are seen at popular vacation spots and amusement megaparks. Camps for technology-dependent children exist in several locations in the continental United States. Moreover, children with chronic lung disease travel by plane with increasing frequency. Commercial airplanes fly at altitudes of 30,000 feet or more. The cabin is adjusted to a barometric pressure equivalent to 6,000–8,000 feet in altitude. The ambient oxygen at such pressures falls considerably below that at sea level. The partial pressure of oxygen in blood of individuals who are already hypoxemic at sea level can become dangerously low during air travel.

Patients who receive ongoing oxygen therapy must ensure its continuance both aboard aircrafts and on the ground. Patients with chronic lung disease who are unsure of their need for oxygen can undergo preflight testing by inhaling oxygen-poor air mixtures under supervision in pulmonary function laboratories.

Airline carriers do not provide ground services, as a rule. Patients are expected to make their own arrangements for durable medical equipment to ensure that oxygen is available at the airports of departure and destination. Many companies that supply such equipment have branches or connections with other companies in several states.

Patients are not allowed to take their own oxygen sources aboard planes. Arrangments must be made with the airline at least 2 days in advance of travel to obtain inflight oxygen. Such requests, which are reviewed and cleared by the carrier's medical department, require a medical certificate stating the flow of oxygen required (most devices aboard airlines provide only two settings, flows of 2 or 4 L/min).

Most airlines provide oxygen for only 3 or 4 hours at a time at the flows mentioned above. Larger requirements call for additional tanks and space and may add a prohibitive cost for most travelers. Nonstop, direct flights should be booked whenever possible. Intermediate stops may be necessary during long trips to renew the supply.

With the exception of a modestly stocked emergency kit, airplanes do not carry medical supplies, nor do they have qualified personnel to attend to complex medical issues. It is advisable, therefore, to take along someone who is knowledgeable about the child's care as well as appropriate supplies to ensure the patient's safety and comfort.

Readers interested in more details are referred to the excellent publications listed below:

Gong H Jr: Advising pulmonary patients about commercial air travel. J Respir Dis 11:484–504, 1990.

Liebman J, Lucas R, Moss A, et al: Airline travel for children with chronic pulmonary disease. Pediatrics 57:408–410, 1976.

43

HOME CARE OF VENTILATOR-ASSISTED CHILDREN

Howard B. Panitch, M.D., and Susan M. Kolb, R.N., M.S.N

With the growth of subspecialties in pediatric critical care and neonatology, sicker and younger patients are surviving life-threatening illnesses in greater numbers. For many of these patients, however, recovery is either incomplete or protracted. Often such patients require extended mechanical ventilator assistance and occupy tertiary care beds when the required level of care is no longer acute.

This situation represents not only poor use of a limited resource—the pediatric intensive care bed—but also suboptimal care for the patient. In an intensive care unit a child's life cannot approach normality despite the best efforts of the health care team. To remedy this situation, home care for infants and children requiring extended mechanical ventilation has become an alternative.

To achieve maximal success and safety in home care of a ventilator-assisted patient, a multidisciplinary team, including a hospital-based physician, nurse, social worker, and community-based physician, must work with the family toward a common goal.

The objectives of home care for a ventilator-assisted child are (1) to extend life and enhance its quality; (2) to reduce morbidity; (3) to improve physiologic function; (4) to achieve normal growth and development; and (5) to reduce health care costs. Weaning from mechanical ventilation cannot be a goal of home-based programs if any of the above objectives is compromised. Changes in ventilatory support must be based solely on clinical and physiologic assessment and not influenced by pressures from families or administrative personnel. Often the community practitioner, who may have the most personal contact with the patient, is the best person to determine when the level of support can be decreased. This chapter demystifies home care of ventilator-assisted patients with chronic illnesses.

HISTORICAL OVERVIEW AND PATIENT SELECTION

The practice of sending patients home on mechanical ventilators originated during the polio epidemics of the 1940s and 1950s. The motivation was no different from current concerns: lack of intensive care beds, an unacceptably high cost of care for hospital-bound patients, and a negative impact on psychosocial development associated with prolonged hospitalizaiton. The development of the subspecialties of neonatology and pediatric intensive care in the 1960s resulted in an increased survival rate of critically ill neonates and children with respiratory insufficiency, congenital heart disease, and severe neurologic disease. In 1982 the Surgeon General's Workshop on Children with Handicaps and Their Families recognized the special needs of ventilator-dependent children and called for development of community programs to help families care for their children at home.

Medical conditions for which home mechanical ventilation may be considered are listed in Table 1. Safe and successful discharges depend on various criteria:

TABLE 1. Medical Conditions for Which Home Mechanical Ventilation May Be Used

Congenital abnormalities
Congenital heart defects
Tracheobronchomalacia
Tracheoesophageal malformations
Diaphragmatic hernia
Chest malformations
Pulmonary parenchymal diseases
Chronic respiratory insufficiency
Bronchopulmonary dysplasia
Neuromuscular and neurologic diseases
Primary hypoventilation
Myopathies
Spinal cord injury
Botulism
Metabolic diseases

1. Whatever the underlying disease, the patient must be medically stable and not require frequent ventilator adjustments. Table 2 lists medical criteria that have to be met by patients considered for home ventilation. These are general guidelines; eligibility must be determined individually. Some underlying illnesses (e.g., spinal cord injury or progressive neuromuscular disease) may require lifelong ventilator support, whereas others, such as respiratory insufficiency accompanying bronchopulmonary dysplasia or congenital heart disease, may eventually allow either partial or complete discontinuation of mechanical ventilaton.

TABLE 2. Medical Criteria for Home Ventilator Patients[1,3]

Children with pulmonary (parenchymal) abnormalities
Clinical
Positive trend on growth curve (weight)
Stamina for periods of play
Freedom from frequent respiratory infections and fever
Medically stable with optimal ventilation
Physiologic
Stable airway
$PaO_2 \geq 60$ torr in $FiO_2 < 0.4$
$PaCO_2 < 50$ torr
Frequent ventilator changes not required (unless weaning)
Children with no underlying lung disease
Physiologic
$PaO_2 \geq 70$ torr in room air
$PaCO_2 < 45$ torr

PaO_2 = partial pressure of oxygen in arterial blood; FiO_2 = fractional concentration of oxygen in inspired gas; $PaCO_2$ = partial pressure of carbon dioxide in alveolar gas.

2. The family must desire to take their child home with a ventilator and be willing to learn the details of care necessary for safe home care. It is not necessary that the family consist of two parents. We have successfully discharged patients to single-parent families, guardians, and other caretakers, provided that a second adult has learned to care for the child and serves as a back-up or support person. Family members must have good judgment-making skills and be willing to help with care of the patient at home as well as with discharge planning and selection of other caregivers. Even with 24-hour nursing coverage, illness or inclement weather may result in missed nursing shifts, which require that family members care for the child.

3. The home environment must be adequate, with running water, a working telephone, adequate heat and electricity, and enough space to accommodate the child, the equipment, and all caregivers. When space is scarce, innovative solutions are necessary. A child's room need not be a bedroom. Often the living room or a room near the kitchen is converted into the child's living space so that the child may be present for family activities. In addition, the caretaker can prepare meals or formula or clean equipment while keeping the child in sight, and the family can have privacy while nurses care for the child. If the child is wheelchair-bound, handicapped ramps and accessways must be made.

4. Adequate insurance coverage is mandatory. Without nearly 100% reimbursement for equipment and nursing services, the financial burden on the family becomes an obstacle to home care. Hidden costs—such as the increase in utility and telephone bills, prescription medications, special formulas or nutritional supplements no longer covered by insurance plans, or loss of income of a family member who becomes a caregiver—place heavy, at times prohibitive, financial strain on families.

5. Community support is integral to the successful discharge of a ventilator-assisted patient. Resources necessary to support home care programs include occupational, physical, and speech therapy and early intervention programs. Families should have access to a pharmacy that is open 7 days/week for long hours, to a durable medical equipment company with a short response time for evaluation of equipment

failure, and to a local emergency department where the patient can be stabilized for transfer in case of emergency. In addition, an efficient system for collecting and transporting laboratory samples and a laboratory with a rapid response time are also important in caring for home ventilator patients. Perhaps the most important community link to the tertiary care center for such patients, however, is the community physician.

ROLE OF THE COMMUNITY PHYSICIAN

The involvement of the community physician varies, depending on the needs of the child, the arrangement made with the hospital-based team, and the physician's availability, type of practice, and training.

The child who requires 24-hour ventilator assistance cannot "drop into the office" for well-child care or for acute emergencies; the community physician must make home visits for vaccinations, check-ups, and acute illnesses. Physicians in solo practice commonly cite such demands as a reason not to accept a ventilator-dependent patient into their practice. In addition, physicians participating in health organizations with a fee structure that does not take into account home visits may have to negotiate special reimbursement for home care.

The community physician should be identified early in the discharge planning of any ventilator-assisted patient, not at the last minute when the child is ready to go home. In this way, the community physician may contribute to the discharge plan, add valuable insight into family dynamics, and come to an agreement with the hospital-based team about his or her degree of involvement in the ongoing monitoring and care of the patient. Issues such as who recommends changes in medications, ventilator settings, and feeding regimens should be established and incorporated into a written plan before the patient is discharged. The role of the primary doctor varies among individual patients and programs.

Goldberg and Monahan[2] examined the roles and perceptions of physicians caring for ventilator-assisted children. Of 51 physicians who responded to their questionnaire, all agreed that such patients require a primary care physician; 47 believed that this person should be a community-based physician. The group consisted of general pediatricians, family practitioners, intensivists, pulmonologists, and various other medical and surgical subspecialists. Of the 51, 29 considered themselves to be the primary care physician; they included among their responsibilities acute care (11/29), ventilator management (7/29), and well-child care (5/29).

The community physician should receive a discharge summary of the patient's hospitalization along with a written home care plan. A summary also should be sent to the child's local emergency department when it is not located in the tertiary care center of origin. Nursing, physical therapy, and respiratory care summaries also are sent to the appropriate agencies.

Although a child's parents are the ultimate caregivers, all families must receive some degree of support from nursing or other trained personnel. In our program, all families receive 24-hour nursing services for the first week that the child is at home after discharge. Most irregularities in the child's medical routine are likely to surface during this transition period. The added help and reassurance of professional caregivers may mean the difference between a successful discharge or prompt readmission into the hospital. After the first week, nursing coverage is cut back to 8–16 hours/day, depending on the patient's needs. Thus, parents are completely responsible for the care of their child as well as the running of the household for the remainder of the day. Although other programs foster complete independence from outside nursing care, we have found this to be an unrealistic goal. Providing at least 8 hours of care helps the family to assume a semblance of normal life and guarantees safety for the child.

Nursing agencies and equipment companies are responsible for supplying competent professionals who are familiar with the care of technology-dependent children. The nursing agency coordinates nursing coverage and facilitates communication with other disciplines. Nurses and respiratory therapists from the equipment company provide ongoing assessments and services as set forth in a written plan of treatment. The care plan, which also includes medication schedules, ventilator settings, and parameters for changing therapy, is reviewed periodically by the physician. Any changes to the care plan, whether by verbal or written order, must be documented and signed by the treating physician. In a typical protocol, orders taken by telephone are written by the nurse, mailed to the physician for his or her signature, and returned to the home medical chart. The respiratory therapist checks all equipment to ensure proper working order and assesses the respiratory status of the patient. Reports are sent to the treating physician, including the type of equipment used by the patient, respiratory rate, a description of the breath sounds, and results of oximetry or capnography.

A challenge of home-based care is to monitor the patient adequately without creating a "mini-ICU" in the home environment. With careful planning and a few pieces of equipment, this goal can be achieved. For instance, a pulse oximeter is preferable to an apnea monitor, because more information about the patient can be obtained. The oximeter can be used for three purposes: (1) as a routine monitoring device when the patient is stable; (2) as an aid in adjusting ventilator settings during acute illnesses; and (3) as a device to monitor weaning of the patient if appropriate. Unless the patient is actively weaning or "sprinting" off the ventilator for periods of time, a PCO_2 monitor (end-tidal capnograph) need not remain in the home. Instead, capnography may be performed on a weekly or biweekly basis by a respiratory therapist, as the patient's stability warrants.

Because ventilator-assisted children are often not mobile, laboratory evaluation must be done at home. The family should be provided with needles, syringes, and tubes for blood sampling, as well as suction traps for obtaining samples of sputum or nasal washings. A system of sample collection and transportation as well as prompt notification of the appropriate caregivers must be organized; typically the nurse or a phlebotomist from an outside laboratory serves this function. Frequently, the physician in the community will write standing orders for a laboratory at a community hospital to simplify matters.

The degree of the community physician's involvement in interpretation of the laboratory tests and results of oximetry and capnography should be determined for each patient based on the physician's preference. Conversely, the hospital-based specialist must be flexible regarding how closely the ventilator program follows the child. Our involvement ranges from receipt and interpretation of all tests to providing consultation to community physicians in their management of patients. In any case, the hospital-based home ventilation program must be accessible to the community physician, maintaining an active dialogue and providing timely back-up.

WHAT TO DO WHEN A VENTILATOR-ASSISTED PATIENT IS SICK

By the time a ventilator-assisted child is ready for discharge from the hospital, various methods of assessment have been established. Table 3 lists the most common reasons for calls from families about home care problems. Problems relating to equipment malfunctions are handled by the supplying vendor. As a safeguard, however, all patients who require continuous ventilator support should have two complete ventilators and circuits in the home as well as resuscitation equipment.

Changes in the status of the child require that a complete evaluation be performed at home. An accurate history and physical examination should include respiratory and heart rate, current weight, oxyhemoglobin saturation, breath sounds and presence of retractions, and quantity and quality of tracheal secretions. Because such measurements are followed frequently and charted by nurses and parents, acute changes or new trends can be identified quickly. Appropriate laboratory tests can be obtained and treatment instituted. Usually, all this can be done at home. Frequently, ventilator changes are made to increase support during an acute illness without having to readmit the child to the hospital. Adequacy of ventilator support can be followed by oximetry, capnography, and occasionally by blood gas determination. If caregivers or parents become uncomfortable with the child's

TABLE 3. Approach to the Most Common Problems of Mechanically Ventilated Children

Reason	Assessment	Disposition
Fever	? Respiratory involvement	No: Antipyretics ? Home visit Telephone follow-up Yes: See below
Increase or change in secretions	Purulent and increased	Sputum Gram stain and culture Complete blood count with differential Antibiotics Monitor respiratory status (SaO_2, $ETCO_2$)
	Thicker and decreased ? ↑ Work of breathing	Check humidification of system See below
↑ Work of breathing; retractions	? Crackles ? Wheezes	Antibiotics Bronchodilators Check SaO_2, $ETCO_2$ Adjust ventilator settings Consider hospital admission
"Not acting right"	? SaO_2, $ETCO_2$? Electrolytes ? Excessive weight gain ? Drug toxicity	Increase ventilator support Electrolyte replacement Diuretics Dose adjustments
Nutritional	Excessive weight gain Hepatomegaly, tachypnea, tachycardia, ↓ SaO_2	Reduce caloric intake Diuretics
	Inadequate weight gain	Increase caloric intake Increase ventilator support
Immunization schedules		Complete in timely manner
General pediatric questions		

SaO_2 = oxyhemoglobin saturation; $ETCO_2$ = end-tidal carbon dioxide.

condition, hospital admission should be arranged promptly.

Once treatment has been instituted at home, the child may require frequent home visits by the local physician as well as close telephone contact between the hospital-based team and both the family and the physician. The family and community physician should be assured of the availability of hospitalization at any time during the illness, if the child's condition worsens.

In the patient whose underlying illness and medical progress permit, weaning from mechanical ventilation also can be achieved at home. Whether weaning is achieved by gradual reduction in support (i.e., a decrease in the number of ventilator breaths/minute) or by gradual discontinuation of mechanical ventilation for longer periods of time ("sprinting") must be determined individually. When the patient is already receiving a low number of ventilator breaths, sprinting may be the preferred method of weaning. When ventilator support is decreased, more frequent monitoring is necessary to ensure that the patient can tolerate weaning. Respiratory rate, work of breathing, and oximetry should be assessed and documented. Capnography before and at the end of a sprint is useful in determining adequacy of ventilation. Besides acute changes in ventilation and oxygenation, stamina for periods of play and continued weight gain must be assessed after a decrease in mechanical ventilator support. **Even when a child can maintain normal oximetry and capnography values, decrease in activity, reduction in growth velocity, somnolence, and increased work of breathing are signs that further attempts at weaning should be forestalled and ventilator support should be increased.**

Caring for a ventilator-assisted patient can be extremely rewarding. Helping a ventilator-assisted child achieve independence for daily activities and weaning of a child from ventilatory support provide great satisfaction. A solid partnership among family, professional caregivers, and the hospital-based team enables the community physician to assume a central role in the care of a child with a chronic disease and ensures necessary support in case of emergencies. Conversely, familes can rely on a well-known caregiver, who provides a vital link to the tertiary care system.

SUGGESTED READING

1. Goldberg AI, Faure EAM, Vaughn CJ, et al: Home care for life-supported persons: An approach to program development. J Pediatr 104:785–795, 1984.
2. Goldberg AI, Monahan CA: Home health care for children assisted by mechanical ventilation: The physician's perspective. J Pediatr 114:378–383, 1989.
3. Home mechanical ventilation of pediatric patients: Official statement of the AmericanThoracic Society. Am Rev Respir Dis 141:258–259, 1990.

44

IMMUNIZATIONS

David S. Smith, M.D.

No area of pediatrics is developing more rapidly than immunization. A new wave of vaccine development, due largely to biotechnology, is already a major promise for the next century. Thus, this chapter makes no attempt to be all-inclusive or to forecast the future availability of effective vaccines for cytomegalovirus, respiratory syncytial virus, parainfluenza and rotaviruses, group B streptococci, or mycoplasma. **The purpose is to bring the reader up to date on available and perhaps soon-to-be-available vaccines that have an impact on diseases of the respiratory tract.**

No vaccine is completely safe or completely effective. Benefits range from partial to complete protection. Risks of immunization may be trivial and common; others may be rare but serious. Some vaccines contain highly defined antigens, such as the polysaccharide of *Hemophilus influenzae,* type b; others have complex and incompletely defined antigens, such as killed *Bordetella pertussis* or live attenuated viruses.

Physicians providing immunizations to children should maintain careful and complete records. Familiarity with the package insert is mandatory. Attention to proper storage is crucial. The frequent changes in the schedules for immunizations should be reviewed in reports from the Committee on Infectious Diseases (Red Book) of the American Academy of Pediatrics and the Advisory Committee on Immunization Practices (ACIP) of the United States Public Health Service.

MEASLES

Many physicians have seen measles for the first time during outbreaks in the past few years, despite 20 or more years of practice. Within 5 years of licensure of measles vaccine in 1963, the incidence of the disease was reduced by 95%. In 1983 only 1,500 cases were reported. Since that time, however, the incidence has increased annually. In 1990 nearly 28,000 cases were reported in the United States. During 1989–1991 there were 132 suspected deaths from measles. Most cases of measles have occurred in urban areas among unvaccinated children of preschool age. In 1991 increasing numbers of infants with measles were younger than 15 months of age; some were as young as 6 months of age. Outbreaks of disease also have involved children and young adults from 5–19 years of age, most of whom had been previously immunized. Several outbreaks have occurred in high schools and on college campuses. This experience has led to reassessment of previous recommendations for immunization. By 1993, however, as as result either of improved vaccination coverage or the periodic cyclicity noted in the prevaccine era with outbreaks of measles, the incidence had dropped dramatically.

Measles is a highly contagious systemic disease with a striking propensity for producing a predictable pattern of symptoms. The evolution of the rash in a cephalocaudad distribution with conjunctivitis, coryza, cough, and fever accompanied by a pathognomonic enanthem (Koplik spots) results in a classic clinical picture.

Few, if any, children experience measles without a harsh, nonproductive cough that often reflects inflammatory changes of laryngotracheitis with stridor and croup. Complications occur frequently, most often in the middle ear or lungs. Diarrhea is frequently seen in younger patients, and abdominal pain, rarely accompanied by acute appendicitis, is common. Encephalitis is a devastating complication seen in approximately 1 in 1,000 cases. Recent outbreaks within major cities have been complicated by mortality rates greater than 1%. Subacute sclerosing panencephalitis (SSPE), a result of persistent infection with measles virus, has been extremely rare since the measles vaccine was introduced.

Measles virus may be isolated from respiratory secretions, but the technology is difficult and usually not available. Serum IgM antibodies are detectable in most patients for 3–4 weeks after the rash has faded. We have used immunofluorescence and detection of multinucleated giant cells in nasal secretions for rapid diagnosis. Patients should be isolated for 4 days after the onset of rash. Exceptions include immunocompromised patients who shed virus for the duration of the illness, which may be prolonged.

Present evidence suggests that the recent increase in cases of measles is due to poor immunization rates in preschool children in urban areas. In addition, primary vaccine failure occurs in approximately 5% of infants immunized at 15 months or older. Evidence for waning immunity is incompletely substantiated, although most outbreaks in adolescents and college students have occurred in previously immunized individuals. In the prevaccine era the diagnosis of measles in the first 6 months of life was virtually unknown. Measles in an infant aged 6 months to 1 year of life was rare and usually appeared to be modified by incomplete transplacental immunity. **Recent experience suggests that the present generation of women whose immunity to measles is vaccine-related are conferring limited protection to their infants.**

Measles Virus Vaccine

Measles vaccine is a live attenuated virus vaccine (Moraten) developed by multiple passages in chick embryo cells. The reconstituted vaccine should be protected from light, stored at 2–8°C, and used within 8 hours. Effectiveness of the vaccine was enhanced in 1979 with addition of an improved stabilizer. Measles vaccine should be administered subcutaneously.

Until recently measles vaccination was given at 15 months of age. When risk of exposure is low, initiating immunization at 15 months may still be more effective than beginning at an earlier age. In 1989 the Committee on Infectious Diseases of the American Academy of Pediatrics and the Advisory Committee on Immunization Practices of the United States Public Health Service recommended a change from a one-dose to a two-dose schedule for measles immunization. Moreover, in epidemics immunization of infants may be started at 6 months of age. Infants should be revaccinated at 15 months. Infants vaccinated on or after their first birthday do not need a second dose until entry into elementary, middle, or junior high schools.

Measles vaccine is available as a monovalent preparation (M), in combination with rubella (MR), and in combination with mumps and rubella (MMR). MMR should be used in routine vaccination programs, although monovalent measles vaccine (M) may be used in infants at 6 months of age during an outbreak.

From 5–15% of children receiving measles vaccine develop fever of 39.4°C (103°F) 6 days after immunization. Approximately 1 in 20 children develops a transient rash. Fewer than 1 in a million vaccinees have developed encephalitis, an incidence lower than in control populations with encephalitis of unknown etiology. Recent data suggest that simple febrile seizures occur with increased frequency after vaccination with measles vaccine in children with a history of previous seizures or with first-degree family members with seizure disorders. **No associations have been made with permanent brain damage in children who develop seizures after immunization.**

Indications and contraindications for measles vaccination are outlined in Table 1.

PERTUSSIS

Pertussis vaccine prepared from killed whole-cell *Bordetella pertussis* organisms has been

TABLE 1. Indications and Contraindications for Measles Vaccination*

Group	Remarks
Indications	
Unvaccinated, no history of measles (≥15 mo of age)	A two-dose schedule is recommended for infants born after 1956. The first dose is recommended at 15 mo; the second at entry to middle or junior high school. In localities where revaccination at school entry is mandated by law, such revaccination substitutes for the preceding recommendation.
Children 15 mo of age	Routine immunization with MMR
Children 12–15 mo of age in areas of recurrent measles transmission	Initiate immunization.
Children 6–15 mo of age during epidemics	Immunize; if vaccinated before the first birthday, revaccination at 15 mo is necessary.
Children 11–12 yr of age who have received 1 dose of measles vaccine at ≥12 mo	Reimmunize.
Students in college and other post-high school institutions who have received 1 dose of measles vaccine at 12 mo	Reimmunize.
History of vaccination before 12 mo	Consider unvaccinated and immunize.
Unknown vaccine, 1963–1967	Consider unvaccinated and immunize.
Further attenuated or unknown vaccine given with immunoglobulin	Consider unvaccinated and immunize.
Egg allergy, anaphylactic	Immunize; no reactions likely.
Tuberculosis	Immunize; vaccine does not exacerbate.
Measles exposure within 72 h	Immunization may protect (or immunoglobulin can be given).
HIV seropositive	Immunize.
Contraindications	
Pregnancy	Theoretical risk of fetal damage.
Anaphylactic to egg ingestion	Vaccinate with caution after skin testing.
Anaphylactic allergy to neomycin	Vaccine contains neomycin.
Immunoglobulin within 3 mo	Interference with immune response.
Compromised immunity (except symptomatic HIV infection)	Possibility of severe infection with vaccine virus.

* Report of the Committee on Infectious Diseases, 22nd ed. American Academy of Pediatrics, 1991.
MMR = measles, mumps, and rubella; HIV = human immunodeficiency virus.

widely used and credited with reducing the morbidity and mortality from whooping cough since the early 1950s. An inverse relationship between age and mortality is observed with the clinical disease. Complications include pneumonia, seizures, and encephalopathy. Basic pathology in pertussis is the destruction of ciliated respiratory epithelium. Studies suggest that a major unrecognized reservoir for pertussis infection is present in adolescents and adults. The disease does not produce optimal, long-lasting immunity, although children recovered from culture-proven pertussis do not need further doses of the vaccine. Atypical cases occur in previously immunized individuals. Immunity to the organism has been poorly understood. Components of the present whole-cell vaccine include various antigens that may play a role in the pathogenesis of disease but may not be important in providing immunity to colonization and disease. Thus, the present whole-cell vaccine undoubtedly contains reactive components that are irrevelant to protection

Because pertussis cells in combination with diphtheria and tetanus toxoids are adsorbed onto an aluminum salt, the preparation should be administered intramuscularly, beginning at approximately 8 weeks of age. An additional 4 doses should be given at 4, 6, and 15–18 months and at 4–6 years. Immunization is discontinued in children 7 years or older. Fever after vaccination occurs in nearly 50% of children; administration of acetaminophen (15 mg/kg/dose) may minimize this response. Reduction of the diphtheria-tetanus-pertussis (DTP) dose of 0.5 ml in an attempt to lessen side effects is not recommended, because ultimate protection has not been determined and the effect on incidence of serious reactions is not known.

Adverse reactions following pertussis (DTP) vaccination include:

Seizures. Most seizures occur within 48 hours of vaccination and usually display the characteristics of febrile convulsions, i.e., brevity, generalization, and self-limitation. Incidence of seizures is approximately 1:1,750 immunizations. Sequelae or increased incidence of afebrile seizures in subsequent years has not been noted.

Unusual Crying. Most persistent crying within 48 hours of immunization appears to be related to pain at the site of injection. Rarely (1:1,000) an unusual, high-pitched cry is observed and is poorly understood. Sequelae have not been reported.

Collapse. A shocklike episode with hypotonia and hyporesponsiveness has been recorded in 1:1,750 vaccinations. Recent data derived from children with history of such an event have revealed no neurologic or developmental dysfunction.

Although numerous adverse events temporally related to the administration of pertussis vaccine have had a profound effect on the lives of families, physicians, and manufacturers, most have not been proved. Infantile myoclonic seizures, sudden infant death syndrome, severe acute neurologic illness, and permanent brain damage have been among the most damaging and controversial. Multiple studies in the United States and in England have failed to prove a relationship between pertussis vaccine and these tragic events. Nevertheless, it is recommended that before the administration of pertussis vaccine parents be questioned about possible adverse events following previous doses. Precautions and contraindications to further use of pertussis immunization include:

1. Encephalopathy within 7 days associated with prolonged seizures, alterations of consciousness, or focal neurologic signs
2. Seizure with or without fever within 3 days
3. Inconsolable crying or screaming for 3 or more hours
4. Collapse or shock within 48 hours
5. Fever within 48 hours in excess of 40.5°C
6. Anaphylaxis: extremely rare

In children with progressive neurologic disorders and developmental delay, decisions should be made on an individual basis, but use of DTP vaccine should be deferred. Children and infants with a history of seizures or with conditions that predispose to seizures or neurologic deterioration should not be routinely immunized. At or before the first birthday consideration should be given to use of DTP or DT.

In 1992 concerns for the safety of the whole-cell pertussis vaccine led to the licensing of two acellular pertussis vaccines: (1) ACEL-IMUNE, prepared by Lederle Laboratories, and (2) TRIPEDIA, manufactured by Connaught Laboratories. **Both vaccines are combined with diphtheria and tetanus toxoids and approved only as the fourth and fifth doses; neither is licensed for use as the initial three-dose series for infants and children, regardless of age.** Whole-cell DTP should continue to be used for the initial three-dose series and remains an acceptable alternative for the fourth and fifth doses. Mild systemic reactions, such as drowsiness, irritability, and fever, appear to be less common after use of the acellular product; severe neurologic events, such as prolonged convulsions or encephalopathy, have not been reported after administration of the acellular preparation. Booster responses appear to be equivalent to those observed after use of whole-cell product.

Hemophilus influenzae, type b

Hemophilus influenzae is a small gram-negative coccobacillus that may demonstrate pleomorphism on smear, particularly when exposed to antibiotics. In the prevaccine era approximately 1/200 children experienced meningitis, pneumonia, cellulitis, pyogenic arthritis, pericarditis, epiglottitis, or other serious manifestations of *H. influenzae* infection in the first 5 years of life. Type b organisms account for 95% of all strains responsible for invasive disease. Mucosal infections occur frequently when the organisms spread from colonization

TABLE 2. *Hemophilus influenzae* Type b Conjugate Vaccines

Manufacturer	Abbreviation	Trade Name	Carrier Protein
Connaught Laboratories	PRP-D*	Prohibit	Diphtheria toxoid
Lederle-Praxis	HbOC†‡§	HIBTITER	CRM 197 (a nontoxic mutant diphtheria toxin)
Merck, Sharp & Dohme	PRP-OMP†§	PedvaxHIB	OMP (an outer membrane protein complex of *Neisseria meningitidis*)
Pasteur Merieux Vaccines (distributed by SmithKline Beecham and Connaught Laboratories)	PRP-T†	ActHIB	Tetanus toxoid

* PRP-D is recommended by the American Academy of Pediatrics only for infants 12 mo of age or older.
† The HbOC, PRP-OMP, and PRP-T are recommended for infants beginning at approximately 2 mo of age.
‡ HbOC is also available as a combination vaccine with DPT (TETRAMUNE).
§ Not interchangeable for the primary immunizations series.

of surfaces to contiguous areas, such as the sinuses or middle ear.

Antibodies to the capsular polysaccharide (polyribosylribitol phosphate) play a pivotal role in host defense against infection by *H. influenzae* type b (HIB). Initial attempts at production of a vaccine met with predictably poor antibody response in infants in the first 2 years of life when most cases of serious invasive disease occur in children. Polysaccharides directly activate B-lymphocytes without the stimulation of T-cells. B-lymphocytes in the infant respond poorly to polysaccharide antigens. Thus, the original purified type b capsular polysaccharide vaccine was ineffective in the first 2 years of life when it was needed most.

Because most protein antigens induce T-helper cell regulation of antibody synthesis as the result of T-cell involvement in the maturation, proliferation, and differentiation of subpopulations of B-cells, so-called conjugate vaccines were produced. By linking the *H. influenzae* type b capsular polysaccharide to a carrier protein, researchers were able to document both efficacy and safety in infants. Four vaccines are currently approved for use in infants beginning at 2 months of age (Tables 2 and 3).

H. influenzae type b vaccine may be given at the same time as DTP and oral polio vaccine. Unimmunized children from 12–14 months of age should receive a two-dose regimen at an interval of 2 months. Infants who were not immunized before 15 months or older and who have not reached their fifth birthday should receive a single dose. Children older than 5 years with anatomic or functional asplenia, Hodgkin disease, or other chronic illnesses known to be associated with increased risk of *H. influenzae* type b disease should be immunized with a single injection of vaccine. Unimmunized children who experience invasive

TABLE 3. Recommendations for *Hemophilus* Conjugate Vaccination in Children Immunized Beginning at 2–6 Months of Age

Vaccine Product at Initiation	Total No. of Doses to Be Administered	Currently Recommended Vaccine Regimens*
HbOC or PRP-T	4	3 doses at 2-mo intervals When feasible, same vaccine for doses 1–3 Fourth dose at 12–15 mo of age Any conjugate vaccine for dose 4†
PRP-OMP	3	2 doses at 2-mo intervals When feasible, same vaccine for doses 1–2 Third dose at 12–15 mo of age Any conjugate vaccine for dose 3†

* The HbOC, PRP-T, or PRP-OMP should be given in a separate syringe and at a separate site from other immunizations. HbOC is also available as a combination vaccine with DTP (HbOC-DTP). This combination can be used in infants scheduled to receive separate injections of DTP and HbOC.
† The safety and efficacy of PRP-OMP, PRP-D, PRP-T, and HbOC are likely to be equivalent in children 12 mo of age and older.

H. influenzae type b disease in the first 2 years of life should receive the vaccine according to the age-appropriate schedule, beginning 1–2 months after the acute illness.

Administration of conjugate vaccines has not been accompanied by serious reactions. No increased incidence of invasive disease has been observed in the first 2 weeks following administration of the vaccine.

BACILLE CALMETTE-GUÉRIN VACCINE

Two bacille Calmette-Guérin (BCG) vaccines are available in the United States: (1) the Tice strain for percutaneous administration (Bionetics Research, Chicago, IL, and Antigen Supply House, Northridge, CA) and (2) the Glaxo strain for intradermal use (Quad Pharmaceuticals, Indianapolis, IN). Each of the vaccines is a live attenuated derivative of the original *Mycobacterium bovis* strain (first used by Calmette and Guérin) from a cow with tuberculous mastitis. The live vaccine was first administered orally to infants in 1921. Controversy concerning its use increased in 1930 when 72 children in Germany died of tuberculosis after receiving an oral BCG vaccine contaminated with virulent tubercle bacilli. Although over 2 billion individuals have received BCG and its use continues to be standard procedure throughout the world, neither the United States nor the Netherlands has adopted the vaccine on a widespread basis.

Although the immunologic mechanisms affording protection from tuberculosis by the use of BCG are incompletely understood, the vaccine does not prevent infection. Most authorities seem to agree that BCG vaccination of infants and young children offers protection against meningeal, cavitary, bone, and miliary forms of the disease. The duration of the protection is ill-defined but probably wanes over time.

Adverse Reactions and Contraindications for the Use of BCG Vaccine

Local ulceration at the site of injection and regional lymphadenitis occur in 1–10% of individuals. On rare occasions, osteomyelitis has been reported. Disseminated and fatal BCG infections have occurred in immunocompromised patients. Children receiving immunosuppressive drugs, including corticosteroids, should not be vaccinated, nor should children with suspected or known asymptomatic HIV infection. For populations at high risk of tuberculosis, however, the World Health Organization has recommended that asymptomatic infants infected with HIV be given BCG at birth or soon thereafter. BCG should not be given to children with burns or skin infections. Vaccination during pregnancy is not advised, although adverse effects on the fetus have not been described.

Recommendations for BCG Vaccination in the United States

The control of tuberculosis in the United States is still based on modern methods of preventive therapy, chemotherapy, and case detection. BCG vaccine should be considered in selected infants and children who have negative tuberculin skin tests but are at high risk for continuing intimate exposure to active sputum-positive tuberculosis when compliance with isoniazid prophylaxis is unlikely. In addition, vaccination is advised when the child is exposed to persons infected with drug-resistant tubercle bacilli.

BCG vaccination is followed by tuberculin skin test reactivity, usually ranging from 5–9 mm of induration. Reactions of 15 mm or more in diameter are likely to represent active tuberculosis. Reactivity diminishes over time. No reliable criteria differentiate a positive tuberculin reaction of 10 mm or more caused by a previous BCG vaccination from the natural disease.

INFLUENZA A AND B INACTIVATED VACCINE

Influenza viruses A and B are responsible for substantial morbidity and mortality in annual outbreaks of respiratory illness throughout the world. The broad spectrum of disease ranges from simple upper respiratory symptoms to a sepsislike illness in infants and laryngotracheobronchitis, pneumonia, acute myositis, and Reye syndrome in older children. Pulmonary complications are of particular concern in children with chronic lupus, cystic fibrosis, and bronchopulmonary dysplasia and in patients with sickle-cell disease, diabetes, chronic renal disease, and malignancies.

Influenza A viruses are classified by subtypes on the basis of two surface antigens: hemagglutinin (H) and neuraminidase (N). Immunity to the three subtypes of hemagglutinin (H1, H2, H3) appears to be important in modifying or preventing illness. Two subtypes of neuraminidase (N1, N2) contribute to the difficulties in acquiring natural immunity, because infection with a virus of one subtype provides little protection against viruses of another subtype. In addition, major changes (shifts) occur in influenza A antigens at intervals of 10 years or more. Minor alterations (drifts) are recognized almost annually in both influenza A and B viruses; over time, they expose the susceptibility of the population previously immunized by natural disease or by vaccination. Virologic surveillance has identified as many as 17 distinct variants of the two major influenza A subtypes (H1N1 and H3N2) in a community over a 15-year period. Influenza viruses have an uncanny ability to mutate with single amino acid alterations in surface antigens (drifts) or by major shifts resulting from gene rearrangement.

Inactivated influenza vaccine is made from highly purified, egg-grown viruses containing antigenic strains anticipated in the forthcoming epidemic. The vaccine is safe, immunogenic, and has few side effects. Two preparations are available: (1) an inactivated whole-virus vaccine containing intact viral particles and (2) a subvirion or so-called split vaccine, in which the lipid-containing membrane of the virus has been interrupted. The split vaccine is recommended for children younger than 13 years. Two doses are advised, administered with a 1-month interval. Efficacy of vaccination is from 50–95%; effectiveness in the first 6 months of life has not been documented.

Inactivated influenza vaccine is contraindicated in children known to have anaphylactic hypersensitivity to eggs. The vaccine is not recommended during acute febrile illness. Fever, malaise, and myalgia occur infrequently after vaccination, usually within 6–12 hours after administration. No increased frequency of Guillain-Barré syndrome has been noted with vaccines developed after 1976.

Influenza vaccine may be given to high-risk children simultaneously with MMR, *H. influenzae* b, pneumococcal, and oral polio vaccines. Vaccines should be given, however, at different sites. Influenza vaccine should not be given within 3 days after administration of pertussis vaccine.

An attenuated cold recombinant influenza vaccine, given intranasally, has recently been demonstrated to be immunogenic, nontransmissible, genetically stable, and well accepted. The inactivated preparation, however, remains the only currently available influenza virus vaccine.

PNEUMOCOCCAL VACCINES

Eighty-three pneumococcal serotypes have been identified. Fortunately, the 23-valent pneumococcal vaccine contains the serotypes responsible for nearly 100% of cases of meningitis and bacteremia in children and approximately 85% of cases of otitis media. **Unfortunately, as with the use of other polysaccharide antigens in the first 2 years of life, immune responses are limited at a time when infants are at greatest risk of invasive disease. In addition to the presence of serotype-specific antibodies and complement to opsonize the organism, the host depends heavily on functional phagocytes and an efficient spleen for defense against the pneumococcus.** Thus, various conditions affecting one or more of these mechanisms predispose the child to potentially serious disease caused by *Streptococcus pneumoniae.*

Management is complicated further by the emergence of strains of pneumococci that are highly resistant to antibiotic therapy. The development of a vaccine that will effectively immunize infants under 2 years of age rests with techniques such as conjugation of polysaccharide antigens to carrier proteins (e.g., diphtheria toxoid) to initiate T-cell responses.

Use of the present 23-valent polysaccharide pneumococcal vaccine is recommended for children 2 years of age and older who are at increased risk of invasive or serious pneumococcal disease (Table 4).

Pneumococcal vaccine should be given 2 weeks or more before an elective splenectomy.

TABLE 4. Recommendations for Pneumococcal Vaccine

Sickle-cell disease
Asplenia (anatomic or functional)
Conditions associated with immunosuppression
Cerebrospinal fluid leaks
Infection with human immunodeficiency virus (HIV)
Nephrotic syndrome or chronic renal failure

Similar timing should be observed before initiating chemotherapy in patients with cancer or patients receiving immunosuppressant therapy, as in organ transplantation. **Vaccination during chemotherapy or immunosuppression is not advised because of predictably poor antibody response.** Administration of the vaccine should be delayed for at least 3 months after therapy has been discontinued.

Use of pneumococcal polysaccharide vaccine is discouraged for the prevention of otitis media. In addition, no data suggest that upper or lower respiratory tract infections are affected by vaccination of healthy children in the United States. **Revaccination of high-risk children (younger than 10 years) should be considered after 3–5 years. Adverse reactions appear to be more common after revaccination of older children.** Such reactions are usually self-limited and not life-threatening. The risks of rare and infrequent reactions to revaccination should be balanced with risks of life-threatening pneumococcal diseases. **Use of pneumococcal vaccine should not replace daily antimicrobial prophylaxis in children with functional or anatomic asplenia.**

CHICKENPOX

Primary infection with the varicella-zoster virus in normal children most often results in a generalized pruritic vesicular rash with mild systemic symptoms. Complications are infrequent but may include secondary bacterial infection of skin lesions. Infrequently chickenpox is associated with encephalitis and cerebellar ataxia; most cases occur in children under 5 years of age, usually within 2–6 days after onset of rash. Although nearly one-half of children with chickenpox have mildly elevated concentrations of serum aspartate aminotransferase, clinical hepatitis is unusual. In children with higher levels of serum transaminases, differentiation from stage I Reye syndrome is difficult. Primary varicella pneumonia is rare in children, in contrast to adults, and usually resolves in 1–3 days.

Varicella-zoster virus is rarely recovered from respiratory secretions by culture. Fewer than 5% of oropharyngeal samples within 24 hours after onset of rash have been positive. Higher recovery rates have been realized by testing for varicella-zoster virus DNA by polymerase chain reaction. Varicella-zoster virus can be identified readily in vesicular lesions during the first 3–4 days in normal children. Chickenpox remains one of the most contagious diseases of childhood with secondary infection rates in susceptible household contacts approaching 90%.

Major morbidity and significant mortality may occur in older individuals and particularly in children with impaired cell-mediated immune responses. Pneumonia is the most common complication in adolescents and adults. Immunocompromised children are at high risk for a diffuse interstitial nodular pneumonia that usually develops within 3–7 days after onset of rash. Progression to respiratory failure has been reported in up to 25% of children with lymphoproliferative malignancies and solid tumors. Disseminated disease in high-risk children is also accompanied by hepatitis, encephalitis, nephritis, pancreatitis, and myocarditis as well as disseminated intravascular coagulation and thrombocytopenia. Risks of varicella are increased in children after bone marrow and other organ transplantation and in children with primary immunodeficiencies and acquired immunodeficiency syndrome (AIDS). Corticosteroid therapy for conditions other than malignancy or transplantation has not been associated with increased mortality, although fatal varicella has been reported with a dosage of prednisone of 2 mg/kg/day. Corticosteroid therapy, however, may be associated with more extensive eruptions and atypical morphology of lesions.

Varicella is uncommon during pregnancy, although the incidence appears to be increased in pregnant women who have recently emigrated from tropical climates. Fetal malformations, in addition to intrauterine growth retardation, occur with low incidence after first-trimester infections. Risks of second- and third-trimester infections are unknown and may not exist.

Immunizations

Passive immunization with high-titer varicella-zoster immune globulin (VZIG) has been possible for over 20 years. Administration of VZIG, which is available from the American Red Cross Blood Services, should be considered in the following clinical situations:

1. Hospitalized premature infants (<28-week gestation), regardless of maternal history of chickenpox.
2. Newborn infants whose mothers develop varicella within 5 days before or 2 days after delivery
3. Immunocompromised, susceptible children
4. Normal, susceptible adolescents and adults, including pregnant women
5. Hospitalized premature infants (>28-week gestation) born to susceptible mothers.

Further details about the administration of VZIG may be found in the American Academy of Pediatrics Red Book 1991.

A varicella vaccine has been tested for nearly two decades in Japan and for a shorter time in Europe and the United States in healthy children and adults and in children with cancer and chronic renal disease. With use of the live attenuated Oka strain, seroconversion rates of over 94% have been realized in healthy children. Adverse effects have been limited to temperature elevations in 5% or less of vaccinees, local discomfort at the injection site in up to 10%, and a generalized rash or rash surrounding the injection in approximately 5–10%. The eruption simulates mild varicella; usually 50 or fewer lesions are noted.

The major adverse systemic reaction to vaccination of immunosuppressed children has been a maculopapular or papulovesicular rash appearing within a few days to 60 days after vaccination. Eruptions requiring acyclovir therapy have developed in nearly 20% of vaccinees with leukemia. Live vaccine virus has been recovered from vesicular fluid. Transmission of vaccine virus to susceptible children has occurred in vaccinees with leukemia.

Recent data suggest a decreased incidence of herpes zoster after immunization of children with leukemia compared with the incidence in children after natural varicella infection. The administration of varicella vaccine in combination with MMR live attenuated viruses has promise for future use.

SUGGESTED READING

1. American Academy of Pediatrics: Measles: Reassessment of the current immunization policy. Pediatrics 84:1110–1113, 1989.
2. American Academy of Pediatrics: Report of the Committee on Infectious Diseases. 1991.
3. Atkinson WL, Markowitz LE: Measles and measles vaccine. Semin Pediatr Infect Dis 2:100–107, 1991.
4. Centers for Disease Control: Measles—United States, 1990. MMWR 40:369–372, 1991.
5. Centers for Disease Control: Prevention and control of influenza. MMWR 40:1–12, 1991.
6. Centers for Disease Control: Pertussis vaccination: Acellular pertussis vaccine for the fourth and fifth doses of the DTP series. Recommendations of the Advisory Committee on Immunization Practices. MMWR 41:1–5, 1992.
7. Edwards KM, Karzon DT: Pertussis vaccines. Pediatr Clin North Am 37:549–566, 1990.
8. Feldman S, Perry S, Andrew M, et al: Comparison of acellular and whole-cell pertussis-component diphtheria-tetanus-pertussis vaccines as the first booster immunization in 15- to 24-month-old children. J Pediatr 121: 857–861, 1992.
9. Hardy I, Gerson A, Steinberg S, et al: The incidence of zoster after immunization with live attenuated varicella vaccine. N Engl J Med 325:1545–1549, 1991.
10. Mortimer EA Jr: Pertussis and pertussis vaccines: 15 years of change. Semin Pediatr Infect Dis 2:82–90, 1991.
11. Murphy TV: Vaccines for *Haemophilus influenzae* type b. Semin Pediatr Infect Dis 2:120–134, 1991.
12. Piedra PA, Glezen WP: Influenza in children: Epidemiology. Semin Pediatr Infect Dis 2:140–146, 1991.
13. Shapiro ED: Pneumococcal vaccines. Semin Pediatr Infect Dis 2:147–152, 1991.
14. Ward J, Cochi S: *Haemophilus influenzae* vaccines. In Plotkin S, Mortimer EA (eds): Vaccines. Philadelphia, W.B. Saunders, 1988, pp 300–322.

INDEX

Page numbers in **boldface** type indicate complete chapters.